T0211555

Lecture Notes in Computer Science   10008

Commenced Publication in 1973
Founding and Former Series Editors:
Gerhard Goos, Juris Hartmanis, and Jan van Leeuwen

Editorial Board

More information about this series at http://www.springer.com/series/7412

Gustavo Carneiro · Diana Mateus
Loïc Peter · Andrew Bradley
João Manuel R.S. Tavares · Vasileios Belagiannis
João Paulo Papa · Jacinto C. Nascimento
Marco Loog · Zhi Lu
Jaime S. Cardoso · Julien Cornebise (Eds.)

Deep Learning
and Data Labeling
for Medical Applications

First International Workshop, LABELS 2016, and
Second International Workshop, DLMIA 2016
Held in Conjunction with MICCAI 2016, Athens, Greece, October 21, 2016
Proceedings

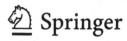 Springer

Editors
Gustavo Carneiro
University of Adelaide
Adelaide, SA
Australia

Diana Mateus
Technical University of Munich
Garching, Germany

Loïc Peter
Technical University of Munich
Garching, Germany

Andrew Bradley
University of Queensland
St Lucia, QLD
Australia

João Manuel R.S. Tavares
Universidade do Porto
Porto, Portugal

Vasileios Belagiannis
University of Oxford
Oxford, UK

João Paulo Papa
Universidade Estadual Paulista
Bauru
Brazil

Jacinto C. Nascimento
Instituto Superior Técnico
Lisbon, Portugal

Marco Loog
Delft University of Technology
Delft, The Netherlands

Zhi Lu
University of South Australia
Adelaide, SA
Australia

Jaime S. Cardoso
Universidade do Porto
Porto, Portugal

Julien Cornebise
Google DeepMind
London, UK

ISSN 0302-9743   ISSN 1611-3349   (electronic)
Lecture Notes in Computer Science
ISBN 978-3-319-46975-1   ISBN 978-3-319-46976-8   (eBook)
DOI 10.1007/978-3-319-46976-8

Library of Congress Control Number: 2016953216

LNCS Sublibrary: SL6 – Image Processing, Computer Vision, Pattern Recognition, and Graphics

Printed on acid-free paper

This Springer imprint is published by Springer Nature
The registered company is Springer International Publishing AG
The registered company address is: Gewerbestrasse 11, 6330 Cham, Switzerland

Preface: DLMIA 2016

After the success of the First Deep Learning in Medical Image Analysis (DLMIA) Workshop, held with MICCAI 2015, where we welcomed hundreds of attendees, we present the proceedings of the Second DLMIA Workshop. Deep learning methods have experienced an immense growth in interest from the medical image analysis community because of their ability to process very large training sets, to transfer learned features between different databases, and to analyze multimodal data. DLMIA is a workshop dedicated to the presentation of work focused on the design and use of deep learning methods in medical image analysis applications. We believe that this workshop is setting the trends and identifying the challenges of the use of deep learning methods in medical image analysis. For the keynote talks, we invited Prof. Dinggang Shen from the Department of Radiology and BRIC at UNC-Chapel Hill, and Prof. Nassir Navab from the Technische Universität München, who are two prominent researchers in the field of deep learning in medical image analysis. We would like to acknowledge the financial support provided by the Butterfly Network for the realization of these keynote talks.

The first call for papers for the Second DLMIA Workshop was released on April 1, 2016, and the last call was on May 24, 2016, with the paper deadline set to July 10, 2016. The submission site of DLMIA received 46 papers registrations, from which 42 papers turned into full paper submissions, where each submission was reviewed by at least three reviewers. The chairs decided to select 21 out of the 42 submissions, based on the scores and comments made by the reviewers (i.e., a 50 % acceptance rate). The top ten papers with the best reviews were selected for oral presentations and the remaining 11 accepted papers had poster presentations. Finally, the workshop chairs voted for the best paper of the workshop based on the reviewers' scores and comments, and the best paper prize of the Second DLMIA Workshop went to Michal Drozdzal, Eugene Vorontsov, Gabriel Chartrand, Samuel Kadoury, and Christopher Pal for the paper "The Importance of Skip Connections in Biomedical Image Segmentation." Nvidia generously offered to sponsor the Best Paper Award. Finally, we would like to acknowledge the support from the Australian Research Council for the realization of this workshop (discovery project DP140102794 and ARC Future Fellowship FT110100623). We would also like to thank the reviewers of DLMIA.

August 2016

Gustavo Carneiro
João Manuel R.S. Tavares
Andrew Bradley
João Paulo Papa
Jacinto C. Nascimento
Jaime S. Cardoso
Vasileios Belagiannis
Zhi Lu

Preface: LABELS 2016

The First Workshop on Large-Scale Annotation of Biomedical Data and Expert Label Synthesis (LABELS) was held during the MICCAI conference on October 21, 2016, in Athens, Greece. With this event, we intended to raise awareness of the importance of training data acquisition in the context of biomedical problems and to promote the development of algorithms that focus on assisting the annotation process.

Our call for papers resulted in ten submissions. Each of them was reviewed in a single-blind fashion by at least three members of the Program Committee. Seven submissions were eventually accepted for a poster presentation at the conference venue and are included in this volume. Following the recommendations of the reviewers, three of these submissions were additionally invited for an oral presentation. We are very enthusiastic about the overall diversity of the final program, which includes topics such as crowdsourcing methods, active learning, transfer learning, semi-supervised learning, or modeling of label uncertainty. In addition to the contribution of the workshop participants, we had the pleasure to invite two keynote speakers who proposed further developments on these topics: Marco Loog from the Technical University of Delft (The Netherlands) and Pascal Fua from the Ecole Polytechnique Federale de Lausanne (Switzerland). We would like to thank them again for their insights and the scientific exchanges fostered by their talks.

To conclude, we would like to thank the reviewers for their contributions and the MICCAI Organizing Committee for encouraging and making possible the holding of this event.

August 2016

Diana Mateus
Loïc Peter
Gustavo Carneiro
Marco Loog
Julien Cornebise

Organization

DLMIA Committee

Workshop Chairs

Gustavo Carneiro	University of Adelaide, Australia
João Manuel R.S. Tavares	Universidade do Porto, Portugal
Andrew Bradley	University of Queensland, Australia
João Paulo Papa	Universidade Estadual Paulista, Brazil
Jacinto C. Nascimento	Instituto Superior Tecnico, Portugal
Jaime S. Cardoso	Universidade do Porto, Portugal
Vasileios Belagiannis	University of Oxford, UK
Zhi Lu	University of South Australia, Australia

Program Committee

Aaron Carass	Gabriel Maicas	Neeraj Dhungel
Adrian Barbu	Ghassan Hamarneh	Patricia Ribeiro
Adrian Johnston	Guosheng Lin	Roger Tam
Amr Abdel-Dayem	Helder Oliveira	Shanghang Zhang
Ana Rebelo	Holger R. Roth	Susana Brandao
Ankush Gupta	Iro Laina	Tiago Veiga
Carlos Santiago	Jianming Liang	Tom Brosch
Daniela Iacoviello	Jianqiao Feng	Vijay Kumar
David Liu	Kelwin Fernandes	Weidong Cai
Dinggang Shen	Le Lu	Yefeng Zheng
Felix Achilles	Manuel Marques	Zhibin Liao

LABELS Committee

Workshop Chairs

Diana Mateus	TU Munich, Germany
Loïc Peter	TU Munich, Germany
Gustavo Carneiro	University of Adelaide, Australia
Marco Loog	TU Delft, The Netherlands
Julien Cornebise	Google Deepmind, UK

Program Committee

Adrian Barbu
Alba Garcia Seco
    de Herrera
Bjoern Menze
Danna Gurari
Daoqiang Zhang
Dinggang Shen
Eugenio Iglesias

Filipe Condessa
Holger Roth
Jaime Cardoso
Joao Papa
Ksenia Konyushova
Le Lu
Lena Maier-Hein
Michael Goetz

Neeraj Dhungel
Rahaf Aljundi
Raphael Sznitman
Roger Tam
Shadi Albarqouni
Weidong Cai
Xue-Cheng Tai

Contents

Large-Scale Annotation of Biomedical Data and Expert Label Synthesis

Deep Learning in Medical Image Analysis

HEp-2 Cell Classification Using K-Support Spatial Pooling in Deep CNNs

Xian-Hua Han[1]([✉]), Jianmei Lei[2], and Yen-Wei Chen[3]

[1] National Institute of Advanced Industrial Science and Technology, Tokyo, Japan
han-xhua@aist.go.jp
[2] State Key Laboratory of Vehicle Noise Vibration and Safe Technology,
Chongqing, China
leijianmei@caeri.com.cn
[3] Ritsumeikan Univeristy, Kusatsu, Shiga, Japan
chen@is.ritsumei.ac.jp

Abstract. This study addresses the recognition problem of the HEp-2 cell using indirect immunofluorescent (IIF) image analysis, which can facilitate the diagnosis of many autoimmune diseases by finding antibodies in the patient serum. Recently, a lot of automatic HEp-2 cell classification strategies including both shallow and deep methods have been developed, wherein the deep Convolutional Neural Networks (CNNs) have been proven to achieve impressive performance. However, the deep CNNs in general requires a fixed size of image as the input. In order to conquer the limitation of the fixed size problem, a spatial pyramid pooling (SPP) strategy has been proposed in general object recognition and detection. The SPP-net usually exploit max pooling strategies for aggregating all activated status of a specific neuron in a predefined spatial region by only taking the maximum activation, which achieved superior performance compared with mean pooling strategy in the traditional state-of-the-art coding methods such as sparse coding, linear locality-constrained coding and so on. However, the max pooling strategy in SPP-net only retains the strongest activated pattern, and would completely ignore the frequency: an important signature for identifying different types of images, of the activated patterns. Therefore, this study explores a generalized spatial pooling strategy, called K-support spatial pooling, in deep CNNs by integrating not only the maximum activated magnitude but also the response magnitude of the relatively activated patterns of a specific neuron together. This proposed K-support spatial pooling strategy in deep CNNs combines the popularly applied mean and max pooling methods, and then avoid awfully emphasizing of the maximum activation but preferring a group of activations in a supported region. The deep CNNs with the proposed K-support spatial pooling is applied for HEp-2 cell classification, and achieve promising performance compared with the state-of-the-art approaches.

1 Introduction

Indirect immunofluorescence (IIF) is widely used as a common methodology to reveal the presence of autoimmune diseases by finding antibodies in the patient

G. Carneiro et al. (Eds.): LABELS 2016/DLMIA 2016, LNCS 10008, pp. 3–11, 2016.
DOI: 10.1007/978-3-319-46976-8_1

serum. Since it is effective for diagnosing autoimmune diseases [1], the demand for applying IIF image analysis in diagnostic tests is increasing. However, manual analysis of IIF images not only leads to heavy burden to the physicians but also subjectively results in the inconsistence across laboratories. Therefore, automatic and reliable HEp-2 cell classification attract a lot of attentions in the computer vision and machine learning fields. Many attempts to achieve the automatic recognition of HEp-2 staining patterns have been made, which mainly includes two procedures: feature extraction and classification. Most works developed recently [2–6] have focused on effective feature extraction, which greatly affects the final performance of the HEp-2 cell classification. Perner et al. [2] proposed the extraction of texture and statistical features for cell image representation and then combined the extraction with a decision tree model for HEp-2 cell image classification. In the first HEp-2 cells classification contest at ICIP2012, the LBP-based descriptor, rotation invariant co-occurrence LBP (RICLBP), was proposed for cell image representation, and achieved promising HEp-2 cell classification performance [3]. In the second HEp-2 cells classification contest at ICIP2013, Qi et al. proposed a pairwise rotation invariant co-occurrence LBP (PRICoLBP) [4], and combined it with Bag-of-Features (BOF) [5] of Sift descriptors [6] for achieving the best recognition results. The other empirically selected hand-crafted features such as histogram of orientation [7], shape index [8] and the statistical features like gray-level. Co-occurrence matrix [9], gray-level size zone matrix [10] have also been developed for giving the comparable and acceptable performances. However, there has still large space for improving the classification performance of HEp-2 cell.

Very recently, the deep learning framework [11–14], have achieved remarkable success in different applications such as generic image classification and recognition, object detection and localization, natural language processing, and so on. Compared with the traditional state-of-the-art methods such as BOW model in image representation, MFCC in speech representation, deep framework can learn the hierarchical features not only including low- and middle- level but also high-level vision ones, and then obtain an end-to-end learned model, which achieved outstanding performance with large-scale labeled dataset and have attracted remarkable attention in both the academic and industrial communities. Therein, deep convolutional neural networks (CNNs) are most popularly used framework, and results in comparable or even better performance than human being on a number of classification benchmarks [15–17]. Several works [18,19] applied deep CNNs for HEp-2 cell classification, and achieved promising performances. Gao et al. [18] exploited three convolutional layers combining two fully connecting layers for HEp-2 cell classification, while Li et al. explored extra cell images to train the CNN model for cross-specimen analysis, which achieved much better results than the utilization of the augmented dataset by only employing affine transformations. However, all the used deep CNNs, in general, needs a fixed size of image as the input, which would cast the deformation and "artificial" effect on the raw images and may reduce the recognition accuracy with the re-scaled images. In order to solve the limitation of the fixed size of images, He et al. proposed a spatial pyramid pooling strategy in the CNNs for generic object classification and detection, called SPP-net [20], which can deal with arbitrary larger size than the fixed size to extract high-level image representation. The SPP-net can in general improve classification performances for a variety of CNN architectures on several image datasets such as the ImageNet 2012, Pascal VOC 2007 and Caltech101 datasets. The SPP-net usually exploit max pooling strategies for aggregating all activated status of a specific neuron in a predefined spatial region by only taking the maximum activation, which achieved superior performance compared with mean pooling strategy in the traditional state-of-the-art coding methods such as sparse coding, linear locality-constrained coding and so on. However, the max pooling strategy in SPP-net only retains the strongest activated pattern, and would completely ignore the frequency: an important signature for identifying different types of images, of the activated patterns. Therefore, this study explores a generalized spatial pooling strategy, called K-support spatial pooling, in deep CNNs by integrating not only the maximum activated magnitude but also the response magnitude of the relatively activated patterns of a specific neuron together. This proposed K-support spatial pooling strategy in deep CNNs combines the popularly applied mean and max pooling methods, and then avoid awfully emphasizing of the maximum activation but preferring a group of activations in a supported region. The deep CNNs with the proposed K-support spatial pooling is applied for HEp-2 cell classification, and achieve promising performance compared with the state-of-the-art approaches.

2   The Deep CNNs with K-Support Spatial Pooling

In the image classification and object detection community, the most popularly used deep CNN models are caffe reference model (denoted as CaffeNet) and Alexnet, which generally include several convolutional layers following two fully connected (fc) layers and an N-way softmax (fc) layer (N is the number of image categories). The convolutional layers in the deep CNNs use the slide window trick by convoluting their input with a much smaller size kernel than the input size, and thus, in principle, there are no requirement for the fixed size of input for these layers. However, the last two fc and the final output layers are fully connected, and are mandatory to have a fixed size of input. This study implements the HEp-2 cell classification based on CaffeNet model, and it is also possible to be extended for other models with any architecture, In order to conquer the limitation the fixed size problem, a spatial pyramid pooling strategy in the CNNs, called SPP-net, has been proposed, which can deal with arbitrary larger size than the fixed size to extract high-level image representation. In SPP-net, the activations of the convolutional layer, also called feature maps, can considered as the encoded coefficients similarly in BOW model using sparse coding, LLC, and GMM on SIFT vectors or image patches, which can be pooled under the global region or spatial pyramids for generating a fixed size of features. The SPP-net analogously pooled the activations of the last convolutional layer in a similar way with BOF model, and thus produce a fixed size output as image representation, which in turn can be used as the input of the fc layer. As we know that the widely used pooling methods for aggregating the encoded coefficient vectors in the traditional BOW model and the SPP-net are mean and max strategies. Mean pooling aggregates all activated coefficients, which are the coded coefficients of a pre-learned word in BOW model and the response output of a neuron in CNN, in a defined region by taking the average value, while max pooling aggregates these by taking the maximum value. In the vision community, the max pooling combining the popularly used coding methods such as SC, LLC manifests promising performance in a variant of image classification applications. Then, SPP-net in general exploit max pooling strategy. However, the max pooling strategy only retains the strongest activated pattern, and would completely ignore the frequency: an important signature for identifying different types of images, of the activated patterns. Therefore, this study explores a generalized spatial pooling strategy in deep CNNs by integrating not only the maximum activated magnitude but also the response magnitude of the relatively activated patterns of a neuron in a spatial region together, also called K-support pooling. This proposed generalized pooling strategy combines the popularly applied mean and max pooling methods and can avoid awfully emphasizing of the maximum activation but preferring a group of activations in a supported region.

Let us denote the activated output of the ith neuron (a convolutional kernel) and the jth location in a convolutional layer as $y_{i,j}$, we aim to aggregate all the activated outputs of the ith neuron in the lth predefined region Φ_l for getting the overall activation degree of this region as the following:

$$z_i^{\Phi_l} = f(\{y_{i,j}\}, j \in \Phi_l) \tag{1}$$

where $z_i^{\phi_l}$ denotes the pooled activation of of the ith neuron in the region Φ_l. We can design different transformation function f for aggregating the set of activations into a indicating value for the lth region. The most simple one just averages the activation of all locations in this region formulated as:

$$z_i^{\Phi_l} = \frac{1}{N_l} \sum_{j \in \Phi_l} y_{i,j} \tag{2}$$

where N_l is location number in the lth region. The mean pooling strategy is generally used in the original BOW model, which assigns a local feature only to a nearest word, and thus produces the coded coefficients with only 1 or 0 value. It eventually creates the representative histogram of the learned words for an image. Motivated by the visual biological study, the maximum activation would be more related to human cortex response than the average one, and can give translation-invariant visual representation. Therefore, the max pooling strategy has widely used accompanied with SC, LLC in BOW model, and also the SPP-net. In our scenario, the max pooling can be formulated as:

$$z_i^{\Phi_l} = \max_{y_{i,j}}(\{y_{i,j}\}, j \in \Phi_l) = y_{i,k}, y_{i,k} >= y_{i,j}, k \neq j, k, j \in \Phi_l \tag{3}$$

Max pooling takes maximum activated value of all locations in the defined region as the overall activation degree, and then completely ignore how many

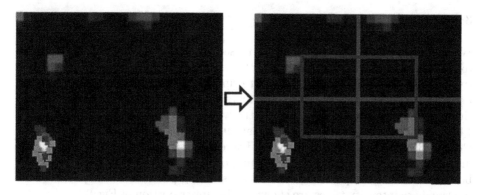

Fig. 1. The used spatial pyramids for aggregating the activation from each divided region.

locations are possibly activated. Figure 1 shows an example of two activation maps. If we equably divided the activation maps into four regions by the blue lines, and it is obvious the aggregated activation degree of the four regions would same, as shown in the bottom of Fig. 1, since the only maximum values are taken. However, from human being the two activation maps are considerably different, where the activation degree should also account for the activation number. Therefore, this study proposes a general spatial pooling strategy.

The proposed general spatial pooling firstly sorts the ith neuron's activated values of all locations from the large to small values in the defined region Φ_l as:

$$y'_{i,j} = \text{sort}\{y_{i,j}\}, \text{with } y'_{i,1} >= y'_{i,2} >= y'_{i,3} >= \cdots >= y'_{i,N_l}, j \in \Phi_l \qquad (4)$$

and then only retains the first K larger activations. The final activation degree of the region is calculated by averaging the retained K-values, which is the mean of the selected K-support locations, then named as K-support pooling. The formula is formed as:

$$z_i^{\Phi_l} = \frac{1}{K} \sum_{j=1}^{K} y'_{i,j} \qquad (5)$$

For each neuron, we repeat the above procedure, and produce the activation degrees of all neurons in a defined regions. For example, there are 256 neuron units (convolutional kernels) of each location (overall $N * N$ 2D-grid locations, which is different according to the size of input images) in the fifth convolutional layer of the CaffeNet, and the aggregated activation degree can be calculated from the ones of $N * N$ locations with the global defined region for each neuron unit. Then the final representation $\mathbf{z}^{\Phi_l} = [z_1^{\Phi_l}, z_2^{\Phi_l}, \ldots, z_{256}^{\Phi_l}]^T$ is a 256-dimensional vector. If we divide the 2D-grid activation maps into different rectangle grid, such as in Fig. 1, which is general called spatial pyramids, the activation vector can be extracted from all grid regions. The concatenated vector $\mathbf{z} = [\mathbf{z}^{\phi_1 T}, \mathbf{z}^{\phi_2 T}, \ldots, \mathbf{z}^{\phi_L T}]^T$, where L is the total number of the divided regions, can be computed for the final image representation.

3   Experimental Results

We applied the deep CNNs with our proposed K-support spatial pooling strategy
to the open ICIP2013 HEp-2 dataset [21], which includes intermediate and positive intensity types. This HEp-2 dataset primarily include the following six staining patterns, with available image numbers for positive and intermediate intensity types shown in parentheses, respectively, for each class: Homogeneous (1087,
1407); Speckled (1457, 1374); Nucleolar (934, 1664); Centromere(1387, 1364);
Golgi(943, 1265); NuMem (347, 377). There are over 10000 images, each showing a single cell, obtained from 83 training IIF images by cropping the bounding
box of the cell. Example images for all six staining patterns of the positive and
intermediate intensity types are shown in the upper portion of Fig. 2.

Since we use the Caffenet architecture as our basic model of deep CNNs, and
then there are five convolutional layers. We consider the feature maps of the
third, fourth and fifth convolutional layers as the encoded vector maps like in
BOW model, and exploit a spatial pyramid pooling as in SPP-net but with the
proposed general spatial pooling strategy instead of the max one. Further, we
spatially divide the feature maps into four (2×2) equally grid regions adding the
center one and the global one as shown in Fig. 1. In the experiments, we randomly divide the HEp-2 cell images in each class into five groups for positive and
intermediate types, respectively, and take four groups from all classes as training, the remainder for test. This procedure is iterated five times and the average
accuracy is calculated as the final performance measure. In our proposed general
spatial pooling strategy, there is a parameter K, which denotes the K locations
with the first K large activation values in the defined region. We set different K
to extract the deep image representation and simply apply SVM shallow model

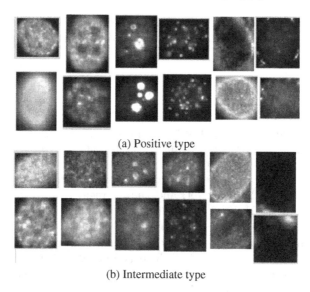

(a) Positive type

(b) Intermediate type

Fig. 2. The sample images of HEp-2 cell.

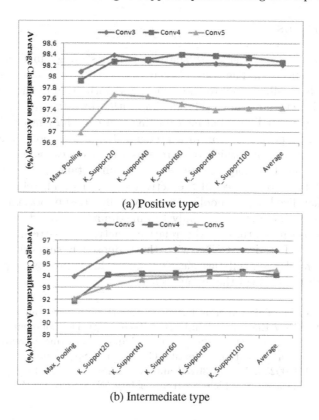

(a) Positive type

(b) Intermediate type

Fig. 3. The compared performances using the deep CNNs with different spatial pooling strategyes.

for classification. The compared results on the three convolutional layers are given in Fig. 3. From Fig. 3, it can be seen that our proposed pooling strategies can improve the classification accuracies in different layers or at least achieve the comparable results. Table 1 shows the compared classification accuracies by our proposed approach without data augmentation, the CNNs w/o data augmentation by Gao et al. [18], and the used features in [22], which manifest our proposed approach can achieve better and comparable performance even without data augmentation. Since [18] only learned a common classification model for both positive and intermediate intensity types, the classification results [18] in Table 1 are the accuracies for both types of intensity.

Table 1. The compared results using our proposed strategy, the used features in [22] and the CNN framework in [18].

%	GLRL	SGLD	Laws	CNN [18]	CNN+Augmentation [18]	Our
Positive	84.91	90.81	97.90	89.04	97.24	**98.41**
Intermediate	49.96	58.45	90.49	*	*	**96.29**

4 Conclusions

This study presented a K-support spatial pooling strategy in deep CNNs for HEp-2 cell classification. The conventional CNNs requires a fixed size of image as input, which possibly leads to the structure deformation of the input image. Therefore, SPP-net were proposed for dealing with arbitrary size of input images. However, SPP-net usually exploit max pooling strategies for aggregating all activated status of a specific neuron in a predefined spatial region by only taking the maximum activation, which only retains the strongest activated pattern, and would completely ignore the frequency: an important signature for identifying different types of images, of the activated patterns. Therefore, this study explores a generalized spatial pooling strategy, called K-support spatial pooling, in deep CNNs by integrating not only the maximum activated magnitude but also the response magnitude of the relatively activated patterns of a specific neuron together. The deep CNNs with the proposed K-support spatial pooling is applied for HEp-2 cell classification, and achieve promising performance compared with the state-of-the-art approaches.

Acknowledgments. This paper is based on results obtained from a project commissioned by the New Energy and Industrial Technology Development Organization (NEDO), and was supported by the Grant-in Aid for Scientific Research from the Japanese Ministry for Education, Scientific Culture and Sports under the Grant No. 15H01130, No. 15K00253, No. 26330212 and No. 25280044, open foundation project from state key laboratory of vehicle NVH and safety (NVHSKL-201414).

References

1. Conrad, K., Schoessler, W., Hiepe, F., Fritzler, M.J.: Utoantibodies in Systemic Autoimmune Diseases. Pabst Science Publishers, Lengerich (2002)
2. Perner, P., Perner, H., Muller, B.: Mining knowledge for HEp-2 cell image classification. J. Artif. Intell. Med. **26**, 161–173 (2002)
3. Nosaka, R., Fukui, K.: Hep-2 cell classification using rotation invariant co-occurrence among local binary patterns. Pattern Recogn. **27**(7), 2428–2436 (2013)
4. Qi, X., Xiao, R., Guo, J., Zhang, L.: Pairwise rotation invariant co-occurrence local binary pattern. In: Fitzgibbon, A., Lazebnik, S., Perona, P., Sato, Y., Schmid, C. (eds.) ECCV 2012, Part VI. LNCS, vol. 7577, pp. 158–171. Springer, Heidelberg (2012)
5. Lazebnik, S., Schmid, C., Ponce, J.: Beyond bags of features: spatial pyramid matching for recognizing natural scene categories. In: Processings of the IEEE Conferenceon Computer Vision and Pattern Recognition, New York, NY, USA, vol. 2, pp. 2169–2178, June 2006
6. Lowe, D.: Distinctive image features from scale-invariant keypoint. Int. J. Comput. Vis. **60**(2), 91–110 (2004)
7. Dala, N., Triggs, B.: Histogram of oriented gradients for human detection. In: Computer Vision and Pattern Recognition (CVPR 2005), vol. 1, pp. 886–893 (2005)
8. Larsen, A.B., Vestergaard, J.S., Larsen, R.: HEp-2 cell classification using shape index histograms with donut-shaped spatial pooling. IEEE Trans. Med. Imaging **33**(7), 1573–1580 (2014)

9. Haralick, M.R., Shanmugam, K., Dinstein, I.: Textural features for image classification. IEEE Trans. Syst. Man Cybern. **SMC-3**(6), 610–621 (1973)
10. Thibault, G., Angulo, J., Meyer, F.: Advanced statistical matrices for texture characterization: application to cell classification. IEEE Trans. Biomed. Eng. **61** 630–637
11. Bengio, Y., Courville, A., Vincent, P.: Representation learning: a review and new perspectives. IEEE Trans. Pattern Anal. Mach. Intell. **35**, 1798–1828 (2013)
12. Krizhevsky, A., Sutskever, I., Hinton, G.E.: Imagenet classification with deep convolutional neural networks. In: Proceedings of the Twenty-Sixth Annual Conference on Neural Information Processing Systems, Lake Tahoe, NY, USA, pp. 1097–1105, December 2012
13. Sermanet, P., Eigen, D., Zhang, X., Mathieu, M., Fergus, R., LeCun, Y.: OverFeat: integrated recognition, localization and detection using convolutional networks. In: Proceedings of the International Conference on Learning Representations, CBLS, Banff, AL, Canada, April 2014
14. Simonyan, K., Zisserman, A.: Very deep convolutional networks for large-scale image recognition. In: Proceedings of the International Conference on Learning Representations, San Diego, CA, USA, May 2015
15. Razavian, A.S., Azizpour, H., Sullivan, J., Carlsson, S.: CNN features off-the-shelf: an astounding baseline for recognition. In: Proceedings of the IEEE Conference on Computer Vision and Pattern Recognition Workshops, Columbus, OH, USA, pp. 512–519, June 2014
16. Fan, H., Xia, G.-S., Jingwen, H.: Transferring deep convolutional neural networks for the scene classification of high-resolution remote sensing imagery. Remote Sens. **7**(11), 14680–14707 (2015)
17. Jia, Y., Shelhamer, E., Donahue, J., Karayev, S., Long, J., Girshick, R., Guadarrama, S., Darrell, T.: Caffe: convolutional architecture for fast feature embedding. In: Proceedings of the ACM International Conference on Multimedia, Orlando, FL, USA, November 2014
18. Gao, Z.M., Zhang, J.J., Zhou, L.P., Wang, L.: HEp-2 cell image classification with convolutional neural networks. In: The 1st Workshop on Pattern Recognition Techniques for Indirect Immunofluorescence Images (I3A), pp. 24–28 (2014)
19. Li, H.W., Zhang, J.G., Zheng, W.-S.: Deep CNNs for HEp-2 cells classification: a cross-specimen analysis, CoRR, vol. abs/1604.05816 (2016). http://arxiv.org/abs/1604.05816
20. He, K., Zhang, X., Ren, S., Sun, J.: Spatial pyramid pooling in deep convolutional networks for visual recognition. In: Fleet, D., Pajdla, T., Schiele, B., Tuytelaars, T. (eds.) ECCV 2014, Part III. LNCS, vol. 8691, pp. 346–361. Springer, Heidelberg (2014)
21. Foggia, P., Percannella, G., Soda, P., Vento, M.: Benchmarking HEp-2 Cells classification methods. IEEE Trans. Med. Imaging **32**(10), 1878–1889 (2013)
22. Agrawal, P., Vatsa, M., Singh, R.: HEp-2 cell image classification: a comparative analysis. In: Wu, G., Zhang, D., Shen, D., Yan, P., Suzuki, K., Wang, F. (eds.) MLMI 2013. LNCS, vol. 8184, pp. 195–202. Springer, Heidelberg (2013)

Robust 3D Organ Localization with Dual Learning Architectures and Fusion

Xiaoguang Lu[✉], Daguang Xu, and David Liu

Medical Imaging Technologies, Siemens Medical Solutions, Inc.,
Princeton, NJ, USA
xiaoguang.lu@siemens.com

Abstract. We present a robust algorithm for organ localization from 3D volumes in the presence of large anatomical and contextual variations. The 3D spatial search space is decomposed into two components: slice and pixel, both are modeled in 2D space. For each component, we adopt different learning architectures to leverage respective modeling power on global and local context at three orthogonal orientations. Unlike conventional patch-based scanning schemes in learning-based object detection algorithms, slice scanning along each orientation is applied, which significantly reduces the number of model evaluations. Object search evidence obtained from three orientations and different learning architectures is consolidated through fusion schemes to lead to the target organ location. Experiments conducted using 499 patient CT body scans show promise and robustness of the proposed approach.

1 Introduction

Automatic 3D organ localization is essential in a wide range of clinical applications. It provides seed points to initialize subsequent segmentation algorithms. It is also useful for visual navigation, automatic windowing, semantic tagging, and organ-based lesion grouping.

Accurate localization of organs still remains a challenging task. From the local contextual perspective, the size, shape, and appearance of organs vary significantly across patients, even more so when there are pathologies or prior surgeries. Global context around each organ also varies significantly, although the context within the entire field of view such as that among multiple anatomical organs provides a cue for individual organ localization. For example, in the abdominal region, organs such as the kidney can "float" around with large degrees of freedom, therefore leading to varying appearance context. Various sizes of field of views and different body regions in clinical practice also increase the variation of global appearance.

Data-driven learning-based approaches have shown success and been widely deployed in object localization tasks. A typical search strategy in such methods uses a scanning window based scheme. A model/classifier is trained based on annotations to determine likelihood of a patch (sub-volume) being the target object. During online testing, the classifier is applied to each sub-volume

© Springer International Publishing AG 2016
G. Carneiro et al. (Eds.): LABELS 2016/DLMIA 2016, LNCS 10008, pp. 12–20, 2016.
DOI: 10.1007/978-3-319-46976-8_2

by scanning through the entire volume. Target location is calculated by consolidating evidence collected from all scanned patches. Conventional scanning window patch-based approach is more suitable for capturing local appearance variations given its limited field of view (voxels within the sub-volume), but not global appearance variations. Many methods have been proposed in this paradigm; some focus on improving the classifiers, while others improve the scanning strategy [11], or integrates other modeling methods such as conditional random field [3] and recursive context propagation network [12].

Another category of method is based on long range regression and voting. In [1], a regression forest is trained to find the non-linear mapping from voxels to the desired anatomy location, which extracts features globally from the volume, and is shown to be effective for resolving local ambiguities. However, it has been shown in [8] that the precision of such regression methods is not as accurate as the patch based classification methods due to large context variations.

We propose a framework which models both local and global context without using patch-based scanning schemes, where two emerging learning architectures are exploited to complement each other. We use the convolution neural network (CNN) [7] to capture global context [13], and the fully convolutional network (FCN) [10] to capture local context. The local context focuses on the localization precision, while the global context helps improve robustness such as resolving ambiguities and eliminating false detections. The global context and local appearance information are integrated through a probabilistic graphical model, and we call such a learning scheme as the dual learning architecture. We show in our experiments that, with explicitly modeling and fusion of both local and global contextual information, our approach is more robust and achieves a higher accuracy compared to the state-of-the-art algorithms. In addition to the object location, a significant amount of positive seeds (within the target organ) are generated, which are useful for subsequent processes such as segmentation using graph-cut methods. Furthermore, because both CNN and FCN support multi-label tasks, our algorithm can be generalized to simultaneous multi-organ localization with limited extra run-time computational cost.

2   Methodology

2.1   Context Modeling with Dual Learning Architectures

The organ localization task is formulated as a probabilistic graphical model [6], as shown in Fig. 1. Random variable I denotes a 2D image, E represents the existence ($E = 1$) or absence ($E = 0$) of the organ of interest within image I, and L is the organ location within image I. Both E and L are hidden variables, while I is an observed variable. The joint distribution factors according to the probabilistic graphical model as follows:

$$P(I, E, L) = P(L|I, E)P(E|I)P(I). \tag{1}$$

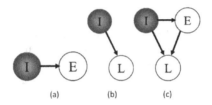

Fig. 1. Probabilistic graphical models describing the relationship between image I, the existence (E) of the organ in the image, and the location (L) of the organ in the image. From left to right: Global image classification (slice-level), local (pixel-level) classification, and the proposed global-local image classification.

Our goal is to query the organ location given the image, i.e., $P(L|I)$. This can be expressed as

$$P(L|I) = P(L,I)/P(I) = \sum_E P(I,E,L)/P(I) = \sum_E P(L|I,E)P(E|I)P(I)/P(I)$$

$$= \sum_E P(L|I,E)P(E|I).$$

$$(2)$$

By definition, $P(L|I,E=0) = 0$ for all valid locations, and $P(L = empty|I, E = 0) = 1$. Therefore

$$P(L|I) = P(L|I,E=1)P(E=1|I) \qquad (3)$$

for all valid pixel locations, and

$$P(L = empty|I)$$
$$= P(L = empty|I, E = 1)P(E = 1|I) + P(L = empty|I, E = 0)P(E = 0|I)$$
$$= P(L = empty|I, E = 0)P(E = 0|I).$$

$$(4)$$

The probability distribution function $P(E = 0 \ or \ 1|I)$ poses an image categorization problem. This function is depicted in Fig. 1(a). This was often implemented by extracting global image features and training a classifier on those features. In recent years, deep Neural Networks have shown superior performance in this task. In this paper, we use the Convolutional Neural Network (CNN) [7].

The probability distribution function $P(L|I, E = 1)$ presents a pixel classification task. In contrast to $P(E|I)$, which is a global image classification problem, $P(L|I, E = 1)$ is a local pixel or patch classification problem, where the patch is centered at pixel location L. One could again use a CNN to classify each patch, but in recent literature it has been shown that the fully convolutional networks (FCN) demonstrate advantages over the CNNs for pixel-level classification. We therefore adopt the FCN for this local image classification problem. To the best of our knowledge, this is the first time an FCN is used in conjunction with a CNN in a "dual learning" architecture for solving the global-local pixel classification problem.

While the FCN is described above as a local pixel classifier, it has been used in the literature to classify pixels into multi-label masks, in which the "background" class is one of the possible labels. This means, we could have used directly the FCN to classify all the pixels without using the global CNN classifier at all. However, as we will show in the experiments, there are significant advantages of combining the FCN with the CNN, where FCN's limited receptive field [9,15] is compensated by CNNs' response. This is also evident from the above probabilistic formulation: a FCN-only pixel classifier would model directly $P(L|I)$ as shown in Fig. 1(b) without considering the hidden variable E. Therefore, our global-local model poses a stronger assumption than a typically FCN-only classifier, which does not have knowledge of the presence of the organ. For multi-organ localization tasks [4], the proposed method can be extended through multi-label training with the same architectures.

Compared with patch-based sub-window scanning in conventional object localization, in our method, one entire slice (not a sub-patch) is used as one input sample to either CNN and FCN. During online testing on a given volume, for each CNN or FCN model, the total number of image samples that are passed through CNN/FCN for evaluation is the number of slices along one orientation.

2.2 Cross-Sectional Fusion and Clustering

The dual learning architectures with respective models operate along each of the three orthogonal orientations, i.e., axial, sagittal, and coronal, resulting in three volumetric probability/score maps. These maps are generated from different orientations with different image context and therefore provide complementary information towards the target localization decision making. Typical ensemble schemes or information fusion approaches can be applied, such as majority voting, or sum rule [5], to lead to a consolidated score for each voxel. We call this scheme cross-sectional fusion.

After the consolidated probability/score map is computed, three-dimensional connected component analysis is conducted. The centroid of the largest cluster is computed as the estimated object location.

3   Experiments

Among all the organs with available expert annotations, the right kidney is one of the most challenging organs [2]. We use the right kidney as an exemplar case in our experiments. We have collected 450 patient CT body scans, one scan from each patient. For each scan, right kidney was manually delineated. At the training stage, 405 scans were selected at random for training and the remaining 45 scans (10 %) for validation. Our training data covers large variations in populations, contrast phases, scanning ranges, and pathologies. The axial slice resolution ranges between 0.5 mm and 1.5 mm. The inter-slice distance varies from 0.5 mm to 7.0 mm. Scan coverage includes abdominal regions, but can extend to head/neck and knees. After all models were trained, we collected another

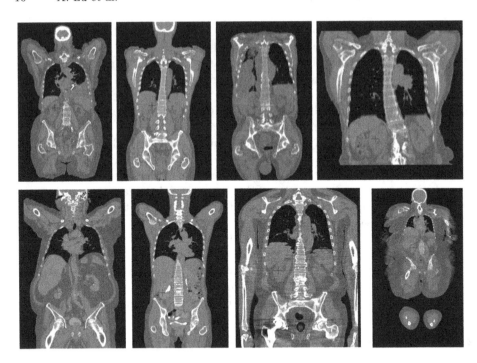

Fig. 2. Coronal slice samples in the test set. Note that the large context variations with respect to the right kidney. Red cross indicates the right kidney location automatically detected by the proposed method. (Color figure online)

49 patient CT scans from clinical sites for independent testing. Right kidney is also manually delineated in these 49 test cases to compute quantitative measurement for algorithm performance evaluation. Typical test scan samples are provided in Fig. 2.

Each CT scan contains a stack of axial slices, which were used to reconstruct a 3D volume at an isotropic resolution of $2 \times 2 \times 2\,mm^3$. All the algorithms/models in our subsequent experiments operate at this resolution. Three orthogonal orientations (axial, sagittal, and coronal) are considered for cross-sectional analysis. Only the right hand side of the body is considered in the experiments (training and testing) as the right kidney is the target object. The centroid of the delineated right kidney was used as ground-truth location. A volumetric mask was generated based on the annotations, where right kidney voxels are labeled

Table 1. Number of training images for each model.

Number of images	Axial	Sagittal	Coronal
CNN	118245	42482	90559
FCN	41276	25938	27378

as ones and all other background was labeled as zeros. This mask was used to provide the labels for FCN training. For CNN training, a two-class classification is defined, i.e., whether or not an image slice contains the right kidney.

Slice-level modeling (CNN): the AlexNet architecture [7], which contains 5 convolution layers and 3 fully connected layers, is adopted. One CNN model is

Table 2. Statistics of Euclidean distance from the automatic localization result to the ground-truth position at $2\,mm$ resolution. Sum rule is applied in cross-sectional fusion. CS: cross-sectional fusion.

Dist. (voxels)	CS-(CNN+FCN)	MSL	CS-CNN	CS-FCN
Mean	3.9	12.8	9.1	9.0
Std	4.7	10.7	11.4	23.0
Median	2.3	10.9	5.4	1.9

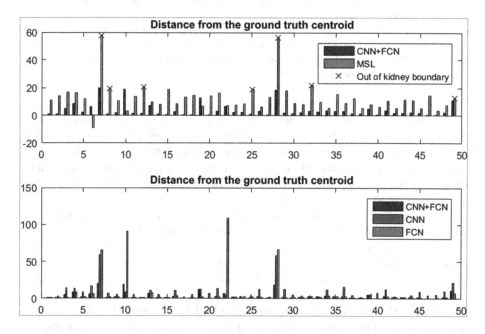

Fig. 3. Euclidean distance between the calculated right kidney location and the ground-truth location for each of the 49 test cases (horizontal axis is case index) in number of voxels at the isotropic $2\,mm$ resolution. Negative distance (case 6 in Top) indicates that the corresponding localization algorithm does not generate any detection results, and the absolute distance value in this case is nominal for visualization purposes. Top: comparison of the proposed method (blue) and MSL (yellow), where a red cross indicates the localization result is out of the actual kidney boundary. Bottom: comparison of the proposed method (blue), CNN only (green), and FCN only (yellow). Results of CNN, FCN, and CNN+FCN are all calculated through cross-sectional fusion. (Color figure online)

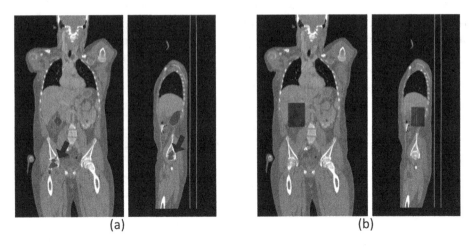

(a)   (b)

Fig. 4. Example of model responses (color overlaid) from FCNs (a) and CNNs (b) after cross-sectional fusion. Responses are presented after fusion across three orientations. Each group contains one sagittal view and one coronal view. Red arrows indicate false alarms detected by FCNs. CNNs response maps show inferior localization precision on the same cluster. Combining both responses through fusion leads to successful right kidney localization. (Color figure online)

trained for each cross-section orientation using the same learning architecture. Pixel-level modeling (FCN): the VGG-FCN8s architecture [10] is adopted, which is an end-to-end network with 7 levels of convolution layers, 5 pooling layers and 3 deconvolution layers. One FCN model is learned for each cross-section orientation with the same network architecture. Table 1 lists the number of training images/slices used for each model.

For comparison, we implemented a 3D patch-based scanning window approach based on the method proposed by Zheng et al. [14], and applied it on the same test set. We refer to their approach as marginal space learning (MSL). Quantitative performance evaluation against the ground-truth is provided in Table 2 and Fig. 3. Figure 4 presents an example to demonstrate complementary information extraction from the dual learning architectures.

Although the focus of the proposed method is on organ localization, one typical use case of organ localization is for organ segmentation. We evaluate the impact of our kidney localization on the accuracy of kidney segmentation. As the MSL method together with active shape models has shown to provide good cardiac segmentation results [14], we adopt it for right kidney segmentation. Our automatic localization led to similar segmentation error rates compared to using the ground-truth locations. Using our automatic localization results as input for segmentation, the [mean, std., median, 80 percentile] of point-to-mesh errors (used in [14]) in mm are [2.32, 1.23, 1.91, 2.22], while the ground-truth locations led to error rates of [2.00, 0.48, 1.85, 2.20].

4   Conclusions

We have presented a robust 3D organ localization algorithm. We approach the 3D localization task through cross-sectional 2D modeling, exploiting two learning architectures that model various context for localizing the target organ. Contextual information extracted by the two learning schemes is complementary and integrated for improved robustness. Because FCN and CNN are capable of learning multiple targets/labels, our method can be extended for simultaneous multi-organ localization. Although CT body scans are used in the experiments, the proposed method is not limited to specific imaging modalities.

References

1. Criminisi, A., Shotton, J., Robertson, D., Konukoglu, E.: Regression forests for efficient anatomy detection and localization in CT studies. In: Menze, B., Langs, G., Tu, Z., Criminisi, A. (eds.) MICCAI 2010. LNCS, vol. 6533, pp. 106–117. Springer, Heidelberg (2011)
2. Cuingnet, R., Prevost, R., Lesage, D., Cohen, L.D., Mory, B., Ardon, R.: Automatic detection and segmentation of kidneys in 3D CT images using random forests. In: Ayache, N., Delingette, H., Golland, P., Mori, K. (eds.) MICCAI 2012, Part III. LNCS, vol. 7512, pp. 66–74. Springer, Heidelberg (2012)
3. Farabet, C., Couprie, C., Najman, L., LeCun, Y.: Learning hierarchical features for scene labeling. IEEE TPAMI **35**(8), 1915–1929 (2013)
4. Gauriau, R., Cuingnet, R., Lesage, D., Bloch, I.: Multi-organ localization combining global-to-local regression and confidence maps. In: Golland, P., Hata, N., Barillot, C., Hornegger, J., Howe, R. (eds.) MICCAI 2014, Part III. LNCS, vol. 8675, pp. 337–344. Springer, Heidelberg (2014)
5. Kittler, J., Hatef, M., Duin, R., Matas, J.: On combining classifiers. IEEE TPAMI **20**(3), 226–239 (1998)
6. Koller, D., Friedman, N.: Probabilistic Graphical Models: Principles and Techniques. Lippincott Williams & Wilkins, Philadelphia (2009)
7. Krizhevsky, A., Sutskever, I., Hinton, G.: Imagenet classification with deep convolutional neural networks. In: Proceedings of the NIPS (2012)
8. Lay, N., Birkbeck, N., Zhang, J., Zhou, S.K.: Rapid multi-organ segmentation using context integration and discriminative models. In: Joshi, S., Pohl, K.M., Wells, W.M., Zöllei, L., Gee, J.C. (eds.) IPMI 2013. LNCS, vol. 7917, pp. 450–462. Springer, Heidelberg (2013)
9. Liu, W., Rabinovich, A., Berg, A.C.: Parsenet: looking wider to see better (2015). arXiv:1506.04579v2
10. Long, J., Shelhamer, E., Darrell, T.: Fully convolutional networks for semantic segmentation. In: Proceedings of the CVPR (2015)
11. Roth, H.R., Lu, L., Farag, A., Shin, H.C., Liu, J., Turkbey, E.B., Summers, R.M.: Deeporgan: multi-level deep convolutional networks for automated pancreas segmentation. In: Navab, N., Hornegger, J., Wells, W.M., Frangi, A. (eds.) MICCAI 2015. LNCS, vol. 9349, pp. 556–564. Springer, Heidelberg (2015)
12. Sharma, A., Tuzel, O., Liu, M.Y.: Recursive context propagation network for semantic scene labeling. In: Proceedings of the NIPS (2014)

13. Sun, Y., Wang, X., Tang, X.: Deep convolutional network cascade for facial point detection. In: Proc. CVPR (2013)
14. Zheng, Y., Barbu, A., Georgescu, B., Scheuering, M., Comaniciu, D.: Four-chamber heart modeling and automatic segmentation for 3D cardiac CT volumes using marginal space learning and steerable features. IEEE TMI **27**(11), 1668–1681 (2008)
15. Zhou, B., Khosla, A., Lapedriza, A., Oliva, A., Torralba, A.: Object detectors emerge in deep scene CNNs. In: Proceedings of the ICLR (2015)

Cell Segmentation Proposal Network
for Microscopy Image Analysis

Saad Ullah Akram[1,2(✉)], Juho Kannala[3], Lauri Eklund[2,4], and Janne Heikkilä[1]

[1] Center for Machine Vision and Signal Analysis, University of Oulu, Finland
[2] Biocenter Oulu, Oulu, Finland
[3] Department of Computer Science, Aalto University, Espoo, Finland
[4] Faculty of Biochemistry and Molecular Medicine,
Oulu Center for Cell-Matrix Research, University of Oulu, Finland
sakram@ee.oulu.fi

Abstract. Accurate cell segmentation is vital for the development of reliable microscopy image analysis methods. It is a very challenging problem due to low contrast, weak boundaries, and conjoined and overlapping cells; producing many ambiguous regions, which lower the performance of automated segmentation methods. Cell proposals provide an efficient way of exploiting both spatial and temporal context, which can be very helpful in many of these ambiguous regions. However, most proposal based microscopy image analysis methods rely on fairly simple proposal generation stage, limiting their performance. In this paper, we propose a convolutional neural network based method which provides cell segmentation proposals, which can be used for cell detection, segmentation and tracking. We evaluate our method on datasets from histology, fluorescence and phase contrast microscopy and show that it outperforms state of the art cell detection and segmentation methods.

Keywords: Cell proposals · Cell segmentation · Cell detection · Convolutional neural network · Deep learning

1 Introduction

In the last few decades advances in automation and optics of microscopes have led to rapid growth in the number and resolution of images being captured, with single experiments in developmental biology producing tera-bytes of data. Often the processes being investigated are subtle and to obtain biologically meaningful quantification, it is necessary to analyze large number of cells in multiple samples. Doing these analyses manually is a very inefficient and tedious use of a biologists time and is dependent on the skill level of biologists leading to very subjective and often non-reproducible results. These factors have increased the importance of automated and semi-automated analysis methods.

Recently, convolutional neural networks (CNNs) have outperformed the state of the art methods in multiple biomedical instance level segmentation challenges [5,13]. These methods either prioritize boundary pixels by increasing their

© Springer International Publishing AG 2016
G. Carneiro et al. (Eds.): LABELS 2016/DLMIA 2016, LNCS 10008, pp. 21–29, 2016.
DOI: 10.1007/978-3-319-46976-8_3

weights [13] or detect them explicitly in addition to binary segmentation [5]. These networks have large receptive fields allowing them to utilize large spatial context and predict very accurate segmentation masks at instance level. However, since these methods provide only one set of segmentations they can still fail in some ambiguous regions. When analyzing microscopy sequences, temporal information can resolve many of these ambiguities. Cell proposals provide a computationally efficient way of exploiting both temporal and spatial context by reducing the number of alternative hypothesis for a region. So far, cell proposals have been used for cell detection [3,4] and tracking [2,14]. These methods rely on MSER [3], superpixels [14] and blob detection [2] for proposal generation and use hand crafted features to score them. Deep learning has also been applied recently for proposing cell candidate bounding boxes [1], however they use thresholding to obtain segmentation masks, which are not very accurate and it is not trivial to obtain segmentation masks using their approach for images from other microscopy modalities.

In this paper, we propose a CNN based method which first proposes cell bounding boxes using a fully convolutional neural network (FCN) [1]. It then uses a second CNN to predict segmentation masks for each proposed bounding box. Recently, [6] have shown the effectiveness of similar idea for general object segmentation. Our novel contributions are: (1) a new network for cell segmentation proposal generation and (2) a single network model which can segment cells from multiple microscopy modalities. We compare our method's proposals with proposals from two state of the art cell detection methods and our cell detections with three state of the art cell segmentation/detection methods and show that our method outperforms them on three different datasets which represent cells with varying appearance and imaging conditions.

2   Method

Our method has two stages, in the first stage (Sect. 2.1) a convolutional neural network (CNN) proposes cell bounding boxes along with their scores, i.e. probability of them being a cell. In the second stage (Sect. 2.2), a second CNN utilizes the proposed bounding boxes to predict segmentation masks for cells.

2.1   Proposal Bounding Boxes

Our first network, shown in the top half of Fig. 1, is modified from the network in [1]. Briefly, it predicts k bounding boxes and their scores at each pixel in the last feature map, removes duplicate proposals using non-maxima suppression and returns the remaining N bounding boxes as the cell proposals. Details of how this network proposes bounding boxes [1,12] and how it is trained are available in [1].

2.2   Proposal Segmentation

Network Structure: Our second network, which is used for predicting segmentation masks is shown in the bottom half of Fig. 1. This network takes the image

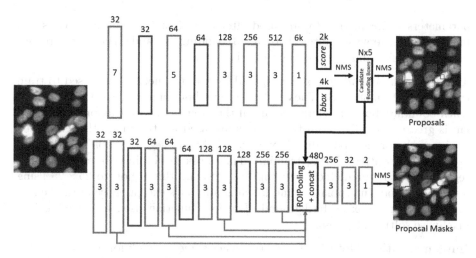

Fig. 1. Cell segmentation proposal network: top half shows the first network, which proposes N bounding boxes and their scores. Bottom half shows the second network which generate segmentation masks for the N proposals. Convolution (filter size is shown in the box), max-pooling, and ROI-Pooling + concatenation layers, with the number of feature maps on top of each layer, are shown. Proposed bounding boxes and segmentation masks after non-maxima suppression (NMS) are shown for a selected area from *Fluo-N2DL-HeLa* dataset.

and N proposed bounding boxes from first network as its inputs and predicts N segmentation masks of size 25×25 each. First part of this network contains eight convolution layers which are applied to the whole image. Second part uses region of interest (ROI) pooling layers [7] to extract fixed size (25×25) features maps from four sets of feature maps as shown in Fig. 1. ROI-Pooling layer uses adaptive max pooling of the region inside the bounding box in a given feature map to extract a fixed sized feature map. The ROI-pooled feature maps are concatenated to obtain a feature map of size $25 \times 25 \times 480$ for each proposed cell bounding box. It is important to select features from layers at different depth so that the network can use both coarse high level information to predict which regions belong to the cell being segmented and fine low level information to predict accurate localization of cell boundaries. The fixed size feature map extracted for each proposed bounding box is used by a small sub-network, consisting of three convolution layers, which picks the appropriate combination of features from different depths so that it can better leverage both fine and coarse information. For each proposed bounding box, this network outputs a 25×25 probability map, which is resized back to the original bounding box size using bicubic interpolation, thresholded and largest connected component is used as the segmentation mask.

All convolutional layers use a stride of 1 pixel and padding to preserve the feature map size. ReLu non-linearities are used after all convolutional layers except the last one. Local contrast normalization layers with same normalization parameters as ZF model [15] are used after first eight convolutional layers. All max-pooling layers use a filter of size 3×3, padding of 1 and stride of 2 to reduce feature map size and increase the receptive field.

Training: The bounding boxes proposed by the first network are used to train the segmentation network. The overlap of these bounding boxes with the ground truth bounding boxes is computed and if the intersection over union (IoU) overlap is greater than 0.5, then these boxes are used for training; otherwise, they are ignored. For each bounding box, a 25×25 binary segmentation mask is used as the target output during training. This mask is obtained by cropping the region inside the predicted bounding box, resizing this region to 25×25 using nearest-neighbor interpolation and labeling all pixels except those of the largest cell within that box as background. The loss function used for training is a pixel-wise softmax log loss.

Implementation Details: To use the exact same network for all datasets, we resize the images in each dataset so that the mean cell bounding box is $\sim 25 \times 25$ pixels. Images in some datasets are quite large so we split these images in equal sized smaller images so that no image dimension is larger than 500 pixels to reduce GPU memory requirement. Since there are very few training images, we use horizontal and vertical flips, and 90 degree rotations to augment training data.

We initialize our segmentation network by picking weights randomly from a Gaussian distribution with zero-mean and 0.01 standard deviation. We use learning rate of 0.0001 for first 40k iterations then it is reduced to 0.00001 for next 10k iterations.

2.3 Cell Detection and Segmentation

There are not many widely used cell proposal generation method which makes it difficult to compare our performance. However, there are few popular cell segmentation and detection methods available publicly. In order to compare our method against these methods, we use stronger non-maxima suppression to remove most duplicate proposals and use the selected proposals (*Ours-Greedy*) as cell detections and their masks as cell segmentations of our method. The IoU and score threshold values which maximize average precision and f-score on the training data are used for each model. Since we use IoU > 0, this can result in some pixels having multiple labels, we assign these pixels the label of the cell (proposal) with the highest score. We would like to point out that these detections can be considered as a weak baseline when using our proposals for cell detection or segmentation. Better performance can be obtained by using dynamic programming [3] or integer linear programming [4], which can select the optimal set of proposals.

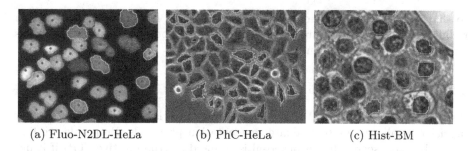

(a) Fluo-N2DL-HeLa   (b) PhC-HeLa   (c) Hist-BM

Fig. 2. Datasets: ground truth cell markers (•) and boundaries are marked. (Color figure online)

3   Experiments

3.1   Data-Sets

We evaluate our method on three datasets *Fluo-N2DL-HeLa* [10], *PhC-HeLa* [3] and *Hist-BM* [8]. Figure 2 shows one sample region from each dataset along with the Ground Truth (GT) segmentation masks and cell markers.

Fluo-N2DL-HeLa data-set is from ISBI cell tracking challenge [10] and it contains 2 time-lapse sequences (92 frames each) of fluorescent HeLa cells cultured and imaged on two dimensional surface. The GT for this data-set contains markers for all 34,060 cells in all frames and segmentation masks for all 874 cells in 4 frames. It also includes segmentation masks for few cells in other frames but since those frames are not exhaustively segmented, we do not use them. Some of the challenges with this data-set are: many cell clusters, frequent cell divisions, low contrast, variation in cell sizes and intensities.

PhC-HeLa data-set [3] consists of 22 phase contrast images of cervical cancer colonies of HeLa cells, split in 2 sets (training and test). The GT for this dataset consists of cell markers for all 2,228 cells. Challenges with this dataset include high variation in cell shapes and sizes, missing cell boundaries, and high cell density.

Ground truth segmentation masks for this dataset are obtained by greedily selecting the largest MSER region for each ground truth marker under the constraints that the selected MSER region contains only one cell marker, has little overlap with previously selected regions and markers which are inside smaller regions are processed first.

Hist-BM data-set [8] consists of 11 images stained with Hematoxylin and Eosin of human bone marrow from eight different patients. The ground truth for this dataset consists of markers for all 4,202 cell nuclei and ambiguous regions. We split this dataset in two sets, with first five images in set 1 and rest in set 2.

Ground truth segmentation masks for this dataset are generated using multi-label graph cuts. Terminal edge costs are set using cell and background Gaussian mixture models, learnt from pixels within radius of 6 from markers and pixels outside radius of 20 from all markers respectively. Cells are divided into 7 sets so that cells adjacent to each other have a different label. Then pixels within radius of 6 from a marker are fixed to the terminal node representing that cell's label to separate cells in contact with each other.

3.2   Evaluation Criteria

Average Precision (AP): We use average precision (AP) - area under precision-recall curve - to evaluate segmentation proposals. Proposals are first sorted by their score, then a proposal is counted as true positive (TP) if it has intersection over union overlap (IoU) > 0.5 with any unmatched ground truth (GT) cell segmentation mask, otherwise it is counted as false positive (FP). GT cells which remain unmatched are counted as false negative (FN). We obtain a pair of recall ($R = \frac{TP}{TP+FN}$) and precision ($P = \frac{TP}{TP+FP}$) values after evaluating each proposal.

F-Score (F1): To evaluate detection performance we use same criteria as above to obtain recall (R) and precision (P) using all cell detections and compute F-Score ($F1 = \frac{2 \cdot P \cdot R}{P+R}$).

SEG: We evaluate accuracy of segmentation masks using the SEG measure, based on Jaccard similarity index, used in ISBI cell tracking challenge [10]. A detection (D) is matched with a GT cell (G) if and only if it contains more than half pixels of that GT cell, i.e. $|D \cap G| > 0.5 \cdot |G|$. For each GT cell and its matched detection, Jaccard similarity index is computed using $J(G, D) = \frac{|D \cap G|}{|D \cup G|}$. SEG is the mean of Jaccard similarity index of all GT cells and ranges between 0 to 1.

We use the SEG measure as defined above to evaluate proposal masks. When evaluating proposals, some pixels can be inside multiple proposals and as a result there might be multiple proposals which satisfy $|D \cap G| > 0.5 \cdot |G|$. We compute Jaccard similarity index for these proposals and match the GT cell with the best proposal, i.e. one having the highest Jaccard similarity index.

Implementation Details: All three datasets are split in two sets as described in Sect. 3.1. One set is used for training the methods and the other for testing; this is repeated for both sets. Same non-maxima suppression settings (IoU=0.5) are used for all methods to remove duplicate proposals. The proposals from both sets are combined, sorted by their score and evaluated as either TP or FP. The detection results are combined similarly and SEG and F-Score computed for the whole dataset.

3.3   Baseline

We compare our method (*Ours*) with two cell proposal generation methods *MSER* [3,11] and *CPN* [1], and three cell detection and segmentation methods, *KTH* [9], *CellDetect*[1][3] and *CPN-Greedy* [1]. **CPN** uses a method similar to

---

[1] http://www.robots.ox.ac.uk/~vgg/software/cell_detection/.

our first stage to propose cell candidates and **CPN-Greedy** uses stronger non-maxima suppression to obtain cell detections from CPN proposals. **CellDetect** uses MSER regions [11] as proposals, represents each proposal using hand crafted features, and uses structured SVM to score them. We use these scores to rank MSER regions during evaluation of **MSER** proposals. CellDetect then selects optimal set of MSER regions using dynamic programming and uses these selected regions as cell detections. **KTH** uses a band pass filter followed by thresholding to segment cells, watershed transform is then used to split cell clusters, and finally tracking is used to correct errors in segmentation. KTH software[2] does not provide access to segmentation results so we use their segmentation masks after the tracking stage during evaluation.

3.4 Results

Figure 3 shows the precision-recall curves for the proposal generation methods and precision-recall values for cell detection methods. Precision-recall curve for our proposals not only remains significantly above the curve for MSER proposals, it is even slightly above the precision-recall values of CellDetect detections for all datasets. For Fluo-N2DL-HeLa dataset, CPN has better precision for all but very high recall values, however it has slightly lower recall than our method. Even though CPN uses simple thresholding, it is able to obtain good performance at IoU=0.5 as thresholding can provide a coarse mask. For higher IoU values, its performance degrades and gap in our method and CPN increases.

Table 1 compares the segmentation quality (SEG) of our method's proposals against other baselines and shows that our method's proposal masks are consistently better than MSER and CPN proposals for all three datasets. Table 1 also lists SEG and F-Score (detection performance) values for all cell detection methods. Our method has better detection and segmentation performance compared to other detection methods. The difference in both detection and segmentation performance of our method and CellDetect is quite large for all three datasets.

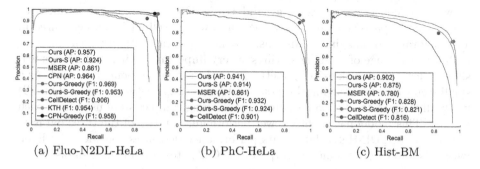

(a) Fluo-N2DL-HeLa   (b) PhC-HeLa   (c) Hist-BM

Fig. 3. Precision vs Recall (at IoU = 0.5) for all three datasets. Average precision (AP) and F-Score (F1) are shown in the legend.

---

[2] http://codesolorzano.com/celltrackingchallenge/Cell_Tracking_Challenge/KTH-SE.html.

Table 1. Cell segmentation (SEG) and detection (F-Score) results.

	Fluo-N2DL-HeLa		PhC-HeLa		Hist-BM	
	SEG	F-Score	SEG	F-Score	SEG	F-Score
Detections						
Ours-Greedy	**0.858**	**0.969**	0.761	**0.932**	**0.804**	**0.828**
Ours-S-Greedy	0.815	0.953	**0.769**	0.924	0.789	0.821
CellDetect [3]	0.734	0.906	0.717	0.901	0.682	0.816
KTH [9]	0.852	0.954	-	-	-	-
CPN-Greedy [1]	0.808	0.958	-	-	-	-
Proposals						
Ours	**0.874**	-	**0.818**	-	**0.823**	-
Ours-S	0.865	-	0.807	-	**0.823**	-
MSER [3]	0.757	-	0.779	-	0.768	-
CPN [1]	0.831	-	-	-	-	-

Our method also outperforms KTH method slightly, which has the best segmentation performance on Fluo-N2DL-HeLa dataset in ISBI cell tracking challenge [10] and uses tracking stage to correct errors in segmentation.

Cell boundaries produced by our method are quite accurate; most segmentation errors are due to (1) errors in localization of bounding boxes, which sometimes clips parts of cells and (2) the failure of segmentation stage to ignore parts of other cells in the proposed bounding box. We tried using a dilated proposal bounding box but it led to lower performance as even though it reduced clipping errors, the errors due to failure to ignore other cells increased. We also experimented with a fully connected layer at the end of the network, which was able to ignore other cells better but it produced coarse masks and did not improve performance.

Two of the challenges of biomedical image analysis are the large variation between sequences and lack of ground truth. Often a method is trained or designed for a particular set of sequences and works well for images captured in a narrow range of imaging conditions. Having a general method which can cope with a wider range of imaging settings is very important as it is not always feasible to design or tweak existing methods for the sequences being analyzed. As a small step towards achieving this goal, we train a single network model (Ours-S) using all three datasets. Equal number of training samples were used from each dataset. This model has slightly lower performance on two of the three datasets but on Fluo-N2DL-HeLa dataset its performance decreases considerably. Even with this lower performance it outperforms CellDetect on all three datasets.

4   Conclusions

In this paper, we have presented a deep learning based method for proposing cell segmentation candidates and demonstrated that it can produce excellent proposals for three different microscopic modalities. We have compared our method against state of the art cell detection and segmentation methods and shown that our method outperform them on common evaluation metrics. We have also presented a single model trained on all three datasets and shown that its performance does not degrade significantly, which is promising and indicates that a single model for cell detection and segmentation can be trained without compromising too much on performance. Performance of such a model may even improve if it is trained on datasets which are imaged in somewhat similar imaging conditions; this is something we plan to investigate in future. We also plan to use our method's proposals for cell detection and tracking. Code is available at https://github.com/SaadUllahAkram/CellProposalNetwork.

References

1. Akram, S.U., Kannala, J., Eklund, L., Heikkilä, J.: Cell proposal network for microscopy image analysis. In: ICIP (2016)
2. Akram, S.U., Kannala, J., Eklund, L., Heikkilä, J.: Joint cell segmentation and tracking using cell proposals. In: ISBI (2016)
3. Arteta, C., Lempitsky, V., Noble, J.A., Zisserman, A.: Learning to detect cells using non-overlapping extremal regions. In: Ayache, N., Delingette, H., Golland, P., Mori, K. (eds.) MICCAI 2012, Part I. LNCS, vol. 7510, pp. 348–356. Springer, Heidelberg (2012)
4. Bise, R., Sato, Y.: Cell detection from redundant candidate regions under nonoverlapping constraints. IEEE Trans. Med. Imaging **34**, 1417–1427 (2015)
5. Chen, H., Qi, X., Yu, L., Heng, P.A.: DCAN: deep contour-aware networks for accurate gland segmentation. In: CVPR (2016)
6. Dai, J., He, K., Sun, J.: Instance-aware semantic segmentation via multi-task network cascades. In: CVPR (2016)
7. Girshick, R.: Fast R-CNN. In: ICCV (2015)
8. Kainz, P., Urschler, M., Schulter, S., Wohlhart, P., et al.: You should use regression to detect cells. In: Navab, N., Hornegger, J., Wells, W.M., Frangi, A.F. (eds.) MICCAI 2015. LNCS, vol. 9351, pp. 276–283. Springer, New York (2015)
9. Magnusson, K.E.G., Jalden, J.: A batch algorithm using iterative application of the viterbi algorithm to track cells and construct cell lineages. In: ISBI (2012)
10. Maška, M., Ulman, V., Svoboda, D., Matula, P., et al.: A benchmark for comparison of cell tracking algorithms. Bioinformatics **30**, 1609–1617 (2014)
11. Matas, J., Chum, O., Urban, M., Pajdla, T.: Robust wide-baseline stereo from maximally stable extremal regions. Image Vis. Comput. **22**, 761–767 (2004)
12. Ren, S., He, K., Girshick, R., Sun, J.: Faster R-CNN: Towards real-time object detection with region proposal networks. In: NIPS (2015)
13. Ronneberger, O., Fischer, P., Brox, T.: U-Net: convolutional networks for biomedical image segmentation. In: MICCAI (2015)
14. Schiegg, M., Hanslovsky, P., Haubold, C., Koethe, U., et al.: Graphical model for joint segmentation and tracking of multiple dividing cells. Bioinformatics (2015)
15. Zeiler, M.D., Fergus, R.: Visualizing and understanding convolutional networks. In: Fleet, D., Pajdla, T., Schiele, B., Tuytelaars, T. (eds.) ECCV 2014, Part I. LNCS, vol. 8689, pp. 818–833. Springer, Heidelberg (2014)

Vessel Detection in Ultrasound Images Using Deep Convolutional Neural Networks

Erik Smistad[1,2(✉)] and Lasse Løvstakken[1]

[1] Norwegian University of Science and Technology, Trondheim, Norway
{erik.smistad,lasse.lovstakken}@ntnu.no
[2] SINTEF Medical Technology, Trondheim, Norway

Abstract. Deep convolutional neural networks have achieved great results on image classification problems. In this paper, a new method using a deep convolutional neural network for detecting blood vessels in B-mode ultrasound images is presented. Automatic blood vessel detection may be useful in medical applications such as deep venous thrombosis detection, anesthesia guidance and catheter placement. The proposed method is able to determine the position and size of the vessels in images in real-time. 12,804 subimages of the femoral region from 15 subjects were manually labeled. Leave-one-subject-out cross validation was used giving an average accuracy of 94.5 %, a major improvement from previous methods which had an accuracy of 84 % on the same dataset. The method was also validated on a dataset of the carotid artery to show that the method can generalize to blood vessels on other regions of the body. The accuracy on this dataset was 96 %.

1 Introduction

Blood vessel segmentation in ultrasound images may be useful in medical applications such as deep venous thrombosis detection [5], anesthesia guidance [12] and catheter placement. The goal of vessel detection in this work, was to identify the position and size of blood vessels in the image. Several segmentation and tracking methods require this as an initialization [1,6]. In [12], a real-time vessel detection method was introduced, removing the need for manual initialization. This method performs an ellipse fitting at each pixel in the image using a graphic processing unit (GPU). However, this method has problems distinguishing vessels from non-vessels when varying user settings, such as gain, on the ultrasound scanner, and on individuals with more subcutaneous fat tissue, due to increased amounts of reverberation artifacts. Also, this method was only made to detect a single vessel for each image.

In this paper, we propose to use a similar ellipse fitting method to find vessel candidate regions which are passed on to a deep neural network classifier which determines if the region contains a vessel or not. As the proposed detection method provides both position and size, it may also be used as a vessel segmentation method, assuming the vessel has an elliptical shape. The proposed method also enables detection of multiple vessels at the same time.

© Springer International Publishing AG 2016
G. Carneiro et al. (Eds.): LABELS 2016/DLMIA 2016, LNCS 10008, pp. 30–38, 2016.
DOI: 10.1007/978-3-319-46976-8_4

2   Methods

The next section will introduce the elliptic vessel model, which was used to find vessel candidate regions in the ultrasound image. Subimages were created from the ultrasound image for each vessel candidate. A deep convolutional network determines if each subimage is of an actual blood vessel. Figure 1 provides an overview of the steps involved in the proposed method.

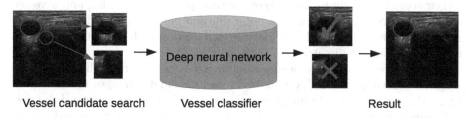

Vessel candidate search   Vessel classifier   Result

Fig. 1. Overview of the proposed method. The first step finds vessel candidates and creates subimages for each. The subimages are then passed on to a deep neural network which identifies the subimages belonging to vessels, and discards those that are not of vessels.

2.1   Vessel Model

Each vessel is modelled as an ellipse with center $c = [c_x, c_y]$ and major and minor radius a and b. The point p_i and its normal n_i of point i on an ellipse of N evenly distributed points can be calculated with the following equations.

$$\alpha_i = \frac{2\pi i}{N} \tag{1}$$

$$d_i = [a\cos(\alpha_i), b\sin(\alpha_i)] \tag{2}$$

$$p_i = c + d_i \tag{3}$$

$$n_i = \frac{[b\cos(\alpha_i), a\sin(\alpha_i)]}{|[b\cos(\alpha_i), a\sin(\alpha_i)]|} \tag{4}$$

2.2   Vessel Candidate Search

First, the image is blurred using convolution with a Gaussian mask ($\sigma = 0.5$mm) and then the image gradients G are calculated using a central difference scheme. For a given radii a and b, the vessel score S is calculated as the average dot product of the outward normal n_i and the corresponding image gradient at N points on the ellipse, as shown in (5).

$$S(c, a, b) = \frac{1}{N} \sum_{i=0}^{N-1} n_i \cdot G(p_i) \tag{5}$$

For each pixel, ellipses of different major radius a ranging from 3.5 to 6 mm, flattening factor f from 0 to 0.5 (minor radius $b = (1 - f)a$) and $N = 32$ samples were used to calculate the vessel score. An increment of 0.25 mm was used for the radius, and 0.1 for the flattening factor. The ellipse with the highest score is selected for each pixel. The best score and the values a and b is stored for each pixel. Any vessel candidate with a score below 1.5 is discarded. This is a low threshold, which will not discard vessels with low contrast, but will also allow several non-vessel regions. Next, the vessel candidates are sorted according to their score from high to low. These are then processed in order, and a vessel candidate is accepted if the center is not inside another vessel candidate structure already accepted. Any vessel candidates which overlap with previously accepted vessel candidates are discarded.

For each vessel candidate, a square subimage is created from the ultrasound images as shown in Fig. 1. Examples of vessel candidates images are shown in Fig. 2. The vessel candidate image is centered at the vessel center c and the size of the image is determined by the major radius a so that the width and height of the image is $4a \times 4a$ converted to pixels. This image size will thus include the vessel as well as some surrounding tissue.

2.3   Vessel Classifier

The next step of the proposed method is to send each vessel candidate image through a deep convolutional neural network classifier to determine if the image belongs to a blood vessel. Caffe [7] was used as the underlying framework both for training and testing of the classifier, while the vessel candidate search was implemented with the FAST medical image computing framework [11].

Data: The data used for training and validation was acquired by first scanning the femoral region of both legs of 15 subjects with varying image quality and different ultrasound acquisition settings. Every tenth frame was run through the vessel candidate search step and the resulting images were stored on disk. This resulted in 12,804 images in total. All images were resized to 128×128, and classified manually as either vessel or non-vessel. Figure 2 show some image examples of both blood vessels and non-vessel structures. The ultrasound system used was an Ultrasonix SonixMDP (Analogic, Boston, USA) with L14-5 linear array probe. To increase the amount of training data, all vessel candidate images were flipped horizontally, effectively doubling the amount of training data.

The Network: The AlexNet [8] network was used initially, and gradually simplified by removing convolution-pooling blocks and reducing the number of convolutions, while maintaining the validation accuracy. The network was simplified mainly to improve the test runtime speed, which was important in order to achieve real-time performance. The final vessel classification network consisted of two convolution layers, one normalization layer, two max pooling layers and three fully connected layers. Additionally, rectified linear units (ReLU), which have shown to improve training [4], was used as non-linear activation units both

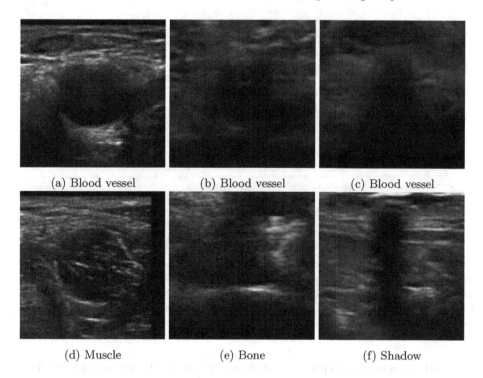

(a) Blood vessel   (b) Blood vessel   (c) Blood vessel

(d) Muscle   (e) Bone   (f) Shadow

Fig. 2. Vessel candidate images of blood vessels and other non-vessel structures used for training the neural network.

for the convolution layers and the fully connected (FC) layers. Thus, including ReLU layers, the network consisted of 13 layers in total, as shown in Fig. 3. Additionally, a softmax loss layer was used for the training of the network. The data layer size was fixed to 110 × 110 pixels. During training, random patches of size 110 × 110 were cropped from the 128 × 128 vessel candidate images to prevent overfitting. This technique increased accuracy with about 1 %. The mean image was calculated from the training data and subtracted from the input image. The first convolution layer had 9 convolutions of size 11 × 11 pixels and the second had 32 convolutions of size 15 × 15. The max pooling was done over patches of 3 × 3. Local response normalization (LRN) [8] was used after the first convolution layer with the same parameters as in [8]. Dropout was used on the fully connected layers with a probability of 0.5. The network was trained with stochastic gradient descent, batch size 128, momentum 0.9 and weight decay 0.0005. The base learning rate was 0.01 with a sigmoid learning rate decay.

2.4   Performance Optimizations

Ultrasound is a real-time imaging modality, delivering typically 10–20 images per second. The proposed method thus have to find vessels in each image in less

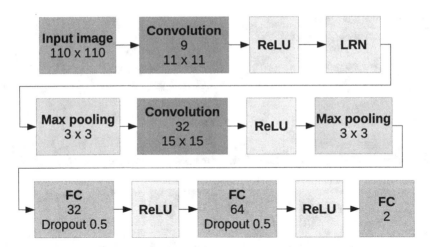

Fig. 3. The vessel detection network. A fixed-size input image of size 110×110 is feed into two convolution-pooling stages with 9 and 32 convolutions respectively. This is followed by three fully connected (FC) layers with dropout to reduce overfitting. A local response normalization (LRN) is performed after the first convolution. Rectified linear units (ReLU) are used as non-linear activation units in all stages.

than 100 ms to be able to process the ultrasound image stream in real-time. The vessel candidate search, subimage creation and resizing were all implemented on the GPU using the FAST framework. Caffe was run in GPU mode and all vessel candidates for a given image frame were batch processed, which significantly boosts performance. Additionally, the vessel candidate search was only performed on every fourth pixel.

3   Results

Figure 4 show the convolutions learned by the neural network. These figures show that the first convolutional layer learns to detect horizontal edges, and the second layer learns to identify different patterns of horizontal edges. The trained neural network does not seem to find vertical edges as important in the ultrasound images. This seems sensible, as vertical edges are often weaker or missing in ultrasound images.

Leave-one-subject-out cross validation was used, thus 14 subjects were used for training and 1 subject kept for validation. The average classification accuracy for the cross validation was 94.5 %, with a standard deviation of 2.9. This was calculated using a discrimination threshold of 0.5 on the softmax output of the vessel classifier. Figure 5a shows the result of the vessel detection on an image of the femoral region.

This dataset was only from a single area of the body, the femoral region covering the femoral artery and vein. To see how well the proposed method can generalize to other parts of the body, a dataset of the left and right carotid

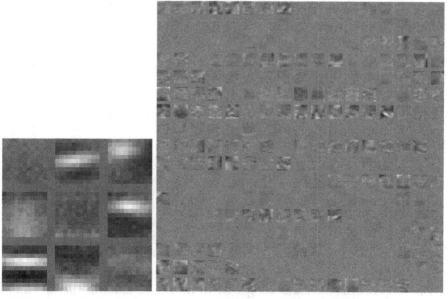

(a) First convolutional layer   (b) Second convolutional layer.

Fig. 4. Features learned by the neural network. The first layer has learned several horizontal edge detectors, while the second convolutional layer has learned to recognize patterns of horizontal edges.

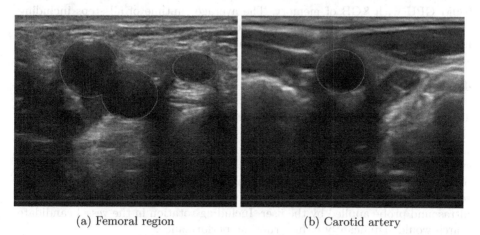

(a) Femoral region   (b) Carotid artery

Fig. 5. Vessel detection result on two ultrasound images.

artery was acquired from two subjects and used as validation data, while the dataset with the 15 subjects of the femoral region was used as training data. The dataset was created with the same method described in Sect. 2.3. With this data, the method achieved an accuracy of 96 %. Figure 5b shows the result of the vessel detection on an image of the carotid artery.

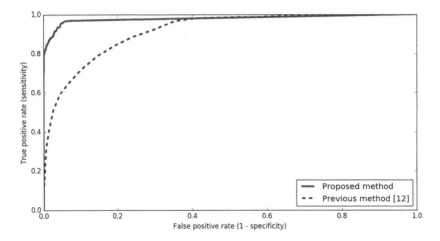

Fig. 6. ROC curve of the proposed method and the method in [12].

The proposed method was compared to a another state of the art vessel detection method [12]. This method achieved an average accuracy of 84 % on the femoral region dataset. The receiver operating characteristics (ROC) curves in Fig. 6 show how the two methods perform when varying the discrimination threshold for the same dataset.

Training time was about 10 min on a laptop computer with an NVIDIA GTX 980M GPU with 8 GB of memory. The average runtime of all steps including the vessel candidate search and vessel classification was 46 ms, enabling the ultrasound images to be processed in real-time.

4   Discussion

The vessel model used in the proposed method assumes that the vessels are elliptical, while this often holds true for arteries, it may not be ideal for veins which often have a more irregular shape. Thus, the proposed method is more suited for arteries than veins. The vessel model also does not consider rotation of the ellipse. However, in our experiments this has not been an issue as vessels usually are compressed in the vertical direction, due to pressure from the ultrasound probe applied by the user. Including rotation in the vessel candidate search would significantly reduce runtime performance.

An alternative to the proposed ellipse fitting method would be to use more general object detection methods, such as R-CNN [3,10]. However, these methods are more complex and bounding boxes would have to be created manually around each vessel in each image, which is time consuming. With the ellipse fitting method, the user only have to choose between the classes "vessel" and "non-vessel" for each vessel candidate subimage. Thus, the proposed ellipse fitting method aids in the labeling of the data.

Another alternative can be to use a fully convolutional neural network [9]. Such as network would provide a classification of each pixel. The ground truth data could be created by a user selecting the center of each blood vessel. Using such as network may be more robust in terms of rotation and deformation of the blood vessels. However, it would not provide the radius of the vessels and a segmentation as shown in Fig. 5.

The validation accuracy was 94.5 %, which is a major improvement from the vessel detection method in [12] which got an accuracy of 84 % on the same validation dataset. The accuracy may be improved by adding more training data, including the temporal dimension of the data with recurrent neural networks, and including Doppler data in a separate image channel. In the proposed network, the weights were initialization using Gaussian noise with standard deviation 0.01. Unsupervised pre-training has shown to be a good way to initialize the weights of deep neural networks [2]. With ultrasound imaging, a large amount of unlabeled data can easily be acquired from the target body regions. Thus, we believe unsupervised pre-training of deep networks will be a useful technique within ultrasound imaging.

5 Conclusion

A robust real-time vessel detection method for ultrasound images was presented. The method uses a deep convolutional neural network to classify subimages. Although the neural network was only trained on images of the femoral artery and vein, it is able to generalize to other vessels such as the carotid artery.

References

1. Abolmaesumi, P., Sirouspour, M., Salcudean, S.: Real-time extraction of carotid artery contours from ultrasound images. In: Proceedings 13th IEEE Symposium on Computer-Based Medical Systems, CBMS 2000, pp. 181–186. IEEE Computer Society (2000)
2. Bengio, Y., Lamblin, P., Popovici, D., Larochelle, H.: Greedy layer-wise training of deep networks. Adv. Neural Inf. Process. Syst. 19(1), 153–160 (2007)
3. Girshick, R.: Fast R-CNN. In: 2015 IEEE International Conference on Computer Vision (ICCV), pp. 1440–1448. IEEE, December 2015
4. Glorot, X., Bordes, A., Bengio, Y.: Deep Sparse rectifier neural networks. In: 14th International Conference on Artificial Intelligence and Statistics, pp. 315–323 (2011)
5. Guerrero, J., Salcudean, S.E., McEwen, J.A., Masri, B.A., Nicolaou, S.: System for deep venous thombosis detection using objective compression measures. IEEE Trans. Biomed. Eng. 53(5), 845–854 (2006)
6. Guerrero, J., Salcudean, S.E., McEwen, J.A., Masri, B.A., Nicolaou, S.: Real-time vessel segmentation and tracking for ultrasound imaging applications. IEEE Trans. Med. Imaging 26(8), 1079–1090 (2007)
7. Jia, Y., Shelhamer, E., Donahue, J., Karayev, S., Long, J., Girshick, R., Guadarrama, S., Darrell, T.: Caffe: convolutional architecture for fast feature embedding. In: Proceedings of the ACM International Conference on Multimedia, pp. 675–678 (2014)

8. Krizhevsky, A., Sutskever, I., Hinton, G.E.: ImageNet classification with deep convolutional neural networks. In: Advances in Neural Information Processing Systems, pp. 1097–1105 (2012)
9. Long, J., Shelhamer, E., Darrell, T.: Fully convolutional networks for semantic segmentation. In: 2015 IEEE Conference on Computer Vision and Pattern Recognition (CVPR), pp. 3431–3440 (2015)
10. Ren, S., He, K., Girshick, R., Sun, J.: Faster R-CNN: Towards real-time object detection with region proposal networks. Advances in neural information processing systems, pp. 91–99, June 2015
11. Smistad, E., Bozorgi, M., Lindseth, F.: FAST: framework for heterogeneous medical image computing and visualization. Int. J. Comput. Assist. Radiol. Surg. **10**(11), 1811–1822 (2015)
12. Smistad, E., Lindseth, F.: Real-time automatic artery segmentation, reconstruction and registration for ultrasound-guided regional anaesthesia of the femoral nerve. IEEE Trans. Med. Imaging **35**(3), 752–761 (2016)

Convolutional Neural Network for Reconstruction of 7T-like Images from 3T MRI Using Appearance and Anatomical Features

Khosro Bahrami, Feng Shi, Islem Rekik, and Dinggang Shen[✉]

Department of Radiology and BRIC, University of North Carolina at Chapel Hill,
Chapel Hill, NC, USA
dinggang_shen@med.unc.edu

Abstract. The advanced 7 Tesla (7T) Magnetic Resonance Imaging (MRI) scanners provide images with higher resolution anatomy than 3T MRI scanners, thus facilitating early diagnosis of brain diseases. However, 7T MRI scanners are less accessible, compared to the 3T MRI scanners. This motivates us to reconstruct 7T-like images from 3T MRI. We propose a deep architecture for Convolutional Neural Network (CNN), which uses the *appearance* (intensity) and *anatomical* (labels of brain tissues) features as input to non-linearly map 3T MRI to 7T MRI. In the training step, we train the CNN by *feeding* it with both appearance and anatomical features of the 3T patch. This outputs the intensity of center voxel in the corresponding 7T patch. In the testing step, we apply the trained CNN to map each input 3T patch to the 7T-like image patch. Our performance is evaluated on 15 subjects, each with both 3T and 7T MR images. Both visual and numerical results show that our method outperforms the comparison methods.

1 Introduction

Magnetic Resonance Imaging (MRI) has widely been used to assist the diagnosis of brain diseases. In the past years, tremendous efforts have been made to improve MR image quality, which is desired for early and more accurate MRI-based disease diagnosis. This has yielded to 7T MRI that has higher resolution and contrast than the conventional 3T MRI. Figure 1 shows the respective axial views of linearly aligned 3T and 7T MR images from the same subject. Due to higher quality imaging, 7T MRI can potentially help in more accurate diagnosis of various brain diseases. For example, cortical lesions and atrophies can be better characterized with higher resolution and contrast in the 7T MRI compared to 3T MRI [1]. Furthermore, partial volume effect (PVE) affects the 3T MRI more than 7T MRI, thus reducing the accuracy of post-processing tasks such as MRI brain tissue segmentation. However, at the current stage, many clinical centers in the world ($\approx$ 20,000) have just 3T MRI scanners, and only a few ($\approx$ 40) have been equipped with 7T MRI scanners due to high expenses [2]. Therefore, an alternative solution is to reconstruct 7T-like images from 3T MR images, which is the main focus of our paper.

© Springer International Publishing AG 2016
G. Carneiro et al. (Eds.): LABELS 2016/DLMIA 2016, LNCS 10008, pp. 39–47, 2016.
DOI: 10.1007/978-3-319-46976-8_5

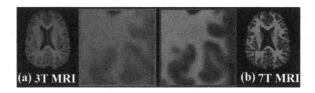

Fig. 1. Axial views, along with zoomed regions, of linearly aligned (a) 3T MRI and (b) 7T MRI of the same subject. 7T MRI has higher resolution and contrast. (Color figure online)

Recently, many methods have been proposed for the reconstruction of high-resolution (HR) images from low-resolution (LR) images. One of the most popular approaches is the learning-based methods, which use pairs of LR and HR training images. In these methods, the LR testing image is first sparsely represented by the LR training images and then the same representation is applied to reconstruct the HR target image by the HR training images. For instance, Rueda et al. [3] presented a sparse representation based method to generate HR brain MRI from LR brain MRI. Burgos et al. [4] proposed a method, namely local image similarity (LIS), for the reconstruction of CT images from MR images. Bahrami et al. [5,6] also proposed a method for the reconstruction of 7T-like images from 3T MRI based on multi-level CCA, called M-CCA.

In the last few years, CNN successfully have been used for reconstruction of HR from LR images by generating a non-linear mapping using paired LR and HR training images. For instance, Dong et al. [7] proposed a super-resolution method by learning an end-to-end mapping between LR and HR images. In another method, Kulkarni et al. [8] proposed a method for reconstruction of HR images from LR images captured by compressive sensing. Although the proposed CNN architectures in the previous methods work for super-resolution of 2D natural images, they may not be suitable for reconstruction of 3D MR images.

However, one main weakness of the previous methods is that they are less reliable when the testing and training 3T MR images come from different MRI scanners. This is most likely to happen when collecting data from multiple imaging centers and thus obtaining MR images with different qualities. Since previous methods often use a predefined set of features (e.g., patch intensities), the representation of new testing images by the training set with different imaging qualities may be affected by quality inconsistency. To alleviate this problem, we propose a novel method based on tailoring a deep Convolutional Neural Network (CNN) architecture. Previously, CNN has been widely proposed to solve many computer vision tasks such as classification and regression and achieved remarkable accuracy compared to other methods, due to the following facts: (1) generating non-linear mapping between input features and target values; (2) incorporating filters for multi-layer representation of features; and (3) learning the features from data without manually designing features. Our proposed framework largely differs from previous methods for HR reconstruction from LR images in several aspects. First, it does not solely rely on appearance features, but also integrates robust anatomical features (labels of brain tissues) to learn the 3T to 7T mapping. This would help ensure a better anatomical consistency between neighboring patches, and achieve more robustness than the previous methods, since the additional anatomical features are less influenced by 3T MR image quality. Second, our proposed deep CNN architecture uses a large number of features (both high-frequency and low-frequency features) via different filters, thus better capturing the variations among 3T MR images with different qualities. Third, we do not need to learn optimal dictionaries or manifolds to map 3T to 7T patches. The convolutional filters are automatically learned during the CNN feed-forward step, while avoiding the need for extra-learning or optimization steps.

2 Proposed Convolutional Neural Network (CNN) Architecture

Overview: Consider a 3T MR image with appearance $\mathbf{X}$ and anatomical features $\mathbf{L}$. Our goal is to learn a mapping function $f(.)$ using CNN that can generate the corresponding 7T-like image $\mathbf{Y} = f(\mathbf{X}, \mathbf{L})$, with quality similar to the ground-truth 7T MRI. Specifically, we propose a CNN architecture with four layers as shown in Fig. 2. Details of our four-layer CNN architecture are given in the following sections.

First Layer Feature Maps. The first layer aims to learn a feature representation of the input 3T MR image. Let $\mathbf{x}$ and $\mathbf{l}$ be the appearance and anatomical maps for a patch of size $m \times m \times m$ extracted from the input 3T MR image. The first layer of our network includes N_1 convolution filters, each with size of $w_1 \times w_1 \times w_1$, followed by ReLU activation function. The convolution filter

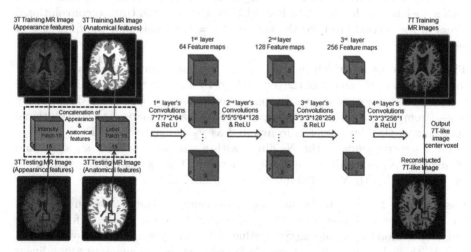

Fig. 2. Our proposed deep CNN architecture for reconstructing 7T-like image from 3T MRI. The testing and training images are indicated in red and blue colors, respectively. (Color figure online)

is the basic component of CNN, which convolves an input patch with a kernel and then outputs a patch generally with a smaller size. For instance, for an image with a size of m (in one dimension) and a kernel with a size of w_1, the size of the output will be $m - w_1 + 1$. In addition to linear convolutions, CNN also includes a non-linear operation encoded by the activation ReLU function. This is desirable for our proposed CNN, since it is used to estimate a non-linear mapping from 3T space to 7T space through our multi-layer convolutional architecture. ReLU is a piecewise linear function, which converts the negative input to zero and retains the positive input, thus introducing sparsity in the network. The input to the first layer is the concatenation of the patch appearance $\mathbf{x}$ and the patch anatomical feature $\mathbf{l}$, denoted as $\mathbf{s}$, while the output $\mathbf{y}_1$ includes N_1 feature maps. Mathematically, our first-layer architecture can be formulated as $\mathbf{y}_1 = \max(0, \mathrm{Conv}(\mathbf{F}_1, \mathbf{s}) + B_1)$, where $\mathbf{F}_1$ corresponds to N_1 filters, and B_1 includes N_1 bias values, each associated with a filter. Conv(.) denotes the convolution operation, which applies each of the N_1 filters to the input to generate the output along with N_1 feature maps, which are then filtered using the ReLU function $\max(0, .)$. By applying the N_1 filters of the first layer to the input 3T MRI, the output $\mathbf{y}_1$, with N_1 feature maps, are generated. Figure 3(a) shows an example of the trained convolutional filters of the first layer with $N_1 = 64$ filters and the filter size of $w_1 = 7$.

Second Layer Feature Maps. In this step, as a part of estimating the cascaded non-linear mapping from 3T to 7T MRI, we estimate the second-level feature maps from the output N_1 feature maps of the first layer. The second layer includes N_2 filters, followed by ReLU operation. It takes as input the N_1 feature maps outputted by the first layer and generates N_2 feature maps. Our second layer is defined as $\mathbf{y}_2 = \max(0, \mathrm{Conv}(\mathbf{F}_2, \mathbf{y}_1) + B_2)$, where $\mathbf{F}_2$ corresponds to the N_2 filters with a size of $N_1 \times w_2 \times w_2 \times w_2$. B_2 includes N_2 bias values, each associated with a filter. In Fig. 3(b), we visualize the trained convolutional filters of the second layer for the case of $N_2 = 128$ filters and the filter size of $w_2 = 5$.

Third Layer Feature Maps. In a similar way, we estimate the third-level feature maps from the output of the second layer. This comprises N_3 filters, followed by ReLU, which are consecutively applied to the previously estimated N_2 feature maps (from the second layer) to output new N_3 feature maps. The convolutional operation in the third layer is formulated as $\mathbf{y}_3 = \max(0, \mathrm{Conv}(\mathbf{F}_3, \mathbf{y}_2) + B_3)$, where $\mathbf{F}_3$ corresponds to the N_3 filters with a size of $N_2 \times w_3 \times w_3 \times w_3$, and B_3 includes N_3 bias values. Figure 3(c) shows the trained convolutional filters of the third layer with $N_3 = 256$ filters and the filter size of $w_3 = 3$.

Last Layer. Finally, in the last layer, we convolve the $N3$ feature maps of the third layer with one filter with a size of $N3 \times w_4 \times w_4 \times w_4$, followed by ReLU operation to output one voxel value, defined as $\mathbf{y} = \max(0, \mathrm{Conv}(\mathbf{F}_4, \mathbf{y}_3) + B_4)$. With such a deep multi-layer CNN architecture, we generate a non-linear mapping from an input 3T MRI patch with a size of $m \times m \times m$ to the voxel intensity at the center of the corresponding 7T MRI patch.

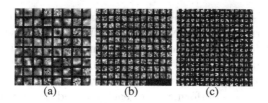

(a)   (b)   (c)

Fig. 3. Examples of the trained convolutional filters. (a) First layer with 64 filters of size $7 \times 7 \times 7$. (b) Second layer with 128 filters of size $5 \times 5 \times 5$. (c) Third layer with 256 filters of size $3 \times 3 \times 3$.

Loss Function. To automatically estimate the network parameters such as the filter weights and biases, we train the end-to-end mapping function $f(.)$. This can be achieved by minimizing the loss, which is defined as a Mean Square Error (MSE) between the reconstructed 7T MRI and ground-truth 7T MRI, as $\mathrm{MSE} = \frac{1}{n}\sum_{i=1}^{n}||\mathbf{Z}_i - \mathbf{Y}_i||^2$, where n is the number of training MR images, $\mathbf{Z}_i$ and $\mathbf{Y}_i$ denote the i-th ground-truth and reconstructed training 7T MR images, respectively. The loss is minimized using stochastic gradient descent with the standard back propagation.

3   Experimental Results

We compare the performance of our proposed CNN with three competing methods including the histogram-matching, local image similarity (LIS) [4], and M-CCA [5]. The histogram-matching method is used as a baseline method, which directly matches the 3T MR image's histogram to the 7T MR image's histogram. We use LIS [4] as a comparison method, which uses patch similarity for reconstruction. We also compare our method with M-CCA [5], since it is based on the sparse representation in multi-level CCA space, which generally outperforms the conventional sparse representation method.

Data and Preprocessing: We used a dataset of 15 pairs of 3T and 7T MRI. This dataset includes 5 healthy subjects, 8 patients with epilepsy, and 2 patients with MCI, which were scanned using both 3T MRI and 7T MRI scanners. These MR images were all linearly aligned and skull-stripped to remove non-brain regions. The 3T and 7T MR images have the resolution of $1 \times 1 \times 1\,\mathrm{mm}^3$ and $0.65 \times 0.65 \times 0.65\,\mathrm{mm}^3$, respectively.

Experimental Settings: We use MatConvNet to implement the CNN architecture. To generate the mapping from 3T MRI to 7T MRI, we use a patch size of $15 \times 15 \times 15$. For CNN, we use a filter size of $w_1 = 7$, $w_2 = 5$, $w_3 = 3$, and $w_4 = 3$, from the first layer to the last layer, respectively. Also, we consider $N_1 = 64$, $N_2 = 128$, $N_3 = 256$, and $N_4 = 1$ filters. For CNN training, we extract overlapping patches with an overlap of 1 voxel. To evaluate our proposed method, we design two experiments. In the first experiment, we only consider the appearance of patches as the input for learning our proposed CNN; while in the second experiment, we consider both appearance and anatomical features of patches to provide richer information for CNN learning. We employed widely-used FAST in FSL package [9] for tissue segmentation to generate anatomical features. Similarly, for the LIS and M-CCA methods, we also consider both appearance and anatomical features of 3T MRI patches to show the contribution of anatomical features in improving the performance of each method. For evaluation, we use a leave-one-out cross-validation by considering one pair of 3T MRI and 7T MRI for testing and the remaining 14 pairs for training.

Numerical Results: In this experiment, we numerically compare our proposed method with three competing methods in terms of peak-signal-to-noise ratio (PSNR), by considering the following two cases:

(1) Training and testing 3T MR images with the same quality. In this case, we use the dataset of 15 pairs of 3T and 7T MR images with the original resolutions, so the testing and training 3T MR images have the same quality. Table 1 compares our proposed method and three competing methods based on the average PSNR across 15 leave-one-out cross-validations. To evaluate the impact of using anatomical features, we independently consider (1) appearance features and (2) both appearance and anatomical features for LIS, M-CCA and our proposed method. Our proposed method has better reconstruction results compared to all three competing methods. Furthermore, these results also clearly show the importance of using anatomical features in improving 7T MRI reconstruction. Figure 4(a) compares the results of different methods in terms of PSNR for 15 leave-one-out cross-validation; for LIS, M-CCA and our proposed method, the reported results are based on both appearance and anatomical features. Compared to all three competing methods, our method has higher PSNR for each leave-one-out case (with $p < 0.01$ in two-sample t-test).

(2) Training and testing 3T MR images with different qualities. In practice, the quality of the testing and training 3T MR images could be different, especially if they are scanned with different imaging protocols and scanners. In this experiment, we simulate this situation by changing the quality of the testing and training 3T MR images using a re-sampling strategy; in this way, the testing images will have a different image quality from the training set. We chart our two simulating scenarios: in the first one we only re-sample the testing images, while in the second one, we only re-sample the training images. We consider two different re-sampling rates to change the quality:

Table 1. Comparison of our proposed method and three competing methods using average PSNR across 15 leave-one-out cross-validations. Two cases, using appearance features or both appearance and anatomical features, are also compared.

Method	Histogram-matching	LIS	LIS	M-CCA	M-CCA	Proposed	Proposed
Feature	Appearance	Appearance	Appearance + Anatomical	Appearance	Appearance + Anatomical	Appearance	Appearance + Anatomical
Average PSNR	21.1	23.9	24.3	25.0	25.4	25.9	**26.5**

• *Re-sampling Rate of 2*. In the first simulating scenario, we re-sample the testing 3T MR image with a factor of 2 (i.e., down-sampling by a factor of 2, followed by up-sampling by a factor of 2), to reduce the quality of 3T MR image. By doing so, down-sampling decreases the number of voxels and also lose image details, while up-sampling increases the number of voxels by interpolation on the existing voxels but will not recover the lost information. Figure 4(b) compares the result of different methods in terms of PSNR for 15 leave-one-out cases. The experimental results show that, after re-sampling, the reconstruction performance by three competing method drops significantly, while our proposed method still achieves good reconstruction quality and regains some lost anatomical details, thus indicating its robustness to image quality changing. This can be explained by two facts. First, we extract many features using various CNN filters from the 3T MR images, thereby obtaining both low-frequency and high-frequency features, which increases robustness to image quality changing. Second, by further incorporating the anatomical features (besides appearance features), our proposed CNN depends less on the resolution and quality of the 3T MR image. In the second simulating scenario, we re-sample the training 3T MR images with a factor of 2. Figure 4(c) compares the result of different

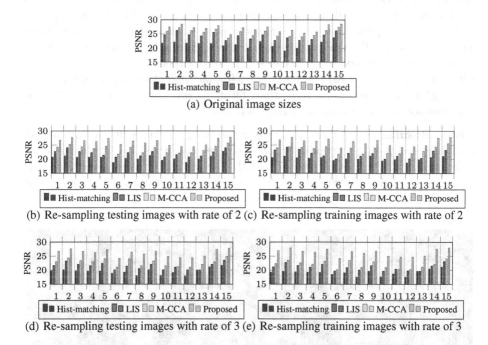

(a) Original image sizes

(b) Re-sampling testing images with rate of 2 (c) Re-sampling training images with rate of 2

(d) Re-sampling testing images with rate of 3 (e) Re-sampling training images with rate of 3

Fig. 4. Comparison of our proposed method and three competing methods, in terms of PSNR, for all 15 leave-one-out cross-validations, for the cases where (a) testing and training 3T MR images have same quality (with no re-sampling); (b) and (c) the testing and training 3T MR images have been re-sampled with a factor of 2, respectively; (d) and (e) the testing and training 3T MR images have been re-sampled with a factor of 3, respectively.

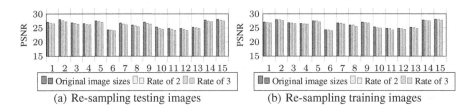

     (a) Re-sampling testing images   (b) Re-sampling training images

Fig. 5. Performance of our method (for 15 subjects), in the cases of (a) same imaging quality for both testing and training 3T MR images (with no re-sampling), and reduced quality of testing 3T MR images by rates of 2 and 3, (b) same imaging quality for both testing and training 3T MR images (with no re-sampling), and reduced quality of training 3T MR images by rates of 2 and 3.

methods in terms of PSNR. Our method shows more robustness to image quality changing compared to the previous methods.

• *Re-sampling Rate of 3*. In this experiment, we further reduce the quality of testing and training 3T MR images by re-sampling by a factor of 3. Figure 4(d) and (e) compares the results of different methods in terms of PSNR for 15 cross-validations, for re-sampling of the testing and training 3T MR images, respectively. Clearly, in the case with extremely poor quality, our proposed method still outperforms all three competing methods. Further, we compare in Fig. 5 the result of our method in three cases: (1) without re-sampling; (2) re-sampling with a factor of 2; and (3) re-sampling with a factor of 3 for (a) testing and (b) training images. The results show that, by increasing the re-sampling rate, the performance of our method does not drop much.

Visual Results: In Fig. 6, we visualize the reconstruction results by our method and three competing methods. Notably, our reconstructed 7T-like image looks more similar to the ground-truth 7T MRI. In addition, our result contains better anatomical details, which were not recovered in the reconstruction by the competing methods.

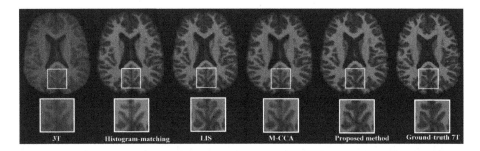

Fig. 6. Comparison of the reconstructed 7T-like images based on histogram-matching, LIS [4], M-CCA [5], and our proposed method.

4   Conclusion and Discussion

In this paper, we have proposed a novel deep Convolutional Neural Network (CNN) architecture for reconstructing 7T-like images from 3T MR images, by exploiting both appearance and anatomical features of MR images. Besides, compared to three competing methods, our method has been shown more robust for the cases with different imaging qualities for the testing and training 3T MR images. Additionally, experimental results, with 15 pairs of 3T and 7T MR images, showed that our proposed method is capable of recovering more structural details than the competing methods.

It should be mentioned that, we used re-sampling to simulate different resolutions for testing and training images for initial experiments. Of course, to claim the robustness against different scanners need acquiring using actual different scanners which is done in the extension of this paper. Since, based on this simulation our method is more robust than other methods, it is potentially be would be better than the previous methods in the case of actual scanning by different method which will remain as our future work.

Of note, the generated brain tissue labels by FAST method are useful in representation of different tissues, which was used together with the appearance features to improve the reconstruction of 7T-like images. However, in the case that the anatomical features are not perfect in representation of different tissues, our reconstruction results may drops but still it would be better than just using appearance features.

References

1. Kolka, A.G., Hendriksea, J., Zwanenburg, J.J.M., Vissera, F., Luijtena, P.R.: Clinical applications of 7T MRI in the brain. Eur. J. Radiol. **82**, 708–718 (2013)
2. DOTmed Daily News (2012). www.dotmed.com/news/story/17820
3. Rueda, A., Malpica, N., Romero, E.: Single-image super-resolution of brain MR images using overcomplete dictionaries. Med. Image Anal. **17**, 113–132 (2013)
4. Burgos, N., Cardoso, M.J., Thielemans, K., Modat, M., Pedemonte, S., Dickson, J., Barnes, A., Ahmed, R., Mahoney, C.J., Schott, J.M., Duncan, J.S., Atkinson, D., Arridge, S.R., Hutton, B.F., Ourselin, S.: Attenuation correction synthesis for hybrid PET-MR scanners: application to brain studies. IEEE Trans. Med. Imag. **33**(12), 2332–2341 (2014)
5. Bahrami, K., Shi, F., Zong, X., Shin, H.W., An, H., Shen, D.: Hierarchical reconstruction of 7T-like images from 3T MRI using multi-level CCA and group sparsity. MICCAI, pp. 1–8 (2015)
6. Bahrami, K., Shi, F., Zong, X., Shin, H.W., An, H., Shen, D.: Reconstruction of 7T-like images from 3T MRI. IEEE Trans. Med Imag. **35**(9), 2085–2097 (2016)
7. Dong, C., Loy, C., He, K., Tang, X.: Image super-resolution using deep convolutional networks. IEEE Trans. Pattern Anal. Mach. Intell. **38**(2), 295–307 (2016)
8. Kulkarni, K., Lohit, S., Turaga, P.K., Kerviche, R., Ashok, A.: ReconNet: non-iterative reconstruction of images from compressively sensed random measurements. arXiv:1601.06892 (2016)
9. Zhang, Y., Brady, M., Smith, S.: Segmentation of brain MR images through Markov random field model and the expectation-maximization algorithm. IEEE Trans. Med. Imag. **20**(1), 45–57 (2001)

Fast Predictive Image Registration

Xiao Yang[1]([✉]), Roland Kwitt[3], and Marc Niethammer[1,2]

[1] Department of Computer Science, UNC Chapel Hill, Chapel Hill, USA
xy@cs.unc.edu
[2] Biomedical Research Imaging Center, UNC Chapel Hill, Chapel Hill, USA
[3] Department of Computer Science, University of Salzburg, Salzburg, Austria

Abstract. We present a method to predict image deformations based on patch-wise image appearance. Specifically, we design a patch-based deep encoder-decoder network which learns the pixel/voxel-wise mapping between image appearance and registration parameters. Our approach can predict general deformation parameterizations, however, we focus on the large deformation diffeomorphic metric mapping (LDDMM) registration model. By predicting the LDDMM momentum-parameterization we retain the desirable theoretical properties of LDDMM, while reducing computation time by orders of magnitude: combined with patch pruning, we achieve a 1500x/66x speed-up compared to GPU-based optimization for 2D/3D image registration. Our approach has better prediction accuracy than predicting deformation or velocity fields and results in diffeomorphic transformations. Additionally, we create a Bayesian probabilistic version of our network, which allows evaluation of deformation field uncertainty through Monte Carlo sampling using dropout at test time. We show that deformation uncertainty highlights areas of ambiguous deformations. We test our method on the OASIS brain image dataset in 2D and 3D.

1 Introduction

Image registration is a critical medical image analysis task to provide spatial correspondences. A prominent application is atlas-to-image registration, commonly used for atlas-based segmentations or population analyses. Image registration is typically cast as an optimization problem, which can be especially computationally demanding for non-parametric diffusive, elastic, or fluid models [11] such as LDDMM [1]. Recently, approaches to *predict* registration parameters have been proposed: resulting deformations can be (i) used directly or (ii) to initialize an optimizer. However, high parameter dimensionality and the non-linearity between image appearance and the registration parameters makes predictions challenging. Chou et al. [3] propose a multi-scale linear regressor, which is restricted to the prediction of affine transformations and low-rank approximations of non-rigid deformations. For complex deformable registrations, Wang et al. [17] use image-template key point matching with sparse learning and a subsequent interpolation to a dense deformation field via radial basis functions. While effective, this method is dependent on proper key point selection. In [2],

© Springer International Publishing AG 2016
G. Carneiro et al. (Eds.): LABELS 2016/DLMIA 2016, LNCS 10008, pp. 48–57, 2016.
DOI: 10.1007/978-3-319-46976-8_6

a semi-coupled dictionary learning technique is used to jointly model image appearance and the deformation parameters; however, assuming a linear relationship between image appearance and deformation parameters only, which is overly restrictive.

Optical flow [4,18] and affine transforms [10] have been computed via deep learning. Here, we explore a deep learning regression model[1] for pixel/voxel-level parameter prediction for non-parametric image-registration from image patches.

Contribution. *Convenient parameterization:* Using the momentum parameterization for LDDMM shooting [16], we retain the mathematical properties of LDDMM under patch-based prediction, e.g., we guarantee diffeomorphic transforms. *Fast computation:* Using a sliding window with a large stride and patch pruning to predict the momentum, we achieve dramatic speed-ups compared to a direct optimization approach, while maintaining high prediction accuracy. *Atlas-based formulation:* In contrast to generic optical flow approaches, we use an atlas-based viewpoint. This allows us to predict the momentum in a fixed atlas coordinate system and hence within a consistent tangent space. *Uncertainty quantification:* We provide a Bayesian model from which estimates for parameter uncertainty and consequentially deformation map uncertainty can be obtained. This information can be used, e.g., for uncertainty-based smoothing [13], surgical treatment planning, or for direct uncertainty isualizations.

Organization. Section 2 reviews the registration parameterization of LDDMM. Section 3 introduces our network structure and our strategy for speeding up deformation prediction. Section 4 presents experimental results for both 2D and 3D brain images from the OASIS [9] brain image data set and discusses the generality of our approach, as well as possible improvements and extensions.

2 Initial Momentum LDDMM Parameterization

Given a source image S and a target image T, a *time-dependent* deformation map $\Phi : \mathbb{R}^d \times \mathbb{R} \to \mathbb{R}^d$, maps between the coordinates of S and T, at time $t = 1$, i.e., $S(\Phi^{-1}(x,1)) = T(x)$; d denotes the spatial dimension. In the LDDMM shooting formulation [16], the initial momentum vector field m_0 is the registration parameter from which Φ (and Φ^{-1}) can be computed. In fact, by integrating the geodesic equations (2), the complete spatio-temporal transformation, $\Phi(x,t)$, is determined. The initial momentum is the dual of the initial velocity v_0, which is an element in the reproducing kernel Hilbert space V, and they are connected by a positive-definite, self-adjoint smoothing operator K as $v = Km$ and $m = Lv$, where $K = L^{-1}$. The energy for the shooting formulation of LDDMM is [14,16]

$$E(m_0) = \langle m_0, Km_0 \rangle + \frac{1}{\sigma^2}||S \circ \Phi^{-1}(1) - T||^2, \quad \text{such that} \quad (1)$$

---

[1] Other regression models could of course be used as well.

$$m_t + \mathrm{ad}_v^* m = 0,$$
$$m(0) = m_0,$$
$$\Phi_t^{-1} + D\Phi^{-1}v = 0, \tag{2}$$
$$\Phi^{-1}(0) = \mathrm{id},$$
$$m - Lv = 0.$$

where id is the identity map, ad^* is the dual of the negative Jacobi-Lie bracket of vector fields: $\mathrm{ad}_v w = Dvw - Dwv$, D denotes the Jacobian, and $\sigma > 0$. *Our goal* is to predict the initial momentum m_0 given the source and target images, in a patch-by-patch manner. We will show, in Sect. 4, that this is a convenient parameterization as (i) the momentum does not need to be smooth, but is compactly supported at image edges and (ii) the velocity is obtained by smoothing the momentum via K. Hence, smoothness does not need to be considered in the prediction step, but is imposed *after* prediction. K governs the theoretical properties of LDDMM: in particular, a strong enough K assures diffeomorphic transformations, Φ [1]. Hence, by predicting m_0, we retain the theoretical properties of LDDMM. Furthermore, patch-wise prediction of alternative parameterizations of LDDMM, such as the initial velocity, or directly predicting displacements, is difficult in homogeneous image regions, as these regions provide no information to guide the registration. As the *momentum* in such regions is zero[2], no such issues arise.

3   Network Structure

Figure 1 shows the structure of our initial momentum prediction network. We first discuss our deterministic version *without* dropout layers, then introduce the probabilistic network using dropout. We focus the discussion on 2D images for notational simplicity, but also implement and experiment with 3D networks by using volumetric layers and adding an additional decoder for the 3rd dimension.

3.1   Deterministic Network

In the 2D version of the network, the input is a two layer 15×15 image patch, where the two layers come from the fixed and the moving image, resp., taken at the same location, and the network output is the initial momentum prediction patch for x and y directions. Our network consists of two parts: the *encoder* and the *decoder*. In the *encoder*, we create a VGG-style [12] network with 2 blocks of three 3×3 convolutional layers with PReLU [7] activations (■), and 2×2 maxpooling layers (■) with a step size of 2 at the end of each two blocks. The number of features in the convolutional layers is 128 for the large image scale block, and 256 for the smaller one. The *decoder* contains two parallel decoders sharing input generated from the encoder; each decoder's structure is the inverse

---

[2] For image-based LDDMM [1,6] the momentum is $m = \lambda \nabla I$, where λ is a scalar-valued momentum field and I is the image. Hence, $m = 0$ in uniform areas of I.

of the encoder, except for using max-unpooling layers with the pooling layers'
indices, and no non-linearity layer at the end ( ). Unpooling layers help retain
image boundary detail, which is important for initial momentum prediction.
During training, we use the L_1 difference for network output evaluation. To
compute a momentum prediction for the *whole* image, we use a sliding window
and patch averaging in the overlapping areas. We use two (three) independent
decoders to predict the initial momentum in 2D (3D) as, experimentally, such a
network structure is much easier to train than a network with one large decoder
to predict the initial momentum in all dimensions simultaneously. In our experiments, such a combined network easily got stuck in poor local minima[3]. Our
independent decoder network can be regarded as a multi-task network, where
each decoder predicts initial momentum for a single dimension.

3.2 Bayesian Probabilistic Network Using Dropout

We extend our network to a Bayesian probabilistic network by using *dropout* [15].
This can be regarded as approximate variational inference for a Bayesian network with Bernoulli distributions over the network's weights [5]. Given a 2-layer
image patch X and the corresponding initial momentum patch Y, we determine
the weights W of the convolutional layers so that given input X, our network
is likely to generate the target output Y. We define the likelihood $p(Y|W, X)$ of
the network output via the L_1 difference. Our goal is to find the posterior of the
weights W, i.e., $p(W|Y, X) \propto (p(Y|W, X)p(W))/p(Y)$, where $p(W) \sim \mathcal{N}(0, I)$ is
the prior of W, and $p(Y)$ is constant. Since this posterior is generally unknown,
we use a variational posterior $q(W)$ to approximate the true posterior by min-
imizing the Kullback-Leibler (KL) divergence $D_{\mathrm{KL}}(q(W) \parallel p(W|X, Y))$. When
using dropout for convolutional layers, the variational posterior $q(W_i)$ for the
ith convolutional layer with $K_i \times K_i$ weight matrix can be written as [5]

$$q(W_i) = W_i \cdot \mathrm{diag}([z_{i,j}]_{j=1}^{K_i}), \quad z_{i,j} \sim \mathrm{Bernoulli}(p_i), \tag{3}$$

where $z_{i,j}$ is a Bernoulli random variable modeling dropout with probability p_i,
randomly setting the jth node in the ith layer to 0. The variational parameter
is the network weight W_i. The variational posterior for all network weights W is
then $q(W) = \prod_i q(W_i)$. According to [5], we minimize KL-divergence by adding
dropout layers (■) after all convolutional layers except for the final output, as
shown in Fig. 1, and train the network using stochastic gradient descent. During
test time, we keep the dropout layers, and evaluate the posterior by Monte Carlo
sampling of the network given fixed input data. We use the sample mean as our
final initial momentum, from which we compute the deformation by integrating
Eq. (2) forward. We calculate the *deformation* variance by integrating Eq. (2) for
each initial momentum sample separately. We set $p_i = 0.3$.

---

[3] It would also be interesting to investigate predicting the scalar field λ, instead of
$m = \lambda \nabla I$, which would require only *one* decoder regardless of image dimension.

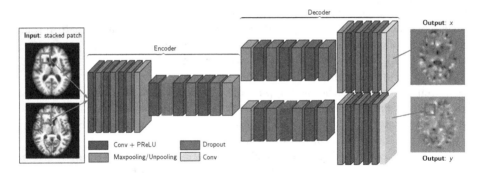

Fig. 1. Bayesian probabilistic network structure (for 2D images): the inputs are 2-layer stacked patches from the moving image and fixed image at the same location. The output is the initial momentum prediction of the patches in x and y spatial directions. For a deterministic version of the network, we simply remove all dropout layers. For a 3D image network, we increase the number of decoders to 3 and use volumetric layers.

3.3 Speeding up Whole Image Deformation Prediction

As we predict the whole-image initial momentum patch-by-patch, computation speed is proportional to the number of patches. We use two techniques to reduce the number of patches/image, thereby increasing computation speed: First, we perform *patch pruning* by ignoring all patches from the background of both the moving and the target image; this can be done, since the initial momentum for the constant background should be zero. Second, we use a large pixel/voxel stride (e.g., 14 for 15×15 patches) for the sliding window. This is reasonable, because of the compact support (around edges) of the initial momentum and the shift-invariance property of pooling/unpooling layers. These two techniques reduce the number of predicted patches/image by 99.5 % for the 128×128 2D images and by 99.97 % for the $128 \times 128 \times 128$ 3D images, at a negligible loss of accuracy (cf. Sect. 4).

4   Experiments

We evaluate our method using 2D (128×128) and 3D ($128 \times 128 \times 128$) images of the OASIS longitudinal dataset [9]. We use the first scan of all subjects, resulting in 150 images. The 2D slices are extracted from the same axial slice of the 3D images after affine registration. We randomly picked 100 images as training target images and used the remaining 50 as testing targets. We created unbiased atlases [8] for 2D and 3D from all the training data using PyCA[4] and use these atlases as our moving image(s). This allows for momentum prediction in a fixed (atlas) tangent space. We used LDDMM-shooting combined with a sum-of-squared intensity difference in PyCA to register the atlases to all 150 images.

---

[4] https://bitbucket.org/scicompanat/pyca.

We chose the regularization kernel for LDDMM as $K = L^{-1} = (a\Delta^2 + b\Delta + c)^{-1}$, and set $[a, b, c]$ as $[0.05, 0.05, 0.005]([1.5, 1.5, 0.15])$ for 2D(3D) images. The obtained initial momenta for registering the atlas to the training data were used to train our network using Torch[5], the ones for the testing data were used for validation. We optimized the network using *rmsprop*, setting the learning rate to 0.0005, the momentum decay to 0.1 and the number of epochs to 10. We fixed the patch size to 15×15 for 2D and to $15 \times 15 \times 15$ for 3D. For generating training patches, we used a 1 pixel stride for the sliding window in 2D and a 7 voxel stride in 3D to keep the number of training patches manageable, resulting in $1,299,600$ 2D patches and $550,800$ 3D patches. For the probabilistic network, we sampled 50 times for each test case to calculate the prediction result and the variation of the deformation fields.

4.1 2D Data

For the 2D experiment, we compare our method with semi-coupled dictionary learning (SCDL), which was used to predict initial momenta for LDDMM in [2]. To compare the deformation prediction accuracy using different parameterizations, we trained networks predicting the *initial velocity*, $v_0 = Km_0$, and the *displacement field*, $\Phi^{-1}(1) - \text{id}$, of LDDMM, respectively. For the initial momentum

Table 1. Test results for 2D (*top*) and 3D (*bottom*). *SCDL*: semi-coupled dictionary learning; *D*: deterministic network; *P*: probabilistic network; *stride*: stride length for sliding window for whole image prediction; *velocity*: predicting initial velocity; *displacement*: predicting displacement field; *PR*: patch pruning. The column $|J| > 0$ shows the ratio of test cases with positive definite Jacobian determinant of the deformation map. Our initial momentum networks (and the best results) are highlighted in **bold**.

	2D test case deformation error [pixel]							$|J| > 0$
Data percentile	0.3 %	5 %	25 %	50 %	75 %	95 %	99.7 %	
Affine	0.0925	0.3779	0.9207	1.4741	2.1717	3.4606	5.4585	N/A
SCDL, 1000 dictionary	0.0819	0.337	0.8156	1.3078	1.9368	3.1285	4.7948	100 %
D, velocity, stride 1	0.0228	0.0959	0.2453	0.4343	0.7354	1.4664	2.9768	100 %
D, velocity, stride 14+PR	0.027	0.1123	0.2878	0.5075	0.8605	1.75	3.6172	76 %
D, displacement, stride 1	0.0215	0.0897	0.2332	0.416	0.7064	1.429	2.9462	90 %
D, displacement, stride 14+PR	0.0252	0.107	0.2786	0.4955	0.8047	1.7298	3.7327	0 %
D, stride 1	0.0194	0.0817	0.2035	0.3436	0.5618	1.1395	2.473	100 %
D, stride 14+PR	0.0221	0.0906	0.2244	0.375	0.6057	1.2076	2.6731	100 %
P, stride 1, 50 samples	**0.0185**	**0.0787**	**0.1953**	**0.3261**	**0.5255**	**1.0745**	**2.3525**	100 %
P, stride 14+PR, 50 samples	0.0209	0.0855	0.2123	0.351	0.5556	1.1133	2.5678	100 %
	3D test case deformation error [voxel]							$|J| > 0$
Data percentile	0.3 %	5 %	25 %	50 %	75 %	95 %	99.7 %	
Affine	0.0821	0.2529	0.5541	0.8666	1.2879	2.1339	3.7032	N/A
D, stride 7	**0.0128**	**0.0348**	**0.0705**	**0.1072**	**0.1578**	**0.2663**	**0.5049**	100 %
D, stride 14+PR	0.0146	0.0403	0.0831	0.1287	0.194	0.351	0.6896	100 %
P, stride 14+PR, 50 samples	0.0151	0.0422	0.0876	0.1363	0.2051	0.3664	0.8287	100 %

---

[5] http://torch.ch.

and the initial velocity parameterizations, the resulting deformation map $\Phi^{-1}(1)$ was computed by integrating Eq. (2). We quantify the deformation errors as the pixel-wise 2-norm of the deformation error with respect to the ground-truth deformation obtained by PyCA LDDMM. Table 1 shows the error percentiles over all pixel and test cases. We observe that our initial momentum networks significantly outperform SCDL and also improve prediction accuracy compared to the initial velocity and the displacement parameterizations in both the 1-stride and the 14-stride + patch pruning cases. In contrast to the initial velocity and the displacement parameterizations, both our deterministic and our probabilistic networks show comparatively small sensitivity to patch pruning and stride, validating our hypothesis that the momentum-based LDDMM parameterization is well-suited for fast predictive image registration. One of the hallmarks of LDDMM registration is that given a sufficiently strong regularization, the obtained deformation maps, $\Phi^{-1}(1)$, will be diffeomorphic. To assess this property, we computed the local Jacobians of the deformation maps. Assuming no coordinate system flips, a diffeomorphic $\Phi^{-1}(1)$ should have a positive definite Jacobian everywhere, otherwise undesirable foldings exist. Column 'det $J > 0$' of Table 1 lists the percentage of test cases with positive definite Jacobian, revealing that our initial-momentum based networks retain this property in all scenarios, even for very large strides and patch pruning. Direct displacement prediction, however, cannot even guarantee diffeomorphic transformations for a stride of 1 (which includes a lot of local averaging) for all our test cases and results in no diffeomorphic transformations at a stride of 14. Velocity prediction performs slightly better, but can also not guarantee diffeomorphic maps at large strides, likely due to more stringent requirements on the numerical integration in this case. Similarly to existing optical flow prediction methods [4,18], a direct prediction of displacements or velocities cannot encode smoothness assumptions or enforce transformation guarantees. Our momentum parameterization encodes these assumptions by design. Figure 2 shows an example of our 2D deformation prediction with uncertainty. The predicted deformation is close to the one generated by costly LDDMM optimization. The uncertainty map shows high uncertainty at the anterior edge of the ventricle and the posterior brain cortex where drastic shape changes occur, which can be seen in the moving and the target image.

4.2   3D Data

Similar to the 2D case, we computed the deformation error for every voxel in all test cases; results are listed in Table 1. Our networks achieve sub-voxel accuracy for about 99.8 % of all the voxels. Figure 2 shows one 3D registration result using the predicted deformation from our probabilistic 3D network using the mean of 50 initial momentum samples, as well as the uncertainty of the deformation field. Our prediction is able to handle large deformations. As in 2D, the uncertainty map highlights areas with drastic and ambiguous deformations.

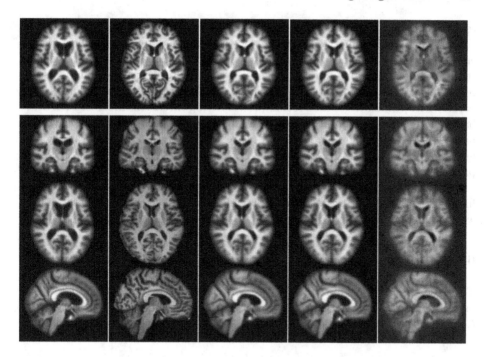

Fig. 2. Test example for 2D (*top*) and 3D (*bottom*). *From left to right*: moving (atlas) image, target image, deformation result by optimizing LDDMM energy, deformation result using 50 samples from probabilistic network with a stride of 14 and patch pruning, and uncertainty as square root of the sum of the variances of deformation in all directions mapped on the predicted registration result. The colors indicates the amount of uncertainty (red = high uncertainty, blue = low uncertainty). Best viewed in color. (Color figure online)

4.3   Computation Speed

On an Nvidia Titan X GPU, it took 9 h to train a 2D network, and 72 h to train a 3D network. By using a 14 pixel stride sliding window + patch pruning, our network (without repeated sampling) predicts the initial momentum for a 2D image in 0.19 s, and in 7.68 s for a 3D image. Compared to the GPU-based optimization in PyCA, we achieve an approximate speedup of 1500x/66x for a 2D/3D image. At a stride of 1, computational cost increases about 200-fold in 2D and 3000-fold in 3D, resulting in runtimes of about half a minute/six hours in 2D/3D. Hence, our momentum representation which is amenable to large strides is essential for achieving fast registration prediction at high accuracy while guaranteeing diffeomorphic transformations.

5   Discussion

Our model is general and directly applicable to many other registration approaches with pixel/voxel-wise registration parameters (e.g., demons or elastic registration). For parametric methods (with less registration parameters) and *local control*, such as B-splines, we could replace the decoders by fully-connected layers. Of course, for methods where parameter locality is not guaranteed, using large stride and patch pruning may no longer be suitable. Future studies should assess registration accuracy in terms of landmarks and/or segmentation overlaps, compared with optimization-based techniques. Exciting extensions are: fast LDDMM-based multi-atlas segmentation; multi-modal image registration (where the input patches are from different modalities); direct image-to-image registration; fast user-interactive registration refinements (requiring prediction for a few localized patches only); and multi-patch-scale networks for better prediction. Furthermore, ambiguous deformations, caused by large deformations or appearance changes, are highlighted by the uncertainty measure, which could detect pathologies in a network trained on normals.

6 Support

This research is supported by NIH R42 NS081792-03A1, NIH R41 NS086295-01 and NSF ECCS-1148870. We gratefully acknowledge the support of NVIDIA Corporation with the donation of the Titan X GPU used for this research.

References

1. Beg, M.F., Miller, M., Trouvé, A., Younes, L.: Computing large deformation metric mappings via geodesic flows of diffeomorphisms. IJCV **61**(2), 139–157 (2005)
2. Cao, T., Singh, N., Jojic, V., Niethammer, M.: Semi-coupled dictionary learning for deformation prediction. In: ISBI, pp. 691–694 (2015)
3. Chou, C.R., Frederick, B., Mageras, G., Chang, S., Pizer, S.: 2D/3D image registration using regression learning. CVIU **117**(9), 1095–1106 (2013)
4. Dosovitskiy, A., Fischery, P., Ilg, E., Hazirbas, C., Golkov, V., van der Smagt, P., Cremers, D., Brox, T.: Flownet: learning optical flow with convolutional networks. In: ICCV, pp. 2758–2766 (2015)
5. Gal, Y., Ghahramani, Z.: Bayesian convolutional neural networks with Bernoulli approximate variational inference. arXiv:1506.02158 (2015)
6. Hart, G.L., Zach, C., Niethammer, M.: An optimal control approach for deformable registration. In: MMBIA, pp. 9–16 (2009)
7. He, K., Zhang, X., Ren, S., Sun, J.: Delving deep into rectifiers: surpassing human-level performance on ImageNet classification. CoRR abs/1502.01852 (2015)
8. Joshi, S., Davis, B., Jomier, M., Gerig, G.: Unbiased diffeomorphic atlas construction for computational anatomy. NeuroImage **23**, 151–160 (2004)
9. Marcus, D.S., Wang, T.H., Parker, J., Csernansky, J.G., Morris, J.C., Buckner, R.L.: Open access series of imaging studies (OASIS): cross-sectional MRI data in young, middle aged, nondemented, and demented older adults. J. Cogn. Neurosci. **19**(9), 1498–1507 (2007)
10. Miao, S., Wang, Z.J., Liao, R.: A CNN regression approach for real-time 2D/3D registration. TMI **35**(5), 1352–1363 (2016)
11. Modersitzki, J.: Numerical Methods for Image Registration. Oxford University Press, Oxford (2004)

12. Simonyan, K., Zisserman, A.: Very deep convolutional networks for large-scale image recognition. CoRR abs/1409.1556 (2014)
13. Simpson, I.J.A., Woolrich, M.W., Groves, A.R., Schnabel, J.A.: Longitudinal brain MRI analysis with uncertain registration. In: Fichtinger, G., Martel, A., Peters, T. (eds.) MICCAI 2011, Part II. LNCS, vol. 6892, pp. 647–654. Springer, Heidelberg (2011)
14. Singh, N., Hinkle, J., Joshi, S., Fletcher, P.T.: A vector momenta formulation of diffeomorphisms for improved geodesic regression and atlas construction. In: ISBI, pp. 1219–1222 (2013)
15. Srivastava, N., Hinton, G., Krizhevsky, A., Sutskever, I., Salakhutdinov, R.: Dropout: a simple way to prevent neural networks from overfitting. JMLR **15**, 1929–1958 (2014)
16. Vialard, F.X., Risser, L., Rueckert, D., Cotter, C.J.: Diffeomorphic 3D image registration via geodesic shooting using an efficient adjoint calculation. IJCV **97**(2), 229–241 (2012)
17. Wang, Q., Kim, M., Shi, Y., Wu, G., Shen, D.: Predict brain MR image registration via sparse learning of appearance and transformation. MedIA **20**(1), 61–75 (2015)
18. Weinzaepfel, P., Revaud, J., Harchaoui, Z., Schmid, C.: DeepFlow: large displacement optical flow with deep matching. In: ICCV, pp. 1385–1392 (2013)

Longitudinal Multiple Sclerosis Lesion Segmentation Using Multi-view Convolutional Neural Networks

Ariel Birenbaum[1](✉) and Hayit Greenspan[2](✉)

[1] Department of Electrical Engineering, Tel-Aviv University, Tel Aviv, Israel
`birenbaum1@mail.tau.ac.il`
[2] Department of Biomedical Engineering, Tel-Aviv University, Tel Aviv, Israel
`hayit@eng.tau.ac.il`

Abstract. Automatic segmentation of Multiple Sclerosis (MS) lesions is a challenging task due to their variability in shape, size, location and texture in Magnetic Resonance (MR) images. A reliable, automatic segmentation method can help diagnosis and patient follow-up while reducing the time consuming need of manual segmentation. In this paper, we present a fully automated method for MS lesion segmentation. The proposed method uses MR intensities and White Matter (WM) priors for extraction of candidate lesion voxels and uses Convolutional Neural Networks for false positive reduction. Our networks process longitudinal data, a novel contribution in the domain of MS lesion analysis. The method was tested on the ISBI 2015 dataset and obtained state-of-the-art Dice results with the performance level of a trained human rater.

Keywords: Multiple Sclerosis · CNN · Segmentation · Longitudinal data

1 Introduction

Multiple Sclerosis is the most common non-traumatic neurological disease in young adults. It is an inflammatory demyelinating disease associated with the formation of lesions in the central nervous system, which are characterized by demyelination, and axonal conduction block. These classically described WM lesions are visible in conventional MRI. Fluid attenuated inversion recovery (FLAIR) images have been shown to be sensitive to WM lesions but can also present other hyper-intensity artifacts [1].

Due to the challenging nature of MS segmentation, several challenges have been organized, such as the MS lesion segmentation challenge in MICCAI 2008 [2] and the Longitudinal MS lesion segmentation challenge in ISBI 2015, where competing teams were able to make use of the longitudinal information between

Electronic supplementary material The online version of this chapter (doi:10. 1007/978-3-319-46976-8_7) contains supplementary material, which is available to authorized users.

© Springer International Publishing AG 2016
G. Carneiro et al. (Eds.): LABELS 2016/DLMIA 2016, LNCS 10008, pp. 58–67, 2016.
DOI: 10.1007/978-3-319-46976-8_7

consecutive MR images. A variety of algorithms have been proposed [3–7]. Top performing methods are based on supervised classification frameworks. Specifically, current state-of-the-art method in both MICCAI 2008 and ISBI 2015 is based on a combination of multi-atlas label fusion (MALF) with a Random Forest classifier for region level lesion refinement [7].

Convolutional Neural Networks (CNNs) have become very popular after Alex Krizhevsky's network won the 2012 ImageNet classification competition [8] by a large margin. Since then, CNNs have been successfully used for additional applications, such as object segmentation. In recent years, they have also been used for medical image analysis. A 2.5D CNN, in which 3D volume-of-interest is decomposed to axial, coronal and sagittal views, achieved state-of-the-art accuracy in lymph node detection. This 2.5D framework, compared to 3D CNNs, reduces the computational burden of training and testing and alleviates the curse-of-dimensionality problem [9]. 2D and 3D CNNs were also proposed for the segmentation of MS lesions [5,6].

In this work, we have trained and tested a Longitudinal Multi-View CNN for MS lesion segmentation. The input are patches from multiple images, multiple views and multiple time points. To the best of our knowledge, this is the first CNN that takes advantage of longitudinal data for MS lesion segmentation. We have evaluated our segmentation method on the dataset provided in the 2015 ISBI challenge, and achieved state-of-the-art accuracy in terms of Dice score on the test set. Our method, trained on a relatively small number of images, was able to achieve human level performance.

The rest of the paper is organized as follows: The proposed method is described in Sect. 2. Experimental evaluation and results on the 2015 ISBI dataset are presented in Sect. 3. A discussion of the network architecture and parameter selection follows at Sect. 4. Finally, Sect. 5 offers concluding remarks.

2 Methods

The proposed segmentation method consists of 3 phases: Pre-Processing, Candidate Extraction and CNN Prediction. In the Pre-Processing phase, multiple operations are applied to the set of MR images, including: Co-Registration, Brain Extraction, Bias Field Correction and Intensity Normalization. In the Candidate Extraction phase, masks based on FLAIR and WM prior are calculated and applied to the MR images. In the CNN Prediction phase, the multi-view CNN outputs a lesion probability for every voxel in the MR image.

2.1 Pre-processing

The input to the segmentation algorithm for every case is a set of MR images: T2-weighted FLAIR, T1-weighted MPRAGE, T2-Weighted and Proton Density weighted. Acquired images are not registered and generally have different spacing and slice thicknesses. Hence, the images are converted to a common space by rigidly registering the MPRAGE image to MNI space and co-registering the rest of the images to it. Secondly, brain extraction is performed on the MPRAGE image and the corresponding brain mask is then applied to the rest of the images. In addition, all images are bias field corrected. The output of these pre-processing steps was supplied by the organizers of the 2015 ISBI challenge.

The final pre-processing operation that we applied to all images is intensity normalization. Intensity normalization of the FLAIR image is required because its values are used for candidate extraction and a single constant FLAIR intensity threshold is used for all cases. In addition, this is an important pre-processing step to CNN prediction when input images have different intensity ranges. Normalization is carried out by histogram matching each image of every case to the corresponding image of a single reference case, after its top 1 and bottom 1 percentiles were clamped and its intensity values were scaled to $[0, 1]$.

2.2 Candidate Extraction

Candidate extraction disqualifies the majority of the image voxels as lesions. This dramatically reduces the computational cost of CNN prediction, which follows this phase. In addition, because candidate extraction operates on the voxel level, while CNN prediction operates on a neighborhood around the voxel, these two phases can be viewed as a multi-scale pipeline where both local (voxel) and semi-global (voxel neighborhood) are incorporated in order to obtain high segmentation accuracy.

Candidate extraction is based on two clinical rules [10]:

1. Lesions appear as hyper-intense in FLAIR images; thus they can be roughly identified by thresholding the FLAIR image.
2. MS lesions tend to be found in the WM or on the border between WM and Gray Matter (GM). To incorporate this information, a probabilistic WM template [11] is registered to the FLAIR image with a mutual information cost function. Due to inter-subject variability, the registered WM template is greyscale dilated isotropically by a radius R.

The candidate mask is thus defined as:

$$Mask(x) = \left\{ \begin{array}{c} 1 \ I_{FLAIR}(x) > \theta_{FLAIR} \cap Dilate_R(WM(x)) > \theta_{WM} \\ 0 \text{ otherwise} \end{array} \right\} \quad (1)$$

Values of the parameters $(\theta_{FLAIR}, \theta_{WM}, R)$ are defined by cross-validation. In our experiments, the optimal parameters, selected as detailed in Sect. 3.1 reduce 97.5 % of the computations from the CNN.

2.3 CNN Prediction

Network Architectures. At this phase, a lesion probability is assigned to each voxel in the image. To determine the contribution of different aspects in the data, 4 CNN models were considered. In all models, patches of 32×32 pixels are extracted from axial, coronal and sagittal views for each evaluated voxel. The principal difference between the various models is the type and number of input patches to the network:

1. Single Image, Single Time Point (*SISTP*): Patches are extracted from the FLAIR image of current time point.
2. Multiple Images, Single Time Point (*MISTP*): Patches are extracted from all images of current time point.
3. Single Image, Multiple Time Points (*SIMTP*): Patches are extracted from the FLAIR image of current and previous time points.
4. Multiple Images, Multiple Time Points (*MIMTP*): Patches are extracted from all images of current and previous time points. Figure 1 illustrates input patches in this model for a single lesion voxel sample.

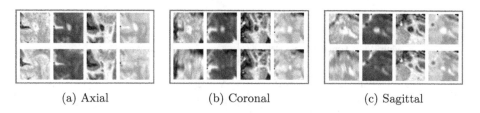

(a) Axial   (b) Coronal   (c) Sagittal

Fig. 1. Input patches to the MIMTP model. In every view, top and bottom rows correspond to previous and current time points respectively. Images from left to right are: FLAIR, T2, MPRAGE and PD

The main building block, common to all 4 models is the Single View CNN (*V-Net*), in which a spatial representation for a single view and time point is generated by a series of convolutions and max pooling layers, as depicted in Fig. 2a. The input to *V-Net* is c input patches, where $c = 1$ for *SISTP* and *SIMTP* and $c = 4$ for *MISTP* and *MIMTP*, corresponding to all 4 available input images. Number and sizes of convolution filters of the V-Net are 24@5 × 5, 32@3 × 3, 48@3 × 3 to the 1st, 2nd and 3rd convolution layers respectively.

For the longitudinal models (*SIMTP*, *MIMTP*) current and previous time points are processed separately and a 48×4×4 spatial representation is generated for each of them. The two temporal representations are then concatenated and processed by a convolution layer with 48@1 × 1 filters and a fully connected layer of 16 neurons, which are the longitudinal representation of a single view. This Longitudinal Network (*L-Net*) is depicted in Fig. 2b.

Axial, coronal and sagittal views are processed by separate *L-Nets* and the 3 corresponding 16 neuron outputs are concatenated and processed by an additional fully connected layer of 16 neurons which yields the full representation of all input patches of a single sample. A final fully connected layer of 2 neurons with Softmax activation yields two output probabilities for non-lesion and lesion voxel at the center of the input patches. This Multi-View Longitudinal network is depicted in Fig. 2c.

In the non-longitudinal (*SISTP*, *MISTP*), V-Net output is processed by a fully connected layer of 16 neurons which are concatenated and processed by

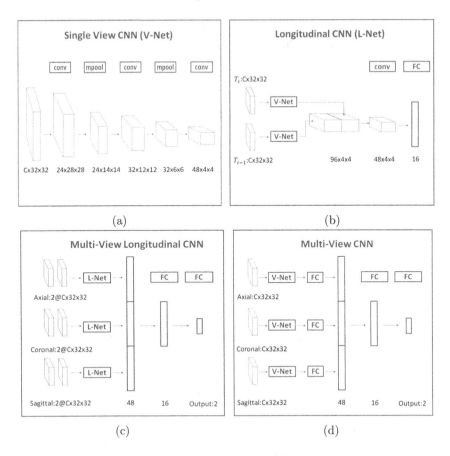

Fig. 2. Network Architectures: (a) V-Net (b) L-Net (c) Multi-View Longitudinal CNN. Represents *SIMTP* with c = 1 and *MIMTP* with c = 4 (d) Multi-View CNN. Represents *SISTP* with c = 1 and *MISTP* with c = 4

two additional fully connected layers as in the longitudinal models. This Multi-View network is depicted in Fig. 2d. The full *MIMTP* network model graph is available in the supplementary materials.

Training Details. In order to avoid overfitting, 3 strategies were employed:

1. Weight sharing: Reducing model complexity is known to be an effective way to generate classifiers that are robust and less prone to overfitting. Hence, *V-Net*s of same view and different time points have identical weights.
2. Dropout: A network layer which prevents large networks from overfitting [12]. We use Dropout with 0.25 probability after all network activation layers.
3. Data Augmentation: Random rotation angles in x-y, y-z and x-z planes are drawn from a Gaussian distribution with $\mu = 0$ and $\sigma = 5$ degrees.

Training was carried out using Keras [13], a modular neural network library running on top of Theano. All convolution and fully connected layers are followed by Leaky ReLU activation layers with $\alpha = 0.3$. Networks weights were optimized using AdaDelta [14] with a Categorical Cross-Entropy objective. Training was completed after accuracy saturated on the validation set, which amounted to 500 epochs. On an NVIDIA GeForce GTX 980 Ti GPU, *MIMTP* model training amounted to 4 h. The average CNN prediction time of all candidate lesion voxels in a time point was 27 s.

3   Experimental Evaluation

Our segmentation algorithms were evaluated on the dataset of the 2015 Longitudinal Multiple Sclerosis Segmentation Challenge. The overall data is composed of two parts: (1) Training data consisting of longitudinal images from 5 patients; (2) Test data consisting of longitudinal images from 14 different patients. For each person, the data includes T1-weighted, T2-weighted, PD-weighted, and T2-weighted FLAIR MRI with 4–6 time points acquired on a 3T MR scanner. T1-weighted images have approximately a 1 mm cubic voxel resolution, while the other scans are 1 mm in plane with 3 mm sections. Training data includes manual delineations performed by 2 trained raters.

Our segmentation algorithm was evaluated by 3 approaches: (1) Cross-Validation; (2) Visual Inspection; (3) Test results submission and analysis.

3.1   Cross-Validation

Cross patient validation on the training dataset is a reliable estimate to segmentation performance on the test set. We trained 5 identical models, corresponding to the 5 available training patients in the dataset. Each model was trained on 4 patients and tested on the remaining 5th patient in the training dataset. This process was repeated for all 4 CNN architectures: *SISTP, MISTP, MISTP* and *MIMTP*. We compared our output segmentation with the delineation of both trained raters. In this evaluation our testing criteria was the Dice score, calculated as:

$$Dice = \frac{2TP}{FP + FN + 2TP} \tag{2}$$

At this stage, we manually optimized lesion mask parameters and the CNN output probability threshold. For each model, we used the parameters that maximize mean Dice score across all 5 patient models.

Our reference score is the mean Dice score between the two manual delineations. Evaluation results are summarized in Table 1. We can note that: (1) Using all scanned images improves segmentation accuracy; (2) Using two consecutive time points improves segmentation accuracy and this improvement is additive to using multiple images; (3) Segmentation accuracy of the *MIMTP* model nearly reaches trained human performance in the cross-validation evaluation.

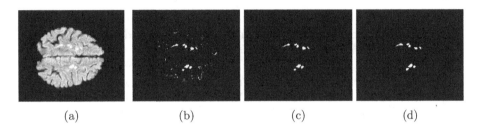

(a)   (b)   (c)   (d)

Fig. 3. Candidate extraction and *MIMTP* prediction. (a) Axial FLAIR (b) Candidate extraction output (c) CNN prediction output (d) Manual rater delineation

3.2   Visual Inspection

Visualizing candidate extraction and CNN prediction outputs, we can note their complementary nature: Candidate extraction phase eliminates most of the volume voxels as possible lesions but has a considerable amount of false positives cases. The subsequent CNN prediction phase processes a small amount of data and eliminates the remaining false positive cases. These results are depicted in Fig. 3.

3.3   Test Results Submission

We applied our segmentation algorithms to the 14 test patients in the following way: (1) 1st time point of each patient was segmented by the *MISTP* model, since there is no previous time point available for these cases; (2) Rest of the time points were segmented by the *MIMTP* model, which was evaluated as our best model in cross validation; (3) All parameters were defined as detailed in Sect. 3.1. The segmentation volumes were uploaded to the ISBI 2015 Challenge's official website, where they were scored and ranked according to:

$$Sc = 0.125 Dice + 0.125 PPV + 0.25 VC + 0.25 LTPR + 0.25(1 - LFPR) \quad (3)$$

Where PPV is the positive predictive value, VC is Pearson's correlation coefficient of the volumes, LTPR is the lesion true positive rate and LFPR is the lesion false positive rate as described in [15]. The score is linearly normalized by the inter-rater scores such that the lower inter-rater score has a rating of 90.

We also compared mean Dice scores, which is the most common metric for medical image segmentation. Table 2 summarizes top 5 submitted methods. We can note that: (1) Our algorithm is ranked 2nd by a small margin; (2) Our algorithm is state-of-the-art in terms of Dice; (3) Our algorithm achieves a score of 90.07, which is comparable to the performance of a trained human rater.

4   Discussion

In addition to the comparison between the four suggested CNN architectures, the selection of different aspects of our method with respect to available alternatives is worth addressing.

Table 1. Cross validation evaluation

Method	Dice(Rater 1)	Dice(Rater 2)
SISTP	0.669	0.649
SIMTP	0.714	0.692
MISTP	0.702	0.672
MIMTP	0.727	0.707
Rater 1	-	0.744

Table 2. ISBI 2015 test results [16]

Rank	Method	Sc	Dice
1	PVG1 [7]	**90.137**	0.579
2	Ours	90.070	**0.627**
3	IMI [3]	89.673	0.573
4	VISAGES2 [4]	89.265	0.560
5	IIT [6]	88.536	0.521

4.1 Patch Based

Fully convolutional networks have shown great success in the task of object segmentation [17]. In our method, candidate extraction eliminates the vast majority of voxels in the volume as lesion candidates. Hence, we considered performing convolutions on the entire volume as a redundancy of computational resources.

4.2 Multi-View

3D CNNs have been applied successfully in the medical field, where volumetric data is available. These models, compared to 2D CNNs, require kernels with a larger amount of coefficients. A multi-view network architecture can make use of the volumetric nature of the data while requiring less weights and thus being less prone to overfitting given a small training dataset.

4.3 Fusion Methods

Different Images. MS lesions appear as hyperintense in FLAIR and hypointense in T1-weighted images [10]. Merging patches from different images at the first convolutional layer enables it to make use of fine-level intensity values before any pooling takes place.

Different Time Points. MS lesions can exhibit change in size between consecutive scans. Such changes are evident when considering sub-patches of the input sample. Merging consecutive time points after two stages of pooling, when each neuron has a receptive field of $8 \times 8\,$mm in each orthogonal view, enables the next layers of the network to process the longitudinal data at an appropriate scale.

Different Views. In standard CNNs, convolutions process neighboring pixels. In our architecture different views belong to orthogonal planes in which voxels are not connected spatially. Hence merging neurons from different views makes sense after fully connected layers, in which each neuron contains information from the entire view rather than spatial information. A similar late fusion strategy was successful in a related work [18].

4.4   Data Augmentation

Subject brain volumes have been registered to an MNI template. Thus, the brain orientation is fixed up to registration inaccuracies in the pre-processing pipeline. Data augmentation with random small angles ($\sigma = 5$) enhances the training dataset while simulating angle errors due to small inaccuracies in registration.

5   Conclusions

In this work we showed that CNNs which make use of longitudinal information can produce better segmentation results than standard CNNs. In addition, by careful design of a pre-processing pipeline, network architecture and training methodology, our algorithm achieved state-of-the-art results on the ISBI 2015 dataset. Finally, it is worth noting that by training on a small dataset of only 5 patients, we have reached trained human level performance on the challenging task of MS lesion segmentation.

Acknowledgement. Part of this work was funded by the INTEL Collaborative Research Institute for Computational Intelligence (ICRI-CI).

References

1. Aït-Ali, L.S., Prima, S., Hellier, P., Carsin, B., Edan, G., Barillot, C.: STREM: a robust multidimensional parametric method to segment MS lesions in MRI. In: Duncan, J.S., Gerig, G. (eds.) MICCAI 2005. LNCS, vol. 3749, pp. 409–416. Springer, Heidelberg (2005)
2. Styner, M., Lee, J., Chin, B., et al.: 3D segmentation in the clinic: a grand challenge II: MS lesion segmentation. MIDAS J. **2008**, 1–5 (2008)
3. Maier, O., Handels, H.: MS-Lesion Segmentation in MRI with Random Forests. In: Proceedings of the 2015 Longitudinal Multiple Sclerosis Lesion Segmentation Challenge, pp. 1–2 (2015)
4. Catanese, L., Commowick, O., Barillot, C.: Automatic graph cut segmentation of multiple Sclerosis lesions. In: Proceedings of the 2015 Longitudinal Multiple Sclerosis Lesion Segmentation Challenge, pp. 1–2 (2015)
5. Ghafoorian, M., Platel, B.: Convolutional neural networks for MS lesion segmentation, method description of DIAG team. In: Proceedings of the 2015 Longitudinal Multiple Sclerosis Lesion Segmentation Challenge, pp. 1–2 (2015)
6. Vaidya, S., et al.: Longitudinal multiple Sclerosis lesion segmentation using 3D convolutional neural networks. In: Proceedings of the 2015 Longitudinal Multiple Sclerosis Lesion Segmentation Challenge, pp. 1–2 (2015)
7. Jesson, A., Arbel, T.: Hierarchical MRF and random forest segmentation of MS lesions and healthy tissues in brain MRI. In: Proceedings of the 2015 Longitudinal Multiple Sclerosis Lesion Segmentation Challenge, pp. 1–2 (2015)
8. Krizhevsky, A., Sutskever, I., Hinton, G.E.: Imagenet classification with deep convolutional neural networks. In: Advances in Neural Information Processing Systems, pp. 1097–1105 (2012)

9. Roth, H.R., et al.: A new 2.5D representation for lymph node detection using random sets of deep convolutional neural network observations. In: Golland, P., Hata, N., Barillot, C., Hornegger, J., Howe, R. (eds.) MICCAI 2014, Part I. LNCS, vol. 8673, pp. 520–527. Springer, Heidelberg (2014)

10. Mechrez, R., Goldberger, J., Greenspan, H.: Patch-based segmentation with spatial consistency: application to MS lesions in brain MRI. Int. J. Biomed. Imaging **2016**, 1–13 (2016)

11. Mazziotta, J., Toga, A., Evans, A., et al.: A probabilistic atlas and reference system for the human brain: International Consortium for Brain Mapping (ICBM). Philos. Trans. Roy. Soc. Lond. Ser. B **356**(1412), 1293–1322 (2001)

12. Srivastava, N., Hinton, G., Krizhevsky, A., Sutskever, I., Salakhutdinov, R.: Dropout: a simple way to prevent neural networks from overfitting. J. Mach. Learn. Res. **15**, 1929–1958 (2014)

13. Chollet, F.: Keras (2015). GitHub. https://github.com/fchollet/keras

14. Zeiler, M.D.: ADADELTA: an adaptive learning rate method. arXiv preprint arXiv:1212.5701

15. Roy, S., et al.: Subject-specific sparse dictionary learning for atlas-based brain MRI segmentation. IEEE J. Biomed. Health Inform. **19**(5), 1598–1609 (2015)

16. ISBI 2015 Longitudinal MS Lesion Segmentation Evaluation Website. https://smart-stats-tools.org/lesion-challenge-2015

17. Long, J., Shelhamer, E., Darrell, T.: Fully convolutional networks for semantic segmentation. In: Proceedings of the IEEE Conference on Computer Vision and Pattern Recognition, pp. 3431–3440 (2015)

18. Setio, A.A.A., et al.: Pulmonary nodule detection in CT images: false positive reduction using multi-view convolutional networks. IEEE Trans. Med. Imaging **35**(5), 1160–1169 (2016)

Automated Retinopathy of Prematurity Case Detection with Convolutional Neural Networks

Daniel E. Worrall$^{(\boxtimes)}$, Clare M. Wilson, and Gabriel J. Brostow

Department of Computer Science, University College London, London, UK
d.worrall@cs.ucl.ac.uk

Abstract. Retinopathy of Prematurity (ROP) is an ocular disease observed in premature babies, considered one of the largest preventable causes of childhood blindness. Problematically, the visual indicators of ROP are not well understood and neonatal fundus images are usually of poor quality and resolution. We investigate two ways to aid clinicians in ROP detection using convolutional neural networks (CNN): (1) We fine-tune a pretrained GoogLeNet as a ROP detector and with small modifications also return an approximate Bayesian posterior over disease presence. To the best of our knowledge, this is the first completely automated ROP detection system. (2) To further aid grading, we train a second CNN to return novel feature map visualizations of pathologies, learned directly from the data. These feature maps highlight discriminative information, which we believe may be used by clinicians with our classifier to aid in screening.

1 Introduction and Background

Retinopathy of Prematurity (ROP) has entered a third global epidemic [1]. Higher neonatal survival rates in developing countries and new clinical practices in the West [2] have led to a sharp increase in the number of premature babies at risk of this iatrogenic, sight-threatening disease. The preterm retina can develop abnormally at any time up to 36 weeks gestational age [3] and is treatable, thus screening plays an important role. However, screening is labour-intensive and challenging, due to insufficient understanding of ROP symptomatology, lack of gold-standard ground-truth data and poor quality fundus imaging. We investigate two methods how CNNs can be used to aid in ROP detection. (1) We detail what we believe to be the first fully automated ROP detector, which can classify per image and per examination. It harnesses traditional deep learning and modern variational Bayesian techniques. We provide information on practical tweaks that did and did not work in achieving our goal. (2) We demonstrate how the feature maps of deep CNNs can be used to create visualizations of the pathologies, indicative of disease, learned directly from the data.

ROP is difficult to detect, but conveniently it co-occurs with *plus-disease* [4], which is easier to diagnose. Plus-disease is characterized by increased *dilation*

The original version of this chapter was revised: Acknowledgement section has been updated. The erratum to this chapter is available at DOI: 10.1007/978-3-319-46976-8_29

© Springer International Publishing AG 2016
G. Carneiro et al. (Eds.): LABELS 2016/DLMIA 2016, LNCS 10008, pp. 68–76, 2016.
DOI: 10.1007/978-3-319-46976-8_8

and *tortuosity* of the retinal vasculature about the posterior pole (central zone about optic disc) [5], together called *plusness*. Figure 1 shows a reference image of plus-disease from [4], which very clearly shows vascular dilation and tortuosity, but has been criticized for showing these quantities as more progressed than usually seen in clinic. In practice, these two quantities prove difficult to measure systematically and repeatably. Some common practical issues are: defining the segmentation boundary for vessel extraction, measuring vessel

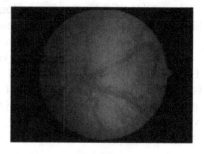

Fig. 1. Standard reference image for identifying plus-disease [4].

dilation/tortuosity, and discerning retinal from choroidal vessels. Other symptoms [6, 7], are known but their use as indicators in screening are limited.

Most semi-automated techniques for ROP case detection rely on measuring plusness via a manual registration followed by semi- or fully-automated vessel segmentation, and by various mechanisms to extract width and tortuousity information [8]. *Jomier et al.* [9] measure width and tortuosity in all four quadrants of a vessel segmentation, which is then fed into a neural network, returning a classification of disease presence. *Wallace et al.* [10] do not seek to build a detection system and differentiate between arteriolar and venular diameter, finding that venular diameter is unimportant in classification. Their system requires significant hand preprocessing to make this work. *Swanson et al.* [11] use a custom vessel segmentation software to semi-automatically measure a tortuosity- and dilation-index for user-selected vessels. They identify plus-positive images as having a tortuosity-index above a certain threshold. In contrast to these methods, we use automated registration and feed the entire registered image into a CNN classifier. We are also able to return per-examination classifications; whereas, existing methods only return per-image classifications.

2   Proposed Method

Neonatal fundus images are usually of poor quality (see Fig. 2), captured from the unsedated premature babies, on a low resolution (640 × 480 px RGB) camera.

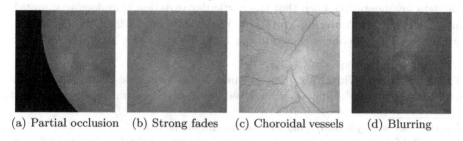

(a) Partial occlusion   (b) Strong fades   (c) Choroidal vessels   (d) Blurring

Fig. 2. Examples factors impeding detection in the neonatal fundus. Only c) is diseased.

They exhibit high levels of variation with different translations and orientations, high levels of motion blur, illumination artifacts, and strongly visible choroidal vessels. Compared with adult fundus images, like in the Kaggle diabetic retinopathy competition[1], these are much degraded and harder to use for classification. The existing techniques mentioned depend on reliable vessel segmentation, which is extremely difficult in the neonatal fundus and sometimes requires some user-intervention to touch up results. Our images are also few in number (~ 1500) with high class-imbalance ($\sim 10\%$). Below we describe our CNN-based classifier and pathology visualization.

2.1 Classifier

The classifier consists of the traditional deep learning pipeline: preprocessing, data augmentation, pretrained CNN, finetuning layers. Presently there are varying gradations of ROP and plus-disease, such as APROP and pre-plus, but we only distinguish 'diseased/healthy', since our dataset was compiled in the late 90s, before these alternatives were used by the mainstream[2].

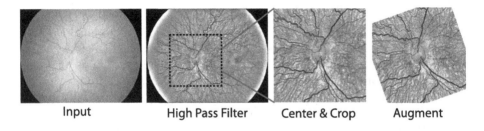

Input   High Pass Filter   Center & Crop   Augment

Fig. 3. Fully automated image registration, preprocessing and augmentation pipeline.

Preprocessing and Data Augmentation. Fundus images are translation registered using [12] and cropped to 240×240 px about the posterior pole, chosen based by cross-validation. The crop size seems small, but biologically reasonable [5]. Post-registration we high pass filter the RGB channels, removing low frequency illumination changes and global color information. This also removes retinal pigmentation, but we assume ethnicity plays a negligible role in plus screening. For variations in the data, which we cannot 'normalize out', we use data augmentation, such that the particular variation is uniformly sampled. In our case we randomly flip, rotate and take subcrops of 96 % of the original image size. The pipeline is shown in Fig. 3.

The Per-Image Classifier. Our per-image classifier consists of a 2-way softmax classifier with affine layer, stacked on top of an ImageNet pretrained

---

[1] https://www.kaggle.com/c/diabetic-retinopathy-detection.

[2] Neonatal fundus imaging quality has not improved since, only the labels are different.

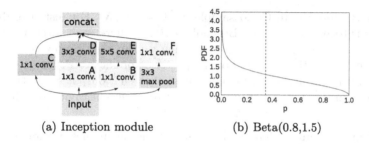

(a) Inception module   (b) Beta(0.8,1.5)

Fig. 4. (a) An inception module consists of a combination of multiscale convolutions. Lettered blocks contain learnable parameters. The GoogLeNet contains 9 inception modules laid end-to-end. (b) The beta distribution is used in the per-exam classifier. It is biased towards healthy images. Solid line: PDF, dashed line: mean.

GoogLeNet [13]. The GoogLeNet is formed of a stack of 9 *inception modules*, which are a combination of convolutional layers and max-pooling (see Fig. 4(a)). Please refer to [13] for more details. For training we minimize a binary cross-entropy loss over the model output and target labels using RMSProp [14].

It is common to just retrain the linear classifier on the end of the network, but we found improved performance, if we included some of the convolutional layers within the 9th inception module. Retraining too many layers led to severe overfitting, however, and so we used an iterative procedure of finetuning the final n layers, and if compared to the previous $n - 1$ layers validation performance increased, then we proceeded to $n + 1$ layers, and so on. With parallel layers, we tried all combinations, for instance A, B and A & B in Fig. 4(a). In the end, we retrained layers ACDEF of inception module 9 with the 2-way softmax classifier.

Bayesian CNNs. CNNs return point-estimate class predictions $\mathbf{y}_* \in \mathbb{R}^D$, where $\sum_{d=1}^{D} y_{*,d} = 1$ given an input image $\mathbf{X}_* \in \mathbb{R}^{N \times M \times C}$. These are overconfident, and a more informative prediction is the posterior predictive distribution $p(\mathbf{y}_*|\mathbf{X}_*, \mathcal{D})$ where $\mathcal{D}$ is the training data. This can be found from the marginal

$$p(\mathbf{y}_*|\mathbf{X}_*, \mathcal{D}) = \int p(\mathbf{y}_*|\mathbf{X}_*, \mathbf{w}) p(\mathbf{w}|\mathcal{D}) \, \mathrm{d}\mathbf{w}, \tag{1}$$

where $p(\mathbf{y}_*|\mathbf{X}_*, \mathbf{w})$ represents the CNN output given image $\mathbf{X}_*$ and weights $\mathbf{w}$, and $p(\mathbf{w}|\mathcal{D})$ is a posterior over the weights, given $\mathcal{D}$. Standard CNN training follows the *maximum likelihood* priniciple, or *maximum a posteriori* when regularlization is involved, so 'traditional' predictions are made with $p(\mathbf{w}|\mathcal{D}) = \delta(\mathbf{w} - \mathbf{w}_{\text{ML}})$ or $p(\mathbf{w}|\mathcal{D}) = \delta(\mathbf{w} - \mathbf{w}_{\text{MAP}})$, where $\delta(x)$ is the Dirac delta function.

Recently it has been shown [15] that training CNNs with sampling behaviour, such as dropout [16], is equivalent to fitting an approximation $q(\mathbf{w}; \boldsymbol{\lambda})$, where $\boldsymbol{\lambda}$ are referred to as the *variational parameters*, to the true Bayesian posterior $p(\mathbf{w}|\mathcal{D})$ over the CNN's weights. Furthermore, these samples are true samples from the approximate posterior. So to approximate Eq. 1, we replace $p(\mathbf{w}|\mathcal{D})$

with $q(\mathbf{w}; \boldsymbol{\lambda})$ and Monte Carlo sample $\mathbf{w}^{(k)} \sim q(\mathbf{w}; \boldsymbol{\lambda})$. For instance, dropout corresponds to $\mathbf{w}_i = z_i \boldsymbol{\lambda}_i$, $z_i \sim \text{Bernoulli}(\mathbf{z}_i; 0.5)$, where $\mathbf{w}_i$ is a set of incoming weights to a neuron. To yield a classification we can then simply threshold the cumulative distribution function of the posterior predictive $\Pr\{y_{*,d} > t\} > s\%$, which in words means, the probability mass of the dth output above threshold t is greater than s%. We can optimize s and t to trade sensitivity–specificity.

Failed Experiments. Here we list some of the techniques, we found to hurt performance. *Vesselness features*: we tried including Frangi vesselness descriptors [17] both as a 4th input channel and as a mask on the input, we presume the network works on a similar representation of the data already. *ADAM solver*: this led to severe overfitting. *Large crops*: increasing the crop size led to underfitting. *More fully-connected layers on output*: this led to overfitting, even with dropout. *Loss function reweighting to remedy class-imbalance*: We found oversampling the smaller class better, because with data augmentation this leads to the network seeing more data per epoch. *Training the softmax classifier from lower layer outputs*: this led to underfitting. Interestingly, one would initially suspect that higher layers are more dataset specific, we found this not to be a problem. *Removing global average pooling (GAP)*: this increased the dimensionality of the output and the number of retrainable parameters, leading to overfitting.

Per-Exam Classifier. Each exam consists of different images of the same eye from differing views and with different artifacts. We build a per-exam classifier by assuming a Beta distribution $p(\pi|a,b) = \text{Beta}(\pi; a, b)$ prior over the probability π that a given eye is diseased in an examination and a Bernoulli distribution $p(c_i|\pi) = c_i^{\pi}(1 - c_i)^{1-\pi}$ on the probability an image i is classified as diseased c_i given π. The posterior over π is $\text{Beta}(\pi; N_1 + a, N_0 + b)$, where N_1 and N_0 are number of images classified as diseased and healthy, respectively, in that examination. When using the Bayesian predictive distribution, we use classifications from the thresholded cumulative distribution. The posterior predictive distribution is $p(c_* = 1|\{c_i\}_{i=1}^{N_0+N_1}) = \frac{N_1 + a}{N_0 + N_1 + a + b}$, where c_* is the diseased/healthy classification for this exam. We found $a = 0.8, b = 1.5$ through Empirical Bayes on the training data, which places a prior on images being healthy.

2.2 Visualization

We visualize diseased regions of the fundus, by examining the CNN feature maps. GoogLeNet feature maps are too small (7×7 px), so we trained a separate 7-layer CNN with 3×3 1-padded kernels and 3×3 stride 2 max-pooling after every even convolution with 31×31 px output feature maps. There is evidence [18] that CNNs trained for the same task learn similar representations at the deepest layers.

For meaningful visualizations, we need to associate activations with a label (diseased/healthy). For this, we manipulate the GAP-layer, found just before

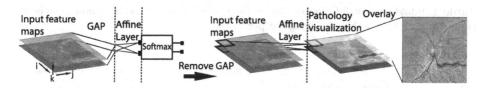

Fig. 5. The linearity of GAP and affine layers means we can swap their order, applying the affine transformation to each stack of pixels in the input.

the softmax classifier. For feature maps $\mathbf{A}_{ijk}$ with spatial indices i, j and channels k, GAP-layers return a spatial mean $a_k = \sum_{i,j} \mathbf{A}_{ijk}$. For GAP-layers feeding directly into a softmax, we need only look at the associated feature maps, but if there is an affine layer between the GAP and the softmax, then we swap the order of the GAP and affine layers,

$$\mathrm{softmax}\left(\mathbf{W}\sum_{i,j}\mathbf{A}_{ij:} + \mathbf{b}\right) = \mathrm{softmax}\left(\sum_{i,j}(\mathbf{W}\mathbf{A}_{ij:} + \mathbf{b})\right),\qquad(2)$$

where $\mathbf{A}_{ij:}$ is the vector with entries a_k. The result is a plusness feature map and a health feature map. A schematic of the process is in Fig. 5 and examples of feature maps overlaid on input images are in Fig. 6.

3   Experiments and Results

Here we run experiments on two large and difficult ROP datasets, comparing results against a baseline and competing methods papers.

Datasets *Canada dataset*: there are 1459 usable images from 35 patients, and 347 *exams* of 2–8 images per eye. There is one label per-exam (plus/no-plus) and per-eye, but *not* per-image. We assume all images from an examination share the same label. We used this dataset for training as well as validation. *London dataset*: there are 106 individually labelled images with 4 expert labels per image. For this dataset we cannot group by exam and use this dataset for testing only.

9-fold validation. Table 1 shows results for 9-fold cross-validation on the Canada dataset for our system and a naïve baseline, a 9-layer scratch-trained CNN. Each patient is assigned to a single fold. We contrast the Bayesian model against the 'traditional' maximum likelihood solution CNN. Key statistics are averaged over the folds. Class-normalized accuracy is the mean of sensitivity and specificity and Fleiss' Kappa (FK) [19] is a measure of agreement. FK of 1.0 is full agreement, 0.0 is random agreement and < 0.0 is no agreement.

Per-exam results are mostly higher than per-image, as expected, since averaging over exams smooths over erroneous per-image labels. For both per-image and per-exam classification, the Bayesian model adds about 5 % class-normalized

Table 1. 9-fold cross-validation results on the Canada dataset. **Bold** denotes the best result for each row within per-image or per-exam.

EXPERIMENT	PER-IMAGE					PER-EXAM		
	BAYES.	TRAD.	BASE.	JOMIER[9]	WALLACE[10]	BAYES.	TRAD.	BASE.
Raw Acc	**0.918**	0.892	0.833	-	-	**0.936**	0.919	0.852
Sensitivity	0.825	0.809	0.598	0.800	**0.950**	**0.954**	0.852	0.625
Specificity	**0.983**	0.909	0.846	0.920	0.780	**0.947**	0.929	0.860
Precision	**0.607**	0.547	0.295	-	-	**0.713**	0.665	0.322
Norm. Acc	**0.904**	0.859	0.722	0.860	0.865	**0.951**	0.890	0.742
Fleiss' Kappa	**0.590**	0.547	0.246	-	-	**0.714**	0.657	0.278

accuracy, with significant gains in sensitivity per-exam. Comparing to other methods, we are competitive, although losing on per-image sensitivity to *Wallace et al.*. We note though that the comparison of results is not straight-forward, since they use smaller test sets (20 images) and *Jomier et al.* use different methodology, testing only non-borderline images. Looking at FK, we see agreement is $0.54 - 0.72$ for our model, considered "moderate" to "substantial".

Multigrader Agreement. With the London dataset there is no groundtruth, so we report the FK score only. For a single prediction, we ensemble the outputs of the 9 cross-validation trained CNNs, taking a mean and thresholding at 50 %, results are in Table 2. Among the experts there is an FK of 0.427, but with our system this drops to 0.366/0.372. It turns out that the system agrees very strongly with one expert and disagrees strongly with another (see Table 2), and that the agreement with the closest expert is stronger than amongst the closest and furthest experts (0.194). For comparison, [20] report an FK of 0.32 for inter-clinician agreement, albeit on a separate dataset.

Table 2. Multigrader agreement is similar to levels found in [20].

EXPERIMENT	EXPERTS ALONE	ALL EXPERTS		CLOSEST EXPERT		FURTHEST EXPERT	
		BAYES.	TRAD.	BAYES.	TRAD.	BAYES.	TRAD.
Fleiss' Kappa	0.427	0.366	0.372	0.551	0.546	−0.118	−0.084

Pre-GAP Visualization. Figure 6 shows the pre-GAP visualization, where red indicates diseased and blue healthy. The blue channel has been intensified for easier visualization. There is a clear indication that the CNN focuses on the vasculature in its decision-making, and that this is by far the most important indicator for plus-disease. This agrees with the current guidance for clinicians as per [4], which focuses on qualitative measurements of the width and tortuosity of retinal blood vessels.

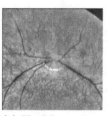 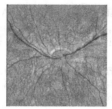 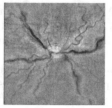 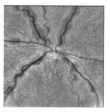

(a) Healthy retina   (b) Healthy retina   (c) Diseased retina   (d) Diseased retina

Fig. 6. Visualizations of learned retinal pathologies with the projected pre-GAP activation layer superimposed. BLUE is healthy tissue and RED is diseased tissue. The CNN has learned that wide and tortuous vessels correlate with plus-disease, as we expect. (Color figure online)

4 Conclusion, Limitations and Future Work

We have presented the first fully automated ROP detection system. We have listed techniques to finetune a GoogLeNet to small datasets, which did and did not work for us. We have also demonstrated a simple Bayesian framework to increase the accuracy of the output of a dropout trained CNN. The system copes with single images or multiple images from a single examination. For understanding we have also demonstrated how to return augmented pathology visualizations from CNNs with large enough feature maps. The code and dataset are available to download upon request.

Our multigrader experiments show that it is possible to train classifiers on subjective labels. These classifiers exhibit good agreement with some of the expert labelers. From a supervised learning perspective, a classifier can only ever be as good as its training data, as such we need to look to less human-dependent training data if we are to surpass human performance. This may involve harnessing unsupervised and semi-supervised learning. It would also be sensible to explore building spatio-temporal models of ROP progression, to see if sequences of images form better predictors of disease than single instances in time.

Acknowledgement. We would like to thank Dr Anna Ells of Alberta Childrens Hospital, Calgary, Canada for the 'Canada dataset', and Alistair Fielder and Philip 'Eddie' Edwards for insightful conversations. Daniel Worrall is supported by Fight for Sight, registered charity number 1111438.

References

1. Zin, A., Gole, G.A.: Retinopathy of prematurity-incidence today. Clin. Perinatol. **40**(2), 185–200 (2013)
2. Fleck, B.W., Stenson, B.J.: Retinopathy of prematurity and the oxygen conundrum: lessons learned from recent randomized trials. Clin. Perinatol. **40**(2), 229–240 (2013)
3. Wilkinson, A., Haines, L., Head, K., Fielder, A., et al.: UK retinopathy of prematurity guideline. Eye (London, England) **23**(11), 2137 (2009)

4. Gole, G.A., Ells, A.L., Katz, X., Holmstrom, G., Fielder, A.R., Capone Jr., A., Flynn, J.T., Good, W.G., Holmes, J.M., McNamara, J., et al.: The international classification of retinopathy of prematurity revisited. JAMA Ophthalmol. **123**(7), 991–999 (2005)

5. Saunders, R.A., Bluestein, E.C., Sinatra, R.B., Wilson, M.E., Rust, P.F.: The predictive value of posterior pole vessels in retinopathy of prematurity. J. Pediatr. Ophthalmol. Strabismus **32**(2), 82–85 (1995)

6. Binenbaum, G.: Algorithms for the prediction of retinopathy of prematurity based on postnatal weight gain. Clin. Perinatol. **40**(2), 261–270 (2013)

7. Oloumi, F., Rangayyan, R.M., Ells, A.L.: Quantification of the changes in the openness of the major temporal arcade in retinal fundus images of preterm infants with plus diseaseanalysis of fundus images of infants with plus disease. Invest. Ophthalmol. Vis. Sci. **55**(10), 6728–6735 (2014)

8. Aslam, T., Fleck, B., Patton, N., Trucco, M., Azegrouz, H.: Digital image analysis of plus disease in retinopathy of prematurity. Acta Ophthalmol. **87**(4), 368–377 (2009)

9. Jomier, J., Wallace, D.K., Aylward, S.R.: Quantification of retinopathy of prematurity via vessel segmentation. In: Ellis, R.E., Peters, T.M. (eds.) MICCAI 2003. LNCS, vol. 2879, pp. 620–626. Springer, Heidelberg (2003)

10. Wallace, D.K., Zhao, Z., Freedman, S.F.: A pilot study using roptool to quantify plus disease in retinopathy of prematurity. J. Am. Assoc. Pediatr. Ophthalmol. Strabismus **11**(4), 381–387 (2007)

11. Swanson, C., Cocker, K., Parker, K., Moseley, M., Fielder, A.: Semiautomated computer analysis of vessel growth in preterm infants without and with ROP. Br. J. Ophthalmol. **87**(12), 1474–1477 (2003)

12. Worrall, D.E., Brostow, G.J., Wilson, C.M.: Automated optic disc (OD) localization in the neonatal fundus image. In: ARVO (2016)

13. Szegedy, C., Liu, W., Jia, Y., Sermanet, P., Reed, S., Anguelov, D., Erhan, D., Vanhoucke, V., Rabinovich, A.: Going deeper with convolutions. In: Proceedings of the IEEE Conference on Computer Vision and Pattern Recognition, pp. 1–9 (2015)

14. Tieleman, T., Hinton, G.: Lecture 6.5-rmsprop. COURSERA: Neural Netw. Mach. Learn. **4**, 2 (2012)

15. Gal, Y., Ghahramani, Z.: Dropout as a bayesian approximation: representing model uncertainty in deep learning. arXiv preprint arXiv:1506.02142 (2015)

16. Hinton, G.E., Srivastava, N., Krizhevsky, A., Sutskever, I., Salakhutdinov, R.R.: Improving neural networks by preventing co-adaptation of feature detectors. arXiv preprint arXiv:1207.0580 (2012)

17. Frangi, A.F., Niessen, W.J., Vincken, K.L., Viergever, M.A.: Multiscale vessel enhancement filtering. In: Wells, W.M., Colchester, A.C.F., Delp, S.L. (eds.) MIC-CAI 1998. LNCS, vol. 1496, p. 130. Springer, Heidelberg (1998)

18. Lenc, K., Vedaldi, A.: Understanding image representations by measuring their equivariance and equivalence. In: Proceedings of the IEEE conference on computer vision and pattern recognition, pp. 991–999 (2015)

19. Fleiss, J.L., Levin, B., Paik, M.C.: Statistical Methods for Rates and Proportions. Wiley, Hoboken (2013)

20. Gschließer, A., Stifter, E., Neumayer, T., Moser, E., Papp, A., Pircher, N., Dorner, G., Egger, S., Vukojevic, N., Oberacher-Velten, I., et al.: Inter-expert and intra-expert agreement on the diagnosis and treatment of retinopathy of prematurity. Am. J. Ophthalmol. **160**(3), 553–560 (2015)

Fully Convolutional Network for Liver Segmentation and Lesions Detection

Avi Ben-Cohen[1]([✉]), Idit Diamant[1], Eyal Klang[2], Michal Amitai[2], and Hayit Greenspan[1]

[1] Medical Image Processing Laboratory, Faculty of Engineering, Department of Biomedical Engineering, Tel Aviv University, 69978 Tel Aviv, Israel
avibenc@mail.tau.ac.il
[2] Sheba Medical Center, Diagnostic Imaging Department, Abdominal Imaging Unit (Affiliated to Sackler School of Medicine) Tel Aviv University, 52621 Tel Hashomer, Israel

Abstract. In this work we explore a fully convolutional network (FCN) for the task of liver segmentation and liver metastases detection in computed tomography (CT) examinations. FCN has proven to be a very powerful tool for semantic segmentation. We explore the FCN performance on a relatively small dataset and compare it to patch based CNN and sparsity based classification schemes. Our data contains CT examinations from 20 patients with overall 68 lesions and 43 livers marked in one slice and 20 different patients with a full 3D liver segmentation. We ran 3-fold cross-validation and results indicate superiority of the FCN over all other methods tested. Using our fully automatic algorithm we achieved true positive rate of 0.86 and 0.6 false positive per case which are very promising and clinically relevant results.

Keywords: Deep learning · Liver lesions · Detection · CT

1 Introduction

Liver cancer is among the most frequent types of cancerous diseases, responsible for the deaths of 745,000 patients worldwide in 2012 alone [14]. The liver is one of the most common organs to develop metastases and CT is one of the most common modalities used for detection, diagnosis and follow-up of liver lesions. The images are acquired before and after intravenous injection of a contrast agent with optimal detection of lesions on the portal phase (60–80 s post injection) images. These procedures require information about size, shape and precise location of the lesions. Manual detection and segmentation is a time-consuming task requiring the radiologist to search through a 3D CT scan which may include multiple lesions. The difficulty of this task highlights the need for computerized analysis to assist clinicians in the detection and evaluation of the size of liver metastases in CT examinations. Automatic detection and segmentation is a very

© Springer International Publishing AG 2016
G. Carneiro et al. (Eds.): LABELS 2016/DLMIA 2016, LNCS 10008, pp. 77–85, 2016.
DOI: 10.1007/978-3-319-46976-8_9

challenging task due to different contrast enhancement behavior of liver lesions and parenchyma. Moreover, the image contrast between these tissues can be low due to individual differences in perfusion and scan time. In addition, lesion shape, texture, and size vary considerably from patient to patient. This research problem has attracted a great deal of attention in recent years. The MICCAI 2008 Grand Challenge [3] provided a good overview of possible methods. The winner of the challenge [11] used the AdaBoost technique to separate liver lesions from normal liver based on several local image features. In more recent works we see a variety of additional methods trying to deal with detection and segmentation of liver lesions [1,9].

In recent years, deep learning has become a dominant research topic in numerous fields. Specially, Convolutional Neural Networks (CNN) have been used for many challenges in computer vision. CNN obtained outstanding performance on different tasks, such as visual object recognition, image classification, handwritten character recognition and more. Deep CNNs introduced by LeCun et al. [5], is a supervised learning model formed by multi-layer neural networks. CNNs are fully data-driven and can retrieve hierarchical features automatically by building high-level features from low-level ones, thus obviating the need to manually customize hand-crafted features. CNN has been used for detection in several medical applications including pulmonary nodule [10], sclerotic metastases, lymph node and colonic polyp [8] and liver tumours [6]. In these works, the CNN was trained using patches taken out of the relevant region of interest (ROI).

In this paper we used a fully convolutional architecture [7] for liver segmentation and detection of liver metastases in CT examinations. The fully convolutional architecture has been recently used for medical purposes in multiple sclerosis lesion segmentation [2]. Fully convolutional networks (FCN) can take input of arbitrary size and produce correspondingly-sized output with efficient inference and learning. Unlike patch based methods, the loss function using this architecture is computed over the entire image segmentation result. Our network processes entire images instead of patches, which removes the need to select representative patches, eliminates redundant calculations where patches overlap, and therefore scales up more efficiently with image resolution. Moreover, there is a fusion of different scales by adding links that combine the final prediction layer with lower layers with finer strides. This fusion helps to combine across different lesion sizes. The output of this method is a lesion heatmap which is used for detection.

Since our dataset is small we use data augmentation by applying scale transformations to the available training images. The variations in slice thickness are large in our data (1.25 to 5 mm) and provides blurred appearance of the lesions for large slice thickness. The scale transformations allows the network to learn alter local texture properties.

We use a fully convolutional architecture for liver segmentation and detection of liver metastases in CT examinations using a small training dataset and compare it to the patch based CNN. To the best of our knowledge, this is the first work that uses fully convolutional neural network for liver segmentation and liver lesions detection.

2   Fully Convolutional Network Architecture

Our network architecture uses the VGG 16- layer net [12]. We decapitate the net by discarding the final classifier layer, and convert all fully connected layers to convolutions. We append a 1×1 convolution with channel dimension 2 to predict scores for lesion or liver at each of the coarse output locations, followed by a deconvolution layer to upsample the coarse outputs to pixel-dense outputs. The upsampling is performed in-network for end-to-end learning by backpropagation from the pixelwise loss. The FCN-8s DAG net was used as our initial network, which learned to combine coarse, high layer information with fine, low layer information as described in [7]. Our initial network architecture is presented in Fig. 1. We also explored the additional value of adding another lower level linking layer creating an FCN-4s DAG net. This was done by linking the Pool2 layer in a similar way to the linking of the Pool3 and Pool4 layers in Fig. 1.

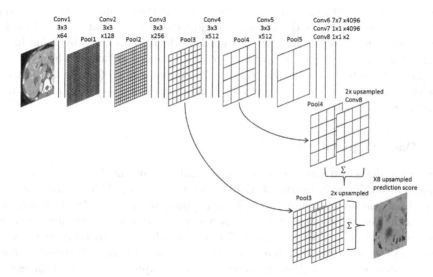

Fig. 1. Initial network architecture. Each convolution layer is illustrated by a straight line with the receptive field size and number of channels denoted above. The ReLU activation function and drop-out are not shown for brevity.

2.1   3D Information

The input in our task are axial CT slices. In order to use the information from z-axis we modified the input image to have three CT slices, the relevant slice and two adjacent slices (above and below). Due to a very high slice spacing in some of our data we had to interpolate the adjacent slices, using linear interpolation, to be with a fixed spacing of 1 mm.

2.2   Training

Input images and their corresponding segmentation maps are used to train the network with the stochastic gradient descent implementation of MatConvNet [13] with GPU acceleration. Two networks were trained, one for the liver segmentation task and one for the lesion detection tasks. For the lesions detection training the areas surrounding the liver including the different organs and tissues were ignored. Note that one network trained on both lesions and liver was not used in our work since we had two different datasets for each task. The softmax log-loss function was calculated pixel-wise with different weights for each class pixels as in Eq. (1):

$$L = - \sum_{ij} w_{ij}(x_{ijc} - \log \sum_{d=1}^{D} \exp(x_{ijd})) \tag{1}$$

Where $c \in [1...D]$ is the ground-truth class and x is the prediction scores matrix (before softmax) and w is the per-pixel weight matrix. As most of the pixels in each image belong to the liver, we balanced the learning process by using fixed weights that are inversely proportional to the population ratios. The learning rate was chosen to be 0.0005 for the first 20 epochs and 0.0001 for the last 30 epochs (total of 50 epochs). The weight decay was chosen to be 0.0005 and the momentum parameter was 0.9.

2.3   Data Augmentation

The lesion detection dataset was much smaller than the liver segmentation dataset since the manual segmentation masks were only in 2D for this dataset so data augmentation was appropriate. Data augmentation is essential to teach the network the desired invariance and robustness properties, when only few training samples are available. We generate different scales from 0.8 to 1.2 as lesion size can change significantly. The scales are sampled using uniform distribution and new images are re-sampled using nearest-neighbour approach. For each image in our dataset, four augmentations were created in different scales.

3   Experiments

3.1   Data

The data used in the current work includes two datasets. The lesion detection dataset includes CT scans from the Sheba medical center, taken during the period from 2009 to 2014. Different CT scanners were used with 0.71–1.17 mm pixel spacing and 1.25–5 mm slice thickness. Each CT image was resized to obtain a fixed pixel spacing of 0.71 mm. The scans were selected and marked by one radiologist. They include 20 patients with 1–3 CT examinations per patient and overall 68 lesion segmentation masks and 43 liver segmentation masks. The data includes various liver metastatic lesions derived from different primary cancers. The liver segmentation dataset includes 20 CT scans with entire liver segmentation masks taken from the SLIVER07 challenge [4] and was used only for training the liver segmentation network.

3.2   Liver Segmentation

We evaluated the liver segmentation network using the lesion detection dataset (43 slices of livers). Two framework variations were used: adding two neighbour slices (above and below), and linking the Pool2 layer for the final prediction (FCN-4s). We evaluated the algorithm's segmentation performance using the Dice index, and calculated the Sensitivity and Positive predictive values (PPV). The results are shown in Table 1. The best results were obtained using the FCN-8s architecture with the addition of the adjacent slices. We obtained an average Dice index of 0.89, an average sensitivity of 0.86 and an average positive predictive value of 0.95. The fusion of an additional low level layer (FCN-4s) did not improve the results, probably since the liver boundary has a smooth shape and there is no need for a higher resolution. Adding the adjacent slices slightly improved the segmentation performance.

Table 1. Liver segmentation performance using algorithm variations

Features	Dice	Sensitivity	PPV
FCN-8s 3 slices	0.89	0.86	0.95
FCN-8s	0.88	0.85	0.95
FCN-4s 3 slices	0.87	0.82	0.95

3.3   Detection-Comparative Evaluation

To evaluate the detection performance independent of the liver segmentation results we constrained the training and the testing sets to the liver area circumscribed manually by a radiologist. One of our goals was to examine the behaviour of the lesion detection network compared to the more classical patch based method. We designed a patch-based CNN similar to the one introduced by Li et al. [6]. The liver area is divided into patches of 17X17 pixels which are fed to the CNN for classification into lesion/normal area. We used a CNN model with seven hidden layers which included three convolutional layers, two max-pooling layers, fully connected layers, ReLU and a softmax classifier. We implemented the CNN model with MatConvNet framework [13] with GPU acceleration. We ran 50 epochs with a learning rate of 0.001. In each epoch a batch of 100 examples is processed simultaneously.

Another comparison made was to a recent work using sparsity based learned dictionaries which achieved strong results [1]. In this method each image was clustered into super-pixels and each super-pixel was represented by a feature vector. The super-pixels are classified using a sparsity based classification method that learns a reconstructive and discriminative dictionary.

As in the liver segmentation evaluation we tried the same two variations by adding two neighbour slices (above and below), and linking the Pool2 layer for the final prediction (FCN-4s). The detection performance was visually assessed considering the following two metrics: True positive rate (TPR)- the total number of detected lesions divided by the total number of known lesions; False positive per case (FPC)- the total number of false detections divided by the number of livers. Each lesion was represented by a 5 mm radius disk in its center of mass for the detection evaluation. The same was done for each connected component in our method results. We define a detected lesion when its center of mass overlap with the system lesion candidate center of mass. A 3-fold cross validation was used (each group containing different patients) using the lesion detection dataset. Results are presented in Table 2. To make this clinically interesting the highest TPR is presented with an FPC lower than 2.

Table 2. FCN, patch based CNN and sparsity based method detection performance given the liver boundary.

Method	TPR	FPC
FCN-4s 3 slices	0.88	0.74
FCN-8s 3 slices	0.86	1.1
FCN-8s	0.85	1.1
Patch based	0.85	1.9
Sparsity Based	0.82	1.1

The FCN-4s with the addition of neighbour slices performed better than the other methods with better TPR and better FPC. Figure 2 shows example results using the FCN. Seem that for lesions the FCN-4s is more appropriate than the FCN-8s because of the lesions size (smaller objects).

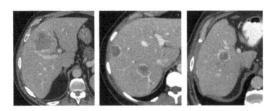

Fig. 2. Example results. In red - false positives; In green - false negatives; in blue - true positives (Color figure online)

3.4 Fully Automatic Detection results

Finally, we tested the combination of the liver segmentation network (FCN-8s with neighbours) and the lesion detection network (FCN-4s with neighbours) to automatically extract the liver and detect the lesions in the liver segmentation result. We achieved a TPR of 0.86 and an FPC of 0.6 using the fully automatic algorithm. These results are close to the detection results achieved using the manual segmentation of the liver with a lower TPR but a better FPC. The liver automatic segmentation output usually did not include some of the boundary pixels which are darker and less similar to the liver parenchyma. These dark boundary pixels can be falsely detected as a lesion. This was the main reason for the improvement in FPC when using the automatic segmentation in comparison to the manual one.

3.5 Synthetic Data Experiments

Trying to understand the FCN discriminative features we created three synthetic images: (1) The lesion filled with a fixed value equal to its mean Hounsfield Units (HU) value; (2)The boundary of the lesion blurred by giving it a fixed value equal to the mean parenchyma HU; (3) The lesion mean HU value equal to the parenchyma mean HU. By using a fixed value to all of the pixels inside the lesion we eliminate the lesion's texture. Figure 3 shows that most of the pixels inside the lesion were misclassified as normal liver tissue. The pixels around the lesion's boundary can look different than normal parenchyma, even if they are not part of the lesion. They are sometimes marked by the experts as part of the lesion and this causes false positives around the boundary of the lesion. The blurred boundary of the lesion reduced the amount of false positives around the lesion's boundary by making it similar to the liver parenchyma. By making the mean HU value of the lesion equal to that of the mean HU value of the parenchyma we eliminate gray levels difference. In that case the lesion was not

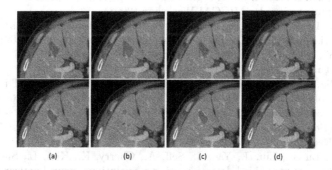

Fig. 3. Synthetic data experiments: (a) Original image; (b) The lesion filled with a fixed value equal to it's mean Hounsfield Units (HU) value; (c) The boundary of the lesion blurred by giving it a fixed value equal to the mean parenchyma HU; (d) The lesion mean HU value equal to the parenchyma mean HU.

detected at all. These results indicate that the network learned the texture of the lesion and mostly relies on the gray level difference between the lesion and the liver parenchyma.

4 Conclusions

To conclude, we showed automated fully convolutional network for liver segmentation and detection of liver metastases in CT examinations. Several approaches were tested including state of the art sparse dictionary classification techniques and patch based CNN. The results indicate that the FCN with data augmentation, addition of neighbour slices, and appropriate class weights provided the best results. Note that we have a small dataset and testing was conducted with 3-fold cross-validation. The detection results are promising. Note that no significant pre-processing or post-processing was implemented in the suggested method. Adding these steps may increase lesion detection accuracy and enable more accurate segmentation as well. Future work entails expanding to 3D analysis on larger datasets.

Acknowledgment. Part of this work was funded by the INTEL Collaborative Research Institute for Computational Intelligence (ICRI-CI).

References

1. Ben-Cohen, A., Klang, E., Amitai, M., Greenspan, H.: Sparsity-based liver metastases detection using learned dictionaries. In: 2016 IEEE 13th International Symposium on Biomedical Imaging (ISBI), pp. 1195–1198 (2016)
2. Brosch, T., Yoo, Y., Tang, L.Y.W., Li, D.K.B., Traboulsee, A., Tam, R.: Deep convolutional encoder networks for multiple sclerosis lesion segmentation. In: Navab, N., Hornegger, J., Wells, W.M., Frangi, A.F. (eds.) MICCAI 2015. LNCS, vol. 9351, pp. 3–11. Springer, Heidelberg (2015)
3. Deng, X., Du, G.: Editorial: 3D segmentation in the clinic: a grand challenge II-liver tumor segmentation. In: MICCAI Workshop (2008)
4. Heimann, T., et al.: Comparison and evaluation of methods for liver segmentation from CT datasets. IEEE Trans. Med. Imaging **28**(8), 1251–1265 (2009)
5. LeCun, Y., Bottou, L., Bengio, Y., Haffner, P.: Gradient-based learning applied to document recognition. Proc. IEEE **86**, 2278–2324 (1998)
6. Li, W., Jia, F., Hu, Q.: Automatic segmentation of liver tumor in CT images with deep convolutional neural networks. J. Comput. Commun. **3**(11), 146 (2015)
7. Long, J., Shelhamer, E., Darrell, T.: Fully convolutional networks for semantic segmentation. In: Proceedings of the IEEE Conference on Computer Vision and Pattern Recognition, pp. 3431–3440 (2015)
8. Roth, H., Lu, L., Liu, J., Yao, J., Seff, A., Cherry, K., Kim, L., Summers, R.: Improving computer-aided detection using convolutional neural networks and random view aggregation. IEEE Trans. Med. Imaging, (2015, pre-print)
9. Rusko, L., Perenyi, A.: Automated liver lesion detection in CT images based on multi-level geometric features. Int. J. Comput. Assist. Radiol. Surg. **9**(4), 577–593 (2014)

10. Setio, A.A., Ciompi, F., Litjens, G., Gerke, P., Jacobs, C., van Riel, S., Wille, M.W., Naqibullah, M., Sanchez, C., van Ginneken, B.: Pulmonary nodule detection in CT images: false positive reduction using multi-view convolutional networks. IEEE Trans. Med. Imaging, (2016, pre-print)
11. Shimizu, A., et al.: Ensemble segmentation using AdaBoost with application to liver lesion extraction from a CT volume. In: Proceedings of Medical Imaging Computing Computer Assisted Intervention Workshop on 3D Segmentation in the Clinic: A Grand Challenge II, New York (2008)
12. Simonyan, K., Zisserman, A.: Very deep convolutional networks for large-scale image recognition. arXiv preprint arXiv:1409.1556 (2014)
13. Vedaldi, A., Lenc, K.: MatConvNet: convolutional neural networks for matlab. In: Proceedings of the 23rd Annual ACM Conference on Multimedia Conference, pp. 689–692 (2015)
14. The World Health Report, World Health Organization (2014)

Deep Learning of Brain Lesion Patterns for Predicting Future Disease Activity in Patients with Early Symptoms of Multiple Sclerosis

Youngjin Yoo[1,2,5]([✉]), Lisa W. Tang[2,3,5], Tom Brosch[1,2,5], David K.B. Li[3,5], Luanne Metz[6], Anthony Traboulsee[4,5], and Roger Tam[2,3,5]

[1] Department of Electrical and Computer Engineering, University of British Columbia, Vancouver, BC, Canada
youngjin.yoo@alumni.ubc.ca
[2] Biomedical Engineering Program, University of British Columbia, Vancouver, BC, Canada
[3] Department of Radiology, University of British Columbia, Vancouver, BC, Canada
[4] Division of Neurology, University of British Columbia, Vancouver, BC, Canada
[5] MS/MRI Research Group, University of British Columbia, Vancouver, BC, Canada
[6] Division of Neurology, University of Calgary, Calgary, AB, Canada

Abstract. Multiple sclerosis (MS) is a neurological disease with an early course that is characterized by attacks of clinical worsening, separated by variable periods of remission. The ability to predict the risk of attacks in a given time frame can be used to identify patients who are likely to benefit from more proactive treatment. In this paper, we aim to determine whether deep learning can extract, from segmented lesion masks, latent features that can predict short-term disease activity in patients with early MS symptoms more accurately than lesion volume, which is a very commonly used MS imaging biomarker. More specifically, we use convolutional neural networks to extract latent MS lesion patterns that are associated with early disease activity using lesion masks computed from baseline MR images. The main challenges are that lesion masks are generally sparse and the number of training samples is small relative to the dimensionality of the images. To cope with sparse voxel data, we propose utilizing the Euclidean distance transform (EDT) for increasing information density by populating each voxel with a distance value. To reduce the risk of overfitting resulting from high image dimensionality, we use a synergistic combination of downsampling, unsupervised pretraining, and regularization during training. A detailed analysis of the impact of EDT and unsupervised pretraining is presented. Using the MRIs from 140 subjects in a 7-fold cross-validation procedure, we demonstrate that our prediction model can achieve an accuracy rate of 72.9 % (SD = 10.3 %) over 2 years using baseline MR images only, which is significantly higher than the 65.0 % (SD = 14.6 %) that is attained with the traditional MRI biomarker of lesion load.

Keywords: Deep learning · Convolutional neural network · Clinical prediction · Multiple sclerosis lesion · Machine learning · MRI

© Springer International Publishing AG 2016
G. Carneiro et al. (Eds.): LABELS 2016/DLMIA 2016, LNCS 10008, pp. 86–94, 2016.
DOI: 10.1007/978-3-319-46976-8_10

1   Introduction

Multiple sclerosis (MS) is an immune mediated disorder characterized by inflammation, demyelination, and degeneration in the central nervous system. There is increasing evidence that early detection and intervention can improve long-term prognosis. However, the disease course of MS is highly variable, especially in its early stages, and it is difficult to predict which patients would progress more quickly and therefore benefit from more aggressive treatment. The McDonald criteria [1,2], which are a combination of clinical and magnetic resonance imaging (MRI) indicators of disease activity, facilitate the diagnosis of MS in patients who present early symptoms suggestive of MS.

However, predicting which patients will meet a given set of criteria for disease activity within a certain time frame remains a challenge. MRI is invaluable for monitoring and understanding the pathology of MS in vivo from the earliest stages of the disease, but the commonly computed MRI biomarkers such as brain and lesion volume are not strongly predictive of future disease activity [3], especially when only baseline measures are available, which is often the case when a patient first presents. Researchers have attempted to define more sophisticated MRI features that are more predictive. Recently, Wottschel *et al.* employed a support vector machine trained on user-defined features to predict the conversion of clinically isolated syndrome (CIS), a prodromal stage of MS, to clinically definite MS [4]. The features included demographic information and clinical measurements at baseline, and also MRI-derived features such as lesion load (also known as burden of disease, BOD) and lesion distance measurements from the center of the brain.

User-defined features typically require expert domain knowledge and a significant amount of trial-and-error, and are subject to user bias. An alternate approach is to automatically learn patterns and extract latent features using machine learning. In recent years, deep learning [5] has received much attention due to its use of automated feature extraction to achieve breakthrough success in many applications, in some cases from high-dimensional data with complex content such as neuroimaging data. For example, deep learning of neuroimaging data has been used to perform various tasks such as the classification between mild cognitive impairment and Alzheimer's disease (*e.g.*, [6]) and to model pathological variability in MS [7].

In this work, using the baseline MRIs of patients with early symptoms of MS but not yet meeting the McDonald 2005 criteria for MS diagnosis, we aim to predict which patients worsened to meet the conversion criteria within two years. MS exhibits a complex pathology that is still not well understood, but it is known that change in spatial lesion distribution may be an indicator of disease activity [8]. Our clinical motivation is to discover white matter lesion patterns that may indicate a faster rate of worsening, so that patients who exhibit such patterns can be selected for more personalized treatment. We investigate whether latent MRI lesion patterns extracted by deep learning can predict disease status conversion to meet the McDonald 2005 criteria with greater accuracy than BOD. The main idea is to employ convolutional neural networks (CNNs) to identify latent lesion pattern features whose variability can maximally distinguish those patients at risk of short-term disease activity from those who will remain relatively stable.

2   Materials and Preprocessing

The baseline T2-weighted (T2w) and proton density-weighted (PDw) MR images of 140 subjects were used to predict each patient's disease status at two years. The dataset consists of 60 non-converters and 80 converters. The image dimensions are $256 \times 256 \times 60$ with a voxel size of $0.937 \times 0.937 \times 3.000$ mm. Preprocessing consisted of skull stripping and linear intensity normalization. The T2w and PDw scans were segmented via a semi-automated multimodal method to produce lesion masks. The mask images were then downsampled to $128 \times 128 \times 30$ with Gaussian pre-filtering as a first dimensionality reduction step.

3   Methods

Prior to feature extraction, all images were spatially normalized to a standard template (MNI152) [9] using affine registration. Our CNN architecture is a 9-layer model (Fig. 1), consisting of three 3D convolutional layers interleaved with three max-pooling layers, followed by two fully connected layers, and finally a logistic regression output layer.

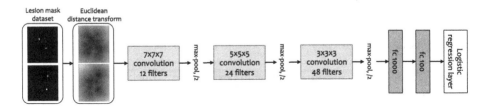

Fig. 1. The proposed convolutional neural network architecture (fc = fully connected layer) for predicting future disease activity in patients with early symptoms of MS. The Euclidean distance transform is used for increasing information density from sparse lesion masks.

3.1   Euclidean Distance Transform of Lesion Masks

MS lesions typically occupy a very small percentage of a brain image, and as a result the binary lesion masks contain mostly zeros. From our preliminary experiments, we observed that the CNN model learns mostly noisy patterns from the binary lesion masks, which is likely due to the fact that sparse lesion voxels can be ignored or deformed into noise spikes by various stages of convolution and pooling operations during training. As described in Sect. 4, the training and test results show that the binary lesion masks are not appropriate as the input to the CNN model. We could have also used raw MR images as the input, but the lesion voxels would almost certainly be lost in the learning process due to their sparsity. To overcome this problem, we propose increasing the density of information in the lesion masks by the Euclidean distance transform (EDT) [10], which measures the Euclidean distance between each voxel and the closest lesion. The EDTs of the binary lesion masks form the input to our CNN model. From Fig. 1, we can see examples of how the spatial distribution of the lesions is densely captured and better amplified than those in the original binary masks. The impact of the transform on training a deep learning network will be presented in Sect. 4. We used the ITK-SNAP's Convert3D tool [11] for applying the EDT.

3.2   CNN Training

It has been shown that pretraining can improve the optimization performance of supervised deep networks when training sets are limited, which often happens in the medical imaging domain [12], but the gains are dependent on data properties. We investigated the impact of using a 3D convolutional deep belief network (DBN) for pretraining to initialize our CNN model. Our convolutional DBN has the same network architecture as the convolutional and pooling layers of our CNN. For our DBN and CNN, we used the leaky rectified non-linearity [13] (negative slope $\alpha = 0.3$), which is designed to prevent the problem associated with non-leaky units failing to reactivate after encountering certain conditions due to large gradient flow. Our convolutional DBN was initialized using a robust method [14] that particularly considers the rectified non-linearity and has been shown to allow successful training of very deep networks on natural images, and trained using contrastive divergence [15]. To analyze the influence of EDT and pretraining on supervised training, we trained our CNN under four conditions: no EDT and no pretraining, no EDT with pretraining, with EDT and no pretraining, with both EDT and pretraining. For all four experiments, we used negative log-likelihood maximization with AdaDelta [16] (conditioning constant $\epsilon = 1e-12$ and decay rate $\rho = 0.95$) and a batch size of 20 for training. Since there are more converters than non-converters in the dataset, the class weights in the cost function (cross entropy) for supervised training were automatically adjusted in each fold to be inversely proportional to the class frequencies observed in the training set. We used Theano [17] and cuDNN [18] for implementing the CNN models.

3.3   Data Augmentation and Regularization

Due to the high dimensionality of the input images relative to the number of samples in the dataset, even after downsampling, the proposed network can suffer from overfitting. Data augmentation is one of the most popular approaches to reduce the risk of overfitting by artificially creating training samples to increase the dataset size. To generate more training samples, we performed data augmentation by applying random rotations (± 3 degrees), translations (± 2 mm), and scaling (± 2 percent) to the mask images, which increased the number of training images by fourfold. To regularize training, we applied dropout [19] with $p = 0.5$, weight decay (L_2-norm regularization) with penalty coefficient 2e−3 and L_1-norm regularization with penalty coefficient 1e−6. Finally, we applied early stopping, which also acts as a regularizer to improve the generalization ability [20], with a convergence target of negative log-likelihood of 0.6. The convergence target was used to stop training when the generalization loss (defined as the relative increase of the validation error over the minimum-so-far during training) started to increase, which was determined by cross-validation.

4   Results and Discussion

To see the impact of EDT on unsupervised pretraining, we computed the root mean squared (RMS) reconstruction error with and without EDT for each epoch during training of the convolutional DBN. The reconstruction error remaining after each epoch during pretraining of the first convolutional layer is shown in Fig. 2. We observed that pretraining with EDT converged faster and produced lower reconstruction error at convergence than pretraining without EDT.

To analyze the impact of EDT and pretraining on supervised training, we compared four different scenarios which were described in Sect. 3.2 and shown in Fig. 3. Without EDT, the CNN converged much faster with pretraining, but the prediction errors at convergence were similar between those obtained with and without pretraining. In both cases, the training made little progress on the prediction error on the training set, and no progress on the test error, which remained high. Using EDT, the optimization did not converge without pretraining even after 500 epochs, but did converge with pretraining. Without pretraining, the prediction errors fluctuated early for both the training and test datasets, but soon remained constant, and training made no further progress. In contrast, with both EDT and pretraining, the prediction errors on both training and test data decreased fairly steadily up to about 200 epochs.

Figure 4 shows visualizations of the manifolds produced by the CNN outputs, reduced to two dimensions using t-distributed stochastic neighbor embedding (t-SNE) [21]. When EDT and pretraining were not used, the two groups

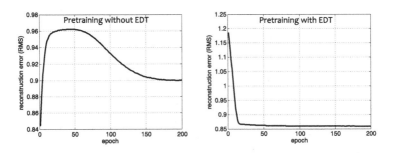

Fig. 2. The influence of EDT on unsupervised pretraining for a convolutional layer. Pretraining with EDT converged faster and produced lower reconstruction error after convergence.

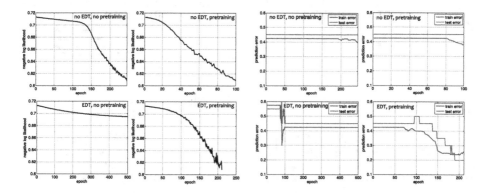

Fig. 3. The influence of EDT and pretraining on supervised training. The left 4 images show training costs and the right 4 images show prediction errors on both training and test datasets for each epoch during supervised training in a selected fold of cross-validation.

(converters and non-converters) showed poor linear separability in the learned manifold space. The two groups were more distinguishable in the manifold space learned from the CNN with EDT and pretraining.

Table 1. Performance comparison (%) between 5 different prediction models for predicting short-term (2 years) clinical status conversion in patients with early MS symptoms. The same training parameters were used for all the CNNs. We performed a 7-fold cross-validation on 80 converters and 60 non-converters and computed the average performance for each prediction model.

Prediction model	Accuracy	Sensitivity	Specificity	AUC
Logistic regression with BOD	65.0 ± 14.6	54.3	80.9	67.6 ± 14.9
CNN (no EDT, no pretraining)	57.9 ± 4.9	94.9	8.3	51.6 ± 4.4
CNN (no EDT, pretraining)	57.9 ± 5.9	98.7	3.6	51.1 ± 4.9
CNN (EDT, no pretraining)	54.3 ± 6.2	71.4	28.6	50.0 ± 0.0
CNN (EDT, pretraining)	72.9 ± 10.3	78.6	65.1	71.8 ± 10.2

For evaluating prediction performance, we used a 7-fold cross-validation procedure in which each fold contained 120 subjects for training and 20 subjects. Note that the number of training images for each fold was increased to 480 by data augmentation. For comparison to the established approach used in clinical studies, a logistic regression prediction model applied to the classic MRI biomarker of BOD was used. The results of the comparison are shown in Table 1. When EDT was not used, the CNN (with and without pretraining) produced lower prediction accuracy rates than those attained by the logistic regression model with BOD. In addition, these cases produced very high sensitivity but

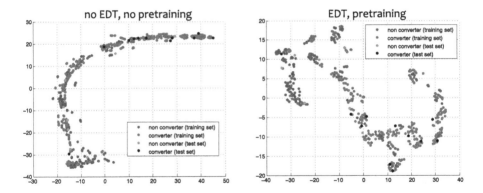

Fig. 4. Visualizations to show the influence of EDT and pretraining on the learned manifold space, reduced to two dimensions using t-SNE [21]. Each subject in the dataset is represented by a two-dimensional feature vector. The axes represent the feature element values of each two-dimensional feature vector in the learned low-dimensional map. The converter and non-converter groups are more linearly separable in the manifold space when using the EDT and pretraining.

low specificity, possibly due to overfitting on the sparse lesion image data. When EDT was used without pretraining, the CNN did not converge for every fold in the cross-validation and also produced lower prediction accuracy rates than lesion volume. The gap between sensitivity and specificity was reduced but still remained large. The CNN with EDT and pretraining improved the prediction performance by approximately 8 % in accuracy and 4 % in AUC when compared to the logistic regression model with BOD. In addition, the SDs for both accuracy and AUC decreased by approximately 4–5%, showing a more consistent performance across folds. This model also achieved the best balance between sensitivity and specificity.

5   Conclusion

We have presented a CNN architecture that learns latent lesion features useful for identifying patients with early MS symptoms who are at risk of future disease activity within two years, using baseline MRIs only. We presented methods to overcome the sparsity of lesion image data and the high dimensionality of the images relative to the number of training samples. In particular, we showed that the Euclidean distance transform and unsupervised pretraining are both key steps to successful optimization, when supported by a synergistic combination of data augmentation and regularization strategies. The final results were markedly better than those obtained by the clinical standard of lesion volume.

Acknowledgements. This work was supported by the MS/MRI Research Group at the University of British Columbia, the Natural Sciences and Engineering Research Council of Canada, the MS Society of Canada, and the Milan and Maureen Ilich Foundation.

References

1. Polman, C., Reingold, S., Edan, G., et al.: Diagnostic criteria for multiple sclerosis: revisions to the McDonald criteria. Ann. Neurol. **58**(2005), 840–846 (2005)
2. Polman, C.H., Reingold, S.C., Banwell, B., et al.: Diagnostic criteria for multiple sclerosis: revisions to the McDonald criteria. Ann. Neurol. **69**(2011), 292–302 (2010)
3. Odenthal, C., Coulthard, A.: The prognostic utility of MRI in clinically isolated syndrome: a literature review. Am. J. Neuroradiol. **36**, 425–431 (2015)
4. Wottschel, V., Alexander, D., Kwok, P., et al.: Predicting outcome in clinically isolated syndrome using machine learning. NeuroImage: Clin. **7**, 281–287 (2015)
5. LeCun, Y., Bengio, Y., Hinton, G.: Deep learning. Nature **521**, 436–444 (2015)
6. Suk, H., Lee, S., Shen, D., et al.: Hierarchical feature representation and multimodal fusion with deep learning for AD/MCI diagnosis. NeuroImage **101**, 569–582 (2014)
7. Brosch, T., Yoo, Y., Li, D.K.B., Traboulsee, A., Tam, R.: Modeling the variability in brain morphology and lesion distribution in multiple sclerosis by deep learning. In: Golland, P., Hata, N., Barillot, C., Hornegger, J., Howe, R. (eds.) MICCAI 2014, Part II. LNCS, vol. 8674, pp. 462–469. Springer, Heidelberg (2014)
8. Giorgio, A., Battaglini, M., Rocca, M.A., et al.: Location of brain lesions predicts conversion of clinically isolated syndromes to multiple sclerosis. Neurology **80**, 234–241 (2013)
9. Mazziotta, J., Toga, A., Evans, A., et al.: A probabilistic atlas and reference system for the human brain: international consortium for brain mapping (ICBM). Philos. Trans. Roy. Soc. B: Biol. Sci. **356**, 1293–1322 (2001)
10. Maurer, C., Qi, R., Raghavan, V.: A linear time algorithm for computing exact Euclidean distance transforms of binary images in arbitrary dimensions. IEEE Trans. Pattern Anal. Mach. Intell. **25**, 265–270 (2003)
11. Yushkevich, P.A., Piven, J., Cody Hazlett, H., et al.: User-guided 3D active contour segmentation of anatomical structures: significantly improved efficiency and reliability. NeuroImage **31**, 1116–1128 (2006)
12. Tajbakhsh, N., Shin, J.Y., Gurudu, S.R., et al.: Convolutional neural networks for medical image analysis: full training or fine tuning? IEEE Trans. Med. Imaging **35**, 1299–1312 (2016)
13. Maas, A., Hannun, A., Ng, A.: Rectifier nonlinearities improve neural network acoustic models. In: International Conference on Machine Learning, vol. 30 (2013)
14. He, K., Zhang, X., Ren, S., et al.: Delving deep into rectifiers: surpassing human-level performance on imagenet classification. In: Proceedings of the IEEE International Conference on Computer Vision, pp. 1026–1034 (2015)
15. Lee, H., Grosse, R., Ranganath, R., et al.: Unsupervised learning of hierarchical representations with convolutional deep belief networks. Commun. ACM **54**, 95–103 (2011)
16. Zeiler, M.: ADADELTA: an adaptive learning rate method. arXiv preprint arXiv:1212.5701 (2012)
17. Theano Development Team: Theano: A Python framework for fast computation of mathematical expressions. arXiv e-prints abs/1605.02688, May 2016
18. Chetlur, S., Woolley, C., Vandermersch, P., et al.: cuDNN: efficient primitives for deep learning. arXiv preprint arXiv:1410.0759 (2014)

19. Srivastava, N., Hinton, G., Krizhevsky, A., et al.: Dropout: a simple way to prevent neural networks from overfitting. J. Mach. Learn. Res. **15**, 1929–1958 (2014)
20. Orr, G.B., Müller, K.R.: Neural networks: tricks of the trade. Springer, Heidelberg (2003)
21. Van Der Maaten, L.: Accelerating t-SNE using tree-based algorithms. J. Mach. Learn. Res. **15**, 3221–3245 (2014)

De-noising of Contrast-Enhanced MRI Sequences by an Ensemble of Expert Deep Neural Networks

Ariel Benou[1,3]([✉]), Ronel Veksler[2,3], Alon Friedman[2,3,4],
and Tammy Riklin Raviv[1,3]

[1] Department of Electrical Engineering,
Ben-Gurion University of the Negev, Beer-Sheva, Israel
[2] Department of Physiology and Cell Biology,
Ben-Gurion University of the Negev, Beer-Sheva, Israel
[3] The Zlotowski Center for Neuroscience,
Ben-Gurion University of the Negev, Beer-Sheva, Israel
[4] Departments of Medical Neuroscience and Brain Repair Centre,
Dalhousie University, Faculty of Medicine, Halifax, NS B3H4R2, Canada
arielbenou@gmail.com

Abstract. Dynamic contrast-enhanced MRI (DCE-MRI) is an imaging protocol where MRI scans are acquired repetitively throughout the injection of a contrast agent. The analysis of dynamic scans is widely used for the detection and quantification of blood brain barrier (BBB) permeability. Extraction of the pharmacokinetic (PK) parameters from the DCE-MRI washout curves allows quantitative assessment of the BBB functionality. Nevertheless, curve fitting required for the analysis of DCE-MRI data is error-prone as the dynamic scans are subject to non-white, spatially-dependent and anisotropic noise that does not fit standard noise models. The two existing approaches i.e. curve smoothing and image de-noising can either produce smooth curves but cannot guaranty fidelity to the PK model or cannot accommodate the high variability in noise statistics in time and space.

We present a novel framework based on Deep Neural Networks (DNNs) to address the DCE-MRI de-noising challenges. The key idea is based on an ensembling of expert DNNs, where each is trained for different noise characteristics and curve prototypes to solve an inverse problem on a specific subset of the input space. The most likely reconstruction is then chosen using a classifier DNN. As ground-truth (clean) signals for training are not available, a model for generating realistic training sets with complex nonlinear dynamics is presented. The proposed approach has been applied to DCE-MRI scans of stroke and brain tumor patients and is shown to favorably compare to state-of-the-art de-noising methods, without degrading the contrast of the original images.

1 Introduction

Dynamic contrast enhanced magnetic resonance imaging (DCE-MRI) of the brain is a noninvasive, *in vivo* tool to detect and quantify pathologies based

© Springer International Publishing AG 2016
G. Carneiro et al. (Eds.): LABELS 2016/DLMIA 2016, LNCS 10008, pp. 95–110, 2016.
DOI: 10.1007/978-3-319-46976-8_11

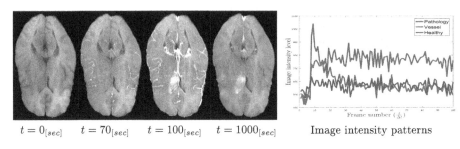

$t = 0_{[sec]}$ $t = 70_{[sec]}$ $t = 100_{[sec]}$ $t = 1000_{[sec]}$ Image intensity patterns

Fig. 1. Left: DCE-MRI scans at different time points of a patient with brain tumor. Right: A plot along 100 frames of the intensity levels of 3 voxels corresponding to the three typical WoCs: vessel (red), pathology (blue) and healthy tissue (green) (Color figure online)

on contrast agent (CA) accumulation [18]. The acquisition technique involves repeated T_1 weighted imaging of tissues before, during and after the injection of a CA. The CA changes the tissue's T_1 relaxation time, which manifests as signal enhancement (see Fig. 1).

Numerous brain pathologies (e.g., stroke, tumor, epilepsy) are associated with the disruption of the blood brain barrier (BBB). The BBB is a tightly-regulated barrier that controls the passage of substances into the central nervous system (CNS). When the BBB does not function well, the CA penetrates the extravascular-extracellular space resulting in a gradual enhancement of the surrounding brain tissues. The voxel-wise variations of the CA concentration over time can be grouped into three different types of washout curves (WoCs), characterizing blood vessels, healthy tissues and pathologies (Fig. 1). The detection of BBB disruption is performed by fitting a pharmacokinetic (PK) model [17] (e.g., Tofts [20], Brix [3], Vexler et al. [21]), to the CA WoCs. Accurate assessment of the disruption is important for various clinical applications [1,21].

Curve fitting required for the analysis of DCE-MRI data is error-prone as the dynamic scans are subject to non-white, spatially-dependent and anisotropic noise that does not fit standard noise models. Current methods either perform curve fitting regardless of the noise (e.g., [14]) or assume a particular noise model [16]. In [13] a low dimensional space using principle component analysis (PCA) is constructed with curves generated by the Tofts model [19]. Then, the PK parameters of the real DCE-MRI are recovered by a projection of the noisy WoCs on this space. Nevertheless, the projection is a linear operation, while the data is non-linear. In [6] a method called dynamic non-local means (DNLM), which extends the algorithm in [4] for spatio-temporal de-noising is suggested. However, the de-noising operation may distort the data due to differences in the PK characteristics of the different image regions.

We propose a new method for noise reduction and reconstruction of the WoCs, without assuming a particular noise distribution and without reducing the quality of the contrast of the original scans. In addition, our approach allows decreasing the temporal resolution of the DCE-MRI scans (and thereby potentially enabling to increase the spatial resolution), while preserving the implicit PK information. This is accomplished by the construction and the training of an ensemble of Deep Neural Networks (DNNs). DNNs are increasingly used for solving regression problems. Recently, it has been used for signal and image de-noising, e.g. [5] for speech recognition and [22] for image processing. A deep learning method was suggested for diffusion weighted imaging (DWI) de-noising [7].

DCE-MRI de-noising introduces several challenges since clean signals cannot be acquired (no ground truth); the spatio-temporal noise model is unknown, and the signal to noise ratio (SNR) spatially varies. These issues are addressed by two key contributions: the construction and the training of an ensemble of expert DNNs for the different signal prototypes and noise levels, and the generation of realistic noisy signals for training. A block diagram of the proposed framework is shown in Fig. 2.

The proposed approach is applied to DCE-MRI sequences of stroke and brain tumor patients. Our method is shown to outperform state-of-the-art de-noising methods, such as the Beltrami filtering (extended for 3D grayscale videos) [12] and the DNLM [6]. Accurate reconstruction of the PK parameters from noisy data, without contrast degradation, is demonstrated for both the original and down-sampled data.

2 Method

2.1 Problem Formulation

Let $\mathcal{I} = \{I_t\}_{t=1}^T$ denote a temporal series of patient-specific MR brain scans, where $I_t \colon \Omega \to \mathbb{R}$ denotes intensities of the scan acquired at a time point t defined on $\Omega \subset \mathbb{R}^3$. We assume that the scans are aligned, equally spaced apart in time, and are acquired after the injection of a CA. Let $c_t \colon \Omega \to \mathbb{R}$ denote the concentration of the CA associated with I_t. A temporal series, $\mathbf{c}(\mathbf{x}) = [c_1(\mathbf{x}), c_2(\mathbf{x}), \dots, c_T(\mathbf{x})]^T$ associated with a voxel $\mathbf{x} \in \Omega$, is called a washout curve (WoC). An *observed* WoC $\mathbf{c}_o(\mathbf{x}) \in \mathbb{R}^T$ is a set of noisy observations of the latent, *clean* signal $\mathbf{c}_c(\mathbf{x}) \in \mathbb{R}^T$, distorted by a noise $\mathbf{n}(\mathbf{x}) \in \mathbb{R}^T$ with an unknown probability density function (PDF). The relation between $\mathbf{c}_o(\mathbf{x})$ and $\mathbf{c}_c(\mathbf{x})$ can be described by: $\mathbf{c}_o(\mathbf{x}) = h(\mathbf{c}_c(\mathbf{x}), \mathbf{n}(\mathbf{x}))$, where $h(\cdot) \colon \mathbb{R}^T \to \mathbb{R}^T$ is an unknown noise model. The de-noising task can be formulated as an inverse problem, as follows:

$$g^* = \arg\min_g E_{\mathbf{c}_o(\mathbf{x})} \left[\|g\left(\mathbf{c}_o(\mathbf{x})\right) - \mathbf{c}_c(\mathbf{x})\|_2^2 \right] \tag{1}$$

where g^* is the function that best approximates $h^{-1}(\cdot)$.

2.2 Deep Neural Network

We use an ensemble of deep neural networks (DNNs) for solving the inverse problem defined by Eq. 1. We denote by $f_l(\cdot)$ the activation function of the artificial neurons (ANs) in layer l and by $\mathbf{w}_i^l$ the vector of weights connecting the i-th AN in layer $l + 1$ to K_l ANs in layer l, where $l \in [0, L-1]$ and K_l is the number of ANs in layer l. The output y_i^{l+1} of the i-th AN in layer $l+1$ is calculated as follows: $y_i^{l+1} = f_l(\sum_{j=1}^{K_l} w_{i,j}^l y_j^l) = f_l(<\mathbf{w}_i^l, \mathbf{y}^l>)$ where $\mathbf{y}^l \triangleq [1, y_1^l, \ldots, y_{K_l}^l]^T$. The DNN's input is the augmented vector $\mathbf{y}^0 = \tilde{\mathbf{c}}_o = [1, \mathbf{c}_o^T]^T$. Given a training set of N input-output pairs $\{\mathbf{c}_o, \mathbf{y}_{GT}\}_n$ we look for a set of weights $\mathbf{W}^*$ that minimizes the cost function: $\mathbf{W}^* \triangleq \arg\min_{\mathbf{W}} E_{\mathbf{c}_o} \left[\|\mathbf{y}^L - \mathbf{y}_{GT}\|_2^2\right]$ where $\mathbf{y}_{GT}$ is synthetically generated, as will be explained in Sect. 2.6. Given $\mathbf{W}^*$ one can solve the inverse problem $g \triangleq (f_L \circ \ldots \circ f_1)(\tilde{\mathbf{c}}_o; \mathbf{W}^*)$ and apply it to new noisy sequences. However, training a clinically applicable de-noising DNN is challenging. First, the SNR level of DCE-MRI changes spatially. In addition, different tissues have different PK patterns. While these issues might be addressed by using an extremely deep network, the number of weights to be optimized and the training examples required, renders the training of such a network impractical. Instead, we suggest using an ensemble of expert DNNs, as we discuss in Sects. 2.3 and 2.4. Second, the usability of the DNN ensemble depends on having an appropriate optimization process, which is unique for each of the expert DNNs. We use a set of stacked restricted Boltzmann machines (RBMs) to facilitate the initialization [9], see Sect. 2.5. The training problem is further complicated since ground truth (GT) data, i.e., clean WoCs, cannot be extracted from real DCE-MRIs and therefore are not available. In Sect. 2.6 we present a model for generating realistic training sets that address this issue.

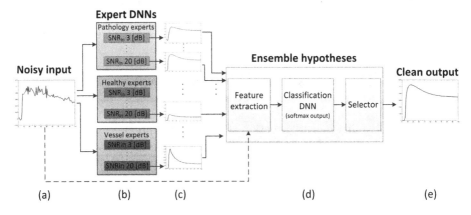

Fig. 2. A block diagram of the proposed DNN ensemble. Given a noisy WoC (a), each expert DNN generates a reconstruction hypothesis (b). The corresponding hypotheses (c) are ensembled using a classification DNN (d) that selects the most likely hypothesis (e).

2.3   Expert DNN: Architecture and Training

We construct a DNN as a non-linear deep autoencoder following [8], which is suitable for de-noising. The architecture and the training process of an expert DNN are illustrated in Fig. 3. The lower $L/2$ layers are designed to expand and

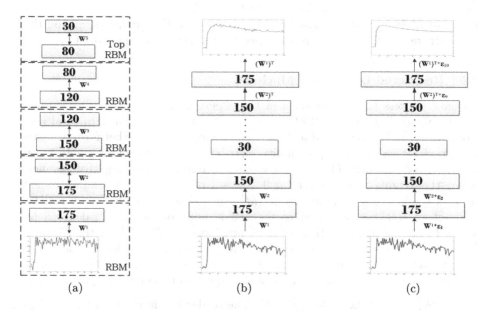

(a)   (b)   (c)

Fig. 3. Training an expert DNN: (a) Pre-training using stacked RBMs, (b) Weights initialization of an expert DNN, (c) Fine tuning using stochastic gradient descent.

then to reduce the dimensionality of the noisy input data. The weights $\{\mathbf{W}^l\}_{l=1}^{L/2}$ are initialized by the stacked RBMs, see Sect. 2.5. The upper $L/2$ layers of the DNN are designed to restore the original dimensionality of the data, allowing reconstruction of a clean observation from the compressed data extracted from layer $l = L/2$. We train the layers of the DNN simultaneously using stochastic gradient descent [15] to minimized the cost $E_{\mathbf{c}_o}\left[\|\mathbf{y}^L - \mathbf{y}_{GT}\|_2^2\right]$.

The entire framework is based on three arrays of DNNs, corresponding to different types of WoCs (healthy, pathology, blood vessel). Each array consists of M expert DNNs that are trained on data with different SNR levels, as is illustrated in Fig. 2b. We next explain how the reconstruction hypotheses provided by the DNNs are ensembled to extract the final output.

2.4 Ensembling Hypotheses

Since each expert DNN is trained on a mutually exclusive subset of the training data (of a specific SNR level and WoC type), the DNN that is trained on data similar to a given test example, is more likely to have the best performance. Therefore, we boost our system confidence by ensembling the experts' hypotheses. Let $g_k(\mathbf{c}_o)$ be the hypothesis of the k-th DNN expert with respect to an observed input $\mathbf{c}_o$. We define five measures that allow the evaluation of the experts' performances as follows: the L_1 and L_2 norms of the deviation from the original WoC $(g_k(\mathbf{c}_o) - \mathbf{c}_o)$, the cosine similarity and correlation between $g_k(\mathbf{c}_o)$ and $\mathbf{c}_o$, and total variation of the hypothesis. We, then, use an additional classification DNN with a softmax activation function [2], that is trained to select the most likely hypothesis based on these measures. For further details on the architecture and the training of the classification DNN see Appendix C[1].

2.5 Restricted Boltzmann Machine

We now address the initialization of the expert DNNs' weights using stacked RBMs [8], see Fig. 3a. An RBM is a generative stochastic artificial neural network with a visible layer and a single hidden layer, that together form a bipartite graph. It can learn a probability distribution over its set of inputs in an unsupervised manner. The process is carried out in an aggregative manner, where the weights of each layer $l = 0 \ldots \frac{L}{2} - 1$ of a given DNN are pre-trained using a single RBM (denoted by RBM^l) such that the hidden units realizations of an RBM^{l-1} are used as the visible units of an RBM^l, denoted by $\mathbf{v}^l$ (see Fig. 3a). The realizations of the input layer of $RBM^{l=0}$ are the N training examples $\{\mathbf{c}_o(i)\}_{i=1}^N$. The RBM training algorithm [10] learns the graph weights $\mathbf{W}_0^l$, for each layer $l = 0 \ldots \frac{L}{2} - 1$, such that the sum of the log likelihood probability of the visible units with respect to training examples is maximized: $\mathbf{W}_0^l = \arg \max_{\mathbf{W}} \sum_{n=1}^N \log \left(p\left(\mathbf{v}_n^l\right) \right)$. The reader is referred to [10, 11] and to Appendix B for further details on RBM and the optimization process. Once the weights of the RBM are learned it can be used to initialize the weights of an expert DNN as follows: $\mathbf{W}^l = \mathbf{W}_0^l$ for $l = 0, \ldots, \frac{L}{2} - 1$ and $\mathbf{W}^l = (\mathbf{W}_0^{L-l-1})^T$ for $l = \frac{L}{2}, \ldots, L - 1$, see Fig. 3b.

2.6 Synthetic Training Data Generation

We train each expert DNN with synthetic data emulating real noisy WoCs as follows. Synthetic WoCs $\{\mathbf{c}_s\}$ are generated according to the Tofts model [19]:

$$c_s(t) = v_p c_p(t) + k_{trans} \int_0^t c_p(\tau) \exp(-k_{ep}(t - \tau)) d\tau, \qquad (2)$$

where $c_s(t)$ is the t-th time point within the curve and the triplet of the PK parameters v_p, k_{ep}, k_{trans} is randomly sampled based on typical values associated with healthy, pathological, and blood vessel WoCs. The value of the arterial input function, $c_p(t)$, is pre-defined. Since noiseless images are not available, we used "signal-less" sequences to construct realizations of the noise. Noise examples $\{\mathbf{n}(\mathbf{x})\}$ are extracted, automatically, from MRI sequences of healthy brains without CA injection. We construct training noisy curves $\mathbf{c}_n = \mathbf{c}_s + A\mathbf{n}(\mathbf{x})$, where A is a constant that simulates different SNR levels. Note that here we assume an additive noise model. Since, $\mathbf{c}_s = \mathbf{0}$, in the absence of CA, even if a multiplicative component exists, it could not be detected. However, the inverse

---

[1] The appendix is avilable in the electronic version of the manuscript and at: https://drive.google.com/file/d/0B_vghaLYgXRKTnAwSU5oLUNDWmc/view? usp=sharing.

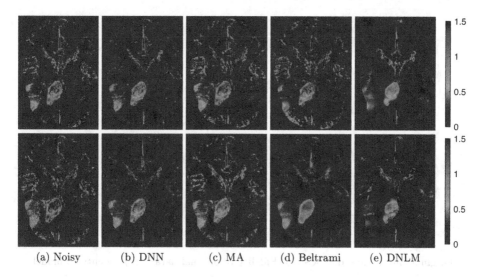

(a) Noisy   (b) DNN   (c) MA   (d) Beltrami   (e) DNLM

Fig. 4. k_{trans} maps reconstructed from: raw (noisy) data (a) and de-noised data (b–e). We compared the k_{trans} reconstruction for proposed de-noising algorithms: (b) the proposed DNN, (c) MA, (d) Beltrami, (e) DNLM. The upper row refers to k_{trans} maps of a single 2D slice generated from the entire dynamic sequence. The lower row presents k_{trans} maps using 2-down-sampled sequence (50 scans).

problem formulation, in Eq. (1), can be applied to a more general noise model for other dynamic imaging sequences.

3   Experimental Results

We tested our method on both synthetic and real data. Synthetic data results are presented in Appendix E. Real data includes 13 DCE-MRI acquisitions (3.0T Philips Ingenia MRI scanner) of stroke and tumor patients (see Appendix G for experimental setup). Videos of the original and cleaned DCE-MRI for all patients can be found at https://www.youtube.com/playlist?list=PLdzBcOOzw1KBz5YOrs97bIZ4qQ_vQ7C68. The proposed DNNs ensemble includes 24 expert DNNs for three WoC types and 8 noise levels (3,5,8,10,13,15,17,20 dB). Each expert DNN consists of 10 layers. The lower layers were pre-trained with five stacked RBMs. The architecture of the expert DNNs are illustrated in Fig. 3.

We compared our algorithm with three different de-noising methods: spatio-temporal Beltrami (st-Beltrami), DNLM, and moving average (MA). The st-Beltrami method is our extension to the Beltrami framework [12], for DCE-MRI (see Appendix D). For 200,000 synthetic curves generated from triplets of randomly samples PK parameters an average mean squared error (MSE) of 2.56×10^{-4} was obtained compare to average MSE of 0.001 for the MA, see Appendix E, Fig. 5. Figure 4a–e visually demonstrates the reconstructed k_{trans} maps using the

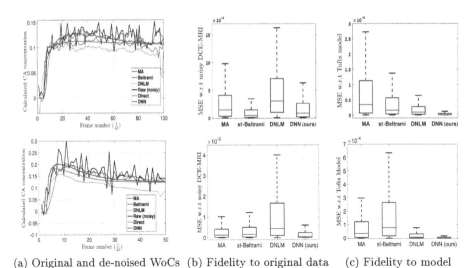

(a) Original and de-noised WoCs (b) Fidelity to original data (c) Fidelity to model

Fig. 5. (a) De-noising of a representative WoC (black) by the proposed DNN-based method (red) versus the st-Beltrami (cyan), DNLM (magenta), MA (green). A WoC with PK parameters that were calculated directly from the noisy WoC is in yellow. (b-c) Box-plot of the MSE between the cleaned WoCs obtained by each of the methods the original noisy WoC. (c) Boxplot of the MSE between the cleaned WoCs and curves which are generated using the PK model based on the PK parameters calculated from the respective de-noised WoCs. The upper panel refers to results obtained from full-length dynamic sequences (100 scans each). The lower panel presents results using 2-down-sampled sequences. (Color figure online)

raw data (a) and de-noised data obtained by the proposed and three other de-noising methods (b–e). The upper row of Fig. 4 refers to k_{trans} maps of a single 2D slice generated from the entire dynamic sequence (100 scans). The lower row of Fig. 4 presents k_{trans} maps using 2-down-sampled sequence (50 scans). It can be seen that the map generated by the proposed DNN framework (Fig. 4b) is less affected by the down-sampling. Figure 5a presents a quantitative comparison of all the de-noising methods for a single representative noisy WoC (pathology). In the absence of GT WoCs, we tested the compatibility of the de-noising methods with the PK model by estimating the PK parameters from the cleaned WoCs and using those parameters to generate synthetic, model-based WoCs (see Appendix E). Box-plots of the MSE of 360,000 WoCs for all the methods are shown on in Fig. 5b. The MSE between the cleaned (de-noised) curves and the input noisy WoCs are shown in Fig. 5c. The upper panel refers to results obtained from full-length dynamic sequences (100 scans each). The lower panel presents results using 2-down-sampled sequences (50 scans each). It can be seen that the DNN-based method demonstrates compatibility with both the PK model and the original (noisy) WoCs. We note that the run-time of the proposed DNN-based method is much shorter than the others, see Table 1 in Appendix F.

4   Summary and Future Work

A method for DCE-MRI de-noising using an ensemble of DNNs is presented. Promising results are demonstrated on both full length and down-sampled data. The latter suggests that the DCE-MRI analysis might be applied to sequences with lower temporal resolution, which can potentially allow finer spatial resolution. The proposed model can be extended to account for voxel-wise spatial dependencies by adding convolutional layers to the DNNs. In addition, the modularity of the ensemble enables combining different PK models. We believe that the key concepts introduced here have great potential for de-noising of other dynamic sequences such as dynamic susceptibility contrast MRI (DSC-MRI) and functional MRI (fMRI).

Acknowledgments. This study was supported by the European Union's Seventh Framework Program (FP7/2007–2013; grant agreement 602102, EPITARGET; A.F.), the Israel Science Foundation (A.F.) and the Binational Israel-USA Foundation (BSF; A.F.).

Appendices

A   Artificial Neuron and Deep neural network

Neural Networks (NNs) are modeled as collections of computational units called *artificial neurons* (ANs) that are connected in an acyclic graph. An AN is a computational unit with multiple inputs, denoted by an augmented input vector $\tilde{\mathbf{c}}_o = \left[1, \mathbf{c}_o^T\right]^T$ and a single output scalar, $y \in \mathbb{R}$, such that $y = f(\mathbf{x}) = f\left(\mathbf{w}^T\mathbf{x}\right)$, where $f : \mathbb{R} \rightarrow \mathbb{R}$ is called the *activation function* of the neuron.

Let $\mathbf{w}_i^l = [w_{i,0}^l, w_{i,1}^l, \dots, w_{i,K_l}^l]^T$ define the weights of the graph edges connecting the $i-$th AN in layer $l+1$ to the K_l ANs in layer l , $l \in [0, L-1]$. Let us also define by $f_l(\cdot)$ the activation function of the ANs in layer l. The output y_i^{l+1} of the $i-$th AN in layer $l+1$ is calculated as follows:

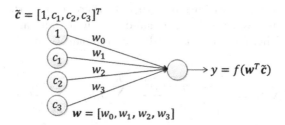

Fig. 6. The output of an Artificial neuron is obtained by applying an activation function, $f(\cdot)$, on the weighted sum of the augmented input $\tilde{c}$.

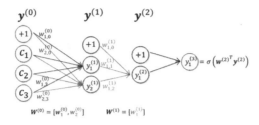

Fig. 7. A Deep neural network with $L = 3$ layers and a sigmoid activation function. Hidden layers are marked in red. (Color figure online)

$$y_i^{l+1} = f_l(\sum_{j=1}^{K_l} w_{i,j}^l y_j^l) = f_l(< \mathbf{w}_i^l, \mathbf{y}^l >) \tag{3}$$

where $\mathbf{y}^l = [1, y_1^l, \ldots, y_{K_l}^l]^T$. The DNN's input is the augmented vector $\mathbf{y}^0 = \tilde{\mathbf{c}}_o = [1, \mathbf{c}_o^T]^T$

B   Expert DNN

We set $L = 10$ layers for each of our expert DNNs. Each layer contains 100-175-150-120-80-30-80-120-150-175-100 neurons, respectively, where the input and output layers are of size $l_0 = l_{10} = 100$. The pre-training process is carried out in an aggregative manner where the weights $\mathbf{W}_0^l$ of each layer $l = 1 \ldots 5$ of a given DNN are pre-trained using a single RBM (denoted by RBM^l) such that the hidden units realizations $\mathbf{h}^{l-1}$ of an RBM^{l-1} are used as the visible units $\mathbf{v}^l$ of an RBM^l, i.e. $\mathbf{h}^{l-1} = \mathbf{v}^l$ (see Fig. 8a). The weights of the DNN are initialized by setting $\mathbf{W}^l = \mathbf{W}_0^l$ for the lower $L/2$ layers ($l = 1 \ldots 5$) and $\mathbf{W}^l = (\mathbf{W}_0^{L-l+1})^T$ for the upper layers ($l = 6, \ldots, 10$) (see Fig. 8b). The calculation of the final weights of the DNN is done simultaneously using stochastic gradient decent (SGD) with linear activation function in the output layer.

For the initialization of the input layer we assume $\{v_i^0\}$ are random variables sampled from a normal distribution $\mathcal{N}(a_i, \sigma_i)$, where a_i, σ_i is the mean and the standard deviation (respectively) associated with unit i and are estimated from the training set. Therefore, it is trained as a Gaussian-Bernoulli RBM, with an energy function:

$$E(\mathbf{v}, \mathbf{h}) = -\sum_{i=1}^{K_{l-1}} \frac{(v_i - a_i)^2}{\sigma_i} - \sum_{j=1}^{K_l} b_j h_j - \sum_{i,j} \frac{v_i}{\sigma_i} h_j w_{ij} \tag{4}$$

The entire training set was scaled such that each entry of input has zero mean and a unit variance. The learning rate of the first RMB^1 was set to 0.001 (0.01 for all the others) and pre-training proceeded for 300 epochs. In addition, we used more binary hidden units than the size of the input vector because real-valued data contains more information than a binary feature activation.

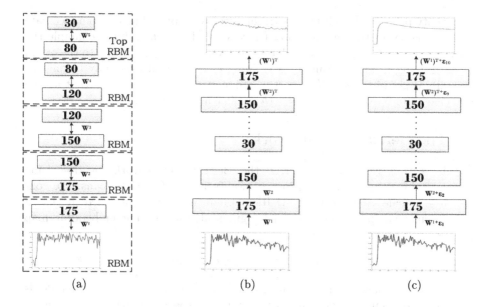

Fig. 8. Training an expert DNN: (a) Pre-training using stacked RBMs, (b) Weights initialization of an expert DNN, (c) Fine tuning using stochastic gradient descent.

C   Classification DNN

The classification DNN contains an input layer, two hidden layers and an output layer; each layer has 120-180-180-24 neurons, respectively. The input of the DNN is defined as follows. Let $g_k(\mathbf{c}_o)$ be the hypothesis of the $k-th$ DNN expert with respect to an observed input $\mathbf{c}_o$, where $k = 1,\ldots,24$. We define five measures that allow the evaluation of the experts' performances as follows: $z_{1;k} = \|g_k(\mathbf{c}_o) - \mathbf{c}_o\|_1$, $z_{2;k} = \|g_k(\mathbf{c}_o) - \mathbf{c}_o\|_2$, are the L_1 and L_2 norm of of the deviation from the original WoC; $z_{3;k} = \frac{<g_k(\mathbf{c}_o),\mathbf{c}_o>}{\|g_k(\mathbf{c}_o)\|\|\mathbf{c}_o\|_2}$, $z_{4;k} = \frac{cov(g_k(\mathbf{c}_o),\mathbf{c}_o)}{var(g_k(\mathbf{c}_o))var(\mathbf{c}_o)}$, are the cosine similarity and correlation between the reconstruction and input signals; and $z_{5;k} = \|\nabla g_k(\mathbf{c}_o)\|_1$ is the hypothesis total variation. The input feature vector is therefore:

$$\mathbf{z} = [z_{1;1}, z_{2;1}, z_{3;1}, z_{4;1}, z_{5;1}, \ldots, z_{1;24}, z_{2;24}, z_{3;24}, z_{4;24}, z_{5;24}]^T \in \mathbb{R}^{120}. \qquad (5)$$

A "softmax" activation function, which is commonly used for multi-class classification problems, was assigned to neurons in the last layer. The softmax activation function takes into account not only the entry value of a specific AN but also the entries to all the other ANs at this layer:

$$f(\alpha_i) = \frac{\exp(\alpha_i)}{\sum_j \exp(\alpha_j)}, \qquad (6)$$

where α_i denotes the entry value at the $i-th$ neuron.

Seventy percent of each DNN's training set were picked at random to create the training set of the classification DNN where for each training example the feature vector $\mathbf{z}$ was calculated and a label $\mathbf{y}$ was assigned according to the origin of the training example. Namely, a training example that originally belongs to the training set of the $k - th$ expert is assigned a label $\mathbf{y} = \mathbf{e}_k$ such that all the coefficients are 0 except for the $k - th$ coefficient which is 1.

D   The Beltrami Framework

In this section we briefly describe the Beltrami framework for de-noising grayscale videos and our extension to modify it to DCE-MRI scans. We consider a grayscale video to be a 3D Riemannian manifold embedded in D $=$ d $+$ 3 dimensional space where d $= 1$ for grayscale images. The embedding map $Q : \Sigma \to M$ is given by:

$$Q(x, y, \tau) = (x, y, \tau, I(x, y, \tau)) \tag{7}$$

where I is the image intensity map. Both Σ and M are Riemannian manifolds and hence are equipped with metrics G and H, respectively, which enable measurement of lengths over each manifold. We require the lengths as measured on each manifold to be the same, i.e.,

$$ds^2 = (dx, dy, d\tau, dI) \, H \, (dx, dy, d\tau, dI)^T = (dx, dy, d\tau) G (dx, dy, d\tau) \tag{8}$$

where $dI = I_x dx + I_y dy + I_\tau d\tau$, according to the chain rule. A natural choice for gray-level videos is a Euclidean space-feature manifold with the metric:

$$H = \begin{pmatrix} 1 & 0 & 0 & 0 \\ 0 & 1 & 0 & 0 \\ 0 & 0 & 1 & 0 \\ 0 & 0 & 0 & \beta^2 \end{pmatrix} \tag{9}$$

where β is the relative scale between the space coordinates and the intensity component. Using (2) the induced metric tensor $G = \{g_{uv}\}$ is:

$$G = \begin{pmatrix} 1 + \beta^2 I_x^2 & \beta^2 I_x I_y & \beta^2 I_x I_\tau \\ \beta^2 I_x I_y & 1 + \beta^2 I_y^2 & \beta^2 I_y I_\tau \\ \beta^2 I_x I_\tau & \beta^2 I_y I_\tau & 1 + \beta^2 I_\tau^2 \end{pmatrix} \tag{10}$$

The Beltrami flow is obtained by minimizing the area of the image manifold:

$$S_{X,G} = \iiint \sqrt{g} dx dy d\tau \tag{11}$$

where $g = det \, (G)$. Using the methods of variational calculus with the resulting Euler-Lagrange relation, the minimization is given by:

$$-\frac{d}{dx}\left(\frac{I_x}{\sqrt{g}}\right) - \frac{d}{dy}\left(\frac{I_y}{\sqrt{g}}\right) - \frac{d}{d\tau}\left(\frac{I_\tau}{\sqrt{g}}\right) = -div\left(\sqrt{g}G^{-1}\nabla I\right) \tag{12}$$

Multiplying both sides by $g^{-1/2}$ we get :

$$I_t = \triangle_g I = -\frac{1}{\sqrt{g}} div \left(\sqrt{g}G^{-1}\nabla I\right) \tag{13}$$

where $\triangle_g$ is the Laplace-Beltrami operator. The discretized version of Eq. (10) allows us to perform iterative traversal through this scale space on a computer and produces a very effective technique for denoising grayscale videos when using the metric in (7):

$$I_{t+1} = I_t + dt \frac{1}{\sqrt{g}}(D_x + D_y + D_\tau) \tag{14}$$

where $D = \sqrt{g}G^{-1}\nabla I$, $div(D) = D_x + D_y + D_\tau$, and $dt \propto \beta^{-2}$. Note that the output depends on two hyper parameters: the number of iterations of the update, and the parameter β.

The above framework assumes similar physical measures of the x, y, and τ coordinates. In reality, the space domain coordinates x and y do not possess the same physical measure as the time domain coordinate τ. Hence, we need to introduce another scaling factor,γ, into the space-time-intensity metric:

$$H = \begin{pmatrix} \mathbf{I}_{2\times2} & 0 & \mathbf{0} \\ 0 & \gamma^2 & \mathbf{0} \\ \mathbf{0} & \mathbf{0} & \beta^2\mathbf{I}_{w^3\times w^3} \end{pmatrix}. \tag{15}$$

The new induced metric tensor for the 3D image manifold is computed using the constraint in Eq. (5) :

$$G = \begin{pmatrix} 1 + \beta^2 I_x^2 & \beta^2 I_x I_y & \beta^2 I_x I_\tau \\ \beta^2 I_x I_y & 1 + \beta^2 I_y^2 & \beta^2 I_y I_\tau \\ \beta^2 I_x I_\tau & \beta^2 I_y I_\tau & \gamma + \beta^2 I_\tau^2 \end{pmatrix} \tag{16}$$

In addition we modified the numerical update step so it would fit the new scaling as follows:

$$I_{t+1} = I_t + dt_1 g^{-1/2}(D_x + D_y) + dt_2 g^{-1/2}D_\tau \tag{17}$$

where $dt_1 \propto \beta^{-2}$ and $dt_2 \propto \gamma^{-2}$.

E   Results on Synthetic Data

The performance evaluation of our DNN-based de-noising method on synthetic data is done using 10-fold cross-validation (10-CV) method. 200,000 noisy WoC were generated using the Tofts model. The training data is randomly divided into ten groups (20,000 training examples in every CV group) such that nine groups are used for training and the remaining set is used for testing. The experiment is performed for different signal to noise ratio (SNR) values independently. Fig. 9 demonstrates successful denoising of a single representative WoC using our DNN-based method (red) and using moving average (MA) method (green) along with the synthetic, clean and noisy WoCs (blue and black, respectively). In Fig. 10 the mean MSE values and standard deviation intervals are plotted for different SNR levels.

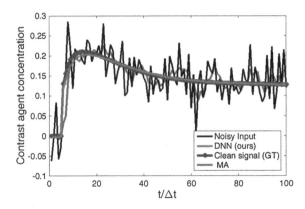

Fig. 9. De-noising of synthetic WoC (black) using DNN (red) and MA (green) $SNR = 10_{[dB]}$. Ground truth (GT) is in blue.

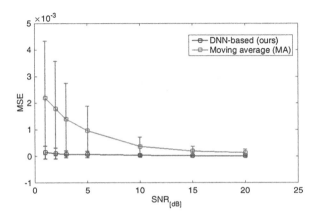

Fig. 10. Mean values and standard deviation intervals of the MSE between the clean (ground-truth) WoC and the cleaned curves using the DNN-based method (red) and MA (green) as a function of the SNR of the simulation (synthetic) curves.

F   Run-time Comparison

We measured the run-time of the different algorithms for the 13 DCE-MRI scans. Table 1 presents the average run-time of each de-noising algorithm in minutes. The measured run-time did not include any pre-processing procedures and measured only the run-time of the de-noiosng algorithms. The algorithms were tested on MatLab 2014b (64-bit) using Intel(R) core(TM) i-7-4470, 3.4 GHz CPU with 16 GB RAM.

Table 1. Average run-time of the different de-noising methods for a single DCE-MRI scan (4D volume with dimentions $255 \times 255 \times 22 \times 100$).

	st-Beltrami	Moving average (MA)	DNLM	DNN-based
Run-time [min]	88.65	1.45	4631.35	3.75

G   Experimental Setup for Real Data

In the absence of ground-truth washout curves, in addition to visual assessment, we estimated the de-noising algorithms' success using two measures: the fidelity of the output of the de-noising methods to the noisy data and to the PK model. Fig. 11 shows a block diagram of our performance assessment method. Given a noisy DCE-MRI scan we apply a de-noising algorithm. The fidelity of the cleaned curves to the noisy data is measured by calculating the mean squared error (MSE) between the noisy curve and the de-noised curve. Then, we extract the PK-parameters from the cleaned curves by applying the standard DCE-MRI curve fitting algorithm. Next, we use the estimated PK-parameters to generate synthetic washout curves according to the Tofts model. The MSE between the model-based synthetic curve and the de-noised curve measure the fidelity of the de-noised curves to the PK-model.

References

1. Abbott, N.J., Friedman, A.: Overview and introduction: the blood-brain barrier in health and disease. Epilepsia **53**(s6), 1–6 (2012)
2. Bridle, J.S.: Probabilistic interpretation of feedforward classification network outputs, with relationships to statistical pattern recognition. In: Soulié, F.F., Hérault, J. (eds.) Neurocomputing. NATO ASI Series, vol. 68, pp. 227–236. Springer, Heidelberg (1990)

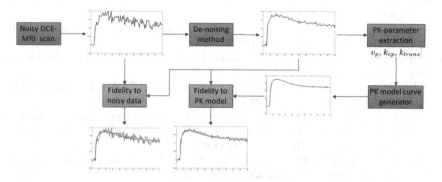

Fig. 11. Block diagram of our performance assessment method for real data.

3. Brix, G., Semmler, W., Port, R., Schad, L.R., Layer, G., Lorenz, W.J.: Pharma-cokinetic parameters in CNS Gd-DTPA enhanced MR imaging. J. Comput. Assist. Tomogr. **15**(4), 621–628 (1991)
4. Buades, A., Coll, B., Morel, J.M.: A non-local algorithm for image denoising. In: Computer Vision and Pattern Recognition, CVPR, vol. 2, pp. 60–65 (2005)
5. Dahl, G.E., Sainath, T.N., Hinton, G.E.: Improving deep neural networks for LVCSR using rectified linear units and dropout. In: ICASSP, pp. 8609–8613. IEEE (2013)
6. Gal, Y., et al.: Denoising of dynamic contrast-enhanced MR images using dynamic nonlocal means. IEEE Trans. Med. Imaging **29**(2), 302–310 (2010)
7. Golkov, V., et al.: q-space deep learning for twelve-fold shorter and model-freediffusion MRI scans. In: Navab, N., Hornegger, J., Wells, W.M., Frangi, A.F. (eds.) MICCAI 2015. LNCS, vol. 9349, pp. 37–44. Springer, Heidelberg (2015)
8. Hinton, G.E., Salakhutdinov, R.R.: Reducing the dimensionality of data with neural networks. Science **313**(5786), 504–507 (2006)
9. Hinton, G., et al.: Deep neural networks for acoustic modeling in speech recognition: the shared views of four research groups. IEEE Sig. Process. Mag. **29**(6), 82–97 (2012)
10. Hinton, G.E.: Training products of experts by minimizing contrastive divergence. Neural Comput. **14**(8), 1771–1800 (2002)
11. Hinton, G.E., Osindero, S., Teh, Y.W.: A fast learning algorithm for deep belief nets. Neural Comput. **18**(7), 1527–1554 (2006)
12. Kimmel, R., Malladi, R., Sochen, N.: Images as embedded maps and minimal surfaces: movies, color, texture, and volumetric medical images. Int. J. Comput. Vis. **39**(2), 111–129 (2000)
13. Martel, A.L.: A fast method of generating pharmacokinetic maps from dynamic contrast-enhanced images of the breast. In: Larsen, R., Nielsen, M., Sporring, J. (eds.) MICCAI 2006. LNCS, vol. 4191, pp. 101–108. Springer, Heidelberg (2006)
14. Murase, K.: Efficient method for calculating kinetic parameters using T1-weighted dynamic contrast-enhanced magnetic resonance imaging. Magn. Reson. Med. **51**(4), 858–862 (2004)
15. Rumelhart, D.E., Hinton, G.E., Williams, R.J.: Learning internal representations by error propagation. Technical report, DTIC Document (1985)
16. Schmid, V.J., et al.: A bayesian hierarchical model for the analysis of a longitudinal dynamic contrast-enhanced MRI oncology study. Magn. Reson. Med. **61**(1), 163–174 (2009)
17. Sourbron, S.P., Buckley, D.L.: Classic models for dynamic contrast-enhanced MRI. NMR Biomed. **26**(8), 1004–1027 (2013)
18. Tofts, P.: Quantitative MRI of the Brain: Measuring Changes Caused by Disease. Wiley, Hoboken (2005)
19. Tofts, P.S.: Modeling tracer kinetics in dynamic Gd-DTPA MR imaging. J. Magn. Reson. Imaging **7**(1), 91–101 (1997)
20. Tofts, P.S., et al.: Estimating kinetic parameters from dynamic contrast-enhanced T1-weighted MRI of a diffusable tracer: standardized quantities and symbols. J. Magn. Reson. Imaging **10**(3), 223–232 (1999)
21. Veksler, R., Shelef, I., Friedman, A.: Blood-brain barrier imaging in human neuropathologies. Arch. Med. Res. **45**(8), 646–652 (2014)
22. Vincent, P., et al.: Stacked denoising autoencoders: learning useful representations in a deep network with a local denoising criterion. J. Mach. Learn. Res. **11**, 3371–3408 (2010)

Three-Dimensional CT Image Segmentation by Combining 2D Fully Convolutional Network with 3D Majority Voting

Xiangrong Zhou[1(✉)], Takaaki Ito[1], Ryosuke Takayama[1],
Song Wang[2], Takeshi Hara[1], and Hiroshi Fujita[1]

[1] Department of Intelligent Image Information, Graduate School of Medicine,
Gifu University, Gifu 501-1194, Japan
zxr@fjt.info.gifu-u.ac.jp
[2] Department of Computer Science and Engineering,
University of South Carolina, Columbia SC 29208, USA

Abstract. We propose a novel approach for automatic segmentation of anatomical structures on 3D CT images by voting from a fully convolutional network (FCN), which accomplishes an end-to-end, voxel-wise multiple-class classification to map each voxel in a CT image directly to an anatomical label. The proposed method simplifies the segmentation of the anatomical structures (including multiple organs) in a CT image (generally in 3D) to majority voting for the semantic segmentation of multiple 2D slices drawn from different viewpoints with redundancy. An FCN consisting of "convolution" and "de-convolution" parts is trained and re-used for the 2D semantic image segmentation of different slices of CT scans. All of the procedures are integrated into a simple and compact all-in-one network, which can segment complicated structures on differently sized CT images that cover arbitrary CT scan regions without any adjustment. We applied the proposed method to segment a wide range of anatomical structures that consisted of 19 types of targets in the human torso, including all the major organs. A database consisting of 240 3D CT scans and a humanly annotated ground truth was used for training and testing. The results showed that the target regions for the entire set of CT test scans were segmented with acceptable accuracies (89 % of total voxels were labeled correctly) against the human annotations. The experimental results showed better efficiency, generality, and flexibility of this end-to-end learning approach on CT image segmentations comparing to conventional methods guided by human expertise.

Keywords: CT images · Anatomical structure segmentation · Fully convolutional network (FCN) · 3D majority voting · End-to-end learning

1 Introduction

Three-dimensional (3D) computerized tomography (CT) images are important resources that provide useful internal information about the human body to support diagnosis, surgery, and therapy [1]. Fully automatic image segmentation is a fundamental part of

© Springer International Publishing AG 2016
G. Carneiro et al. (Eds.): LABELS 2016/DLMIA 2016, LNCS 10008, pp. 111–120, 2016.
DOI: 10.1007/978-3-319-46976-8_12

the applications based on 3D CT images by mapping the physical image signal to a useful abstraction. Conventional approaches to CT image segmentation usually try to transfer human knowledge directly to a processing pipeline, including numerous hand-crafted signal processing algorithms and image features [2–5]. In order to further improve the accuracy and robustness of image segmentation, we need to be able to handle a larger variety of ambiguous image appearances, shapes, and relationships of anatomical structures. It is difficult to achieve this goal by defining and considering human knowledge and rules explicitly. Instead, a data-drive approach using big image data—such as a deep convolutional neural network (deep CNN)—is expected to be better for solving this segmentation problem.

Recently, several studies were reported that applied deep CNNs to medical image analysis. Many of these used deep CNNs for lesion detection or classification [6, 7]. Studies of this type usually divide CT images into numerous small 2D/3D patches at different locations, and then classify these patches into multiple pre-defined categories. Deep CNNs are used to learn a set of optimized image features (sometimes combined with a classifier) to achieve the best classification rate for these image patches. Similarly, deep CNNs have also been embedded into conventional organ-segmentation processes to reduce the FPs in the segmentation results or to predict the likelihoods of the image patches [8–10]. However, the anatomical segmentation of CT images over a wide region of the human body is still challenging because of the image appearance similarities between different structures, as well as the difficulty of ensuring global spatial consistency in the labeling of patches in different CT cases.

This paper proposes a novel approach based on deep CNNs that naturally imitate the thought processes of radiologists during CT image interpretation for image segmentation. Our approach models CT image segmentation in a way that can best be described as "multiple 2D proposals with a 3D integration." This is very similar to the way that a radiologist interprets a CT scan as many 2D sections, and then reconstructs the 3D anatomical structure as a mental image. Unlike previous work on medical image segmentation that labels each voxel/pixel by a classification based on its neighborhood information (i.e., either an image patch or a "super-pixel") [8–10], our work uses rich information from the entire 2D section to directly predict complex structures (multiple labels on images). Furthermore, the proposed approach is based on an end-to-end learning without using any conventional image-processing algorithms such as smoothing, filtering, and level-set methods.

2   Methods

2.1   Overview

As shown in Fig. 1, the input is a 3D CT case (the method can also handle a 2D case, which can be treated as a degenerate 3D case), and the output is a label map of the same size and dimension, in which the labels are a pre-defined set of anatomical structures. Our segmentation process is repeated to sample 2D sections from the CT case, pass them to a fully conventional network (FCN) [11] for 2D image segmentation, and stack the 2D labeled results back into 3D. Finally, the anatomical structure label at each

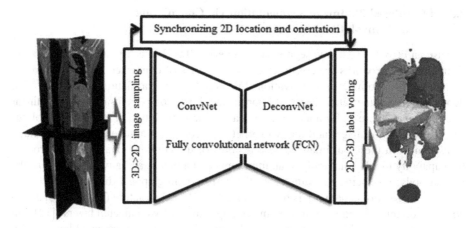

Fig. 1. Pipeline of proposed anatomical structure segmentation for 3D CT scan. See Fig. 2 for the details of FCN structure.

voxel is decided based on majority voting at the voxel. The core part of our segmentation is an FCN that is used for the anatomical segmentation of the 2D sections. This FCN is trained based on a set of CT cases, with the human annotations as the ground truth. All of the processing steps of our CT image segmentation are integrated into an all-in-one network under a simple architecture with a global optimization.

2.2   3D-to-2D Image Sampling and 2D-to-3D Label Voting

In the proposed approach, we decompose a CT case (a 3D matrix, in general) into numerous sections (2D matrices) with different orientations, segment each 2D section, and finally, assemble the outputs of the segmentation (labeled 2D maps) back into 3D. Specifically, each voxel in a CT case (a 3D matrix) can lie on different 2D sections that pass through the voxel with different orientations. Our idea is to use the rich image information of the entire 2D section to predict the anatomical label of this voxel, and to increase the robustness and accuracy by redundantly labeling this voxel on multiple 2D sections with different orientations. In this work, we select all the 2D sections in three orthogonal directions (axial, sagittal, and coronal-body); this ensures that each voxel in a 3D case is located on three 2D CT sections.

After the 2D image segmentation, each voxel is redundantly annotated three times from these three 2D CT sections. The annotated results for each voxel should ideally be identical, but may be different in practice because of mislabeling during the 2D image segmentation. A label fusion by majority voting for the three labels is then introduced to improve the stability and accuracy of the final decision. Furthermore, a *prior* for each organ type (label) is estimated by calculating voxel appearance frequency of the organ region within total image based on training samples. In the case of no consensus between three labels during the majority voting process, our method simply selects the label with the biggest *prior* as the output.

2.3 FCN-Based 2D Image Segmentation via Convolution and de-Convolution Networks

We use an FCN for semantic segmentation in each 2D CT slice by labeling each pixel. Convolutional networks are constructed using a series of connected basic components (convolution, pooling, and activation functions) with translation invariance that depends only on the relative spatial coordinates. Each component acts as a nonlinear filter that operates (e.g., by matrix multiplication for convolution or maximum pooling) on the local input image, and the whole network computes a general nonlinear transformation from the input image. These features of the convolutional network provide the capability to adapt naturally to an input image of any size and any scan range of the human body, producing an output with the corresponding spatial dimensions.

Our convolutional network is based on the VGG16 net structure (16 layers of 3 × 3 convolution interleaved with maximum pooling plus 3 fully connected layers) [12], but with a change in the VGG16 architecture by replacing its fully connected layers (FC6 and 7 in Fig. 2) with convolutional layers (Conv 6 and 7 in Fig. 2). Its final fully connected classifier layer (FC 8 in Fig. 2) is then changed to a 1 × 1 convolution layer (Conv 8 in Fig. 2) whose channel dimension is fixed at the number of labels (the total number of segmentation targets was 20 in this work, including the background). This network is further expanded by docking a de-convolution network (the right-hand side in Fig. 2). Here, we use idea of the de-convolution in [11], and reinforce the network structure by adding five de-convolution layers, each of which consists of up-sampling, convolution, and crop (summation) layers as shown in Fig. 2.

FCN training: The proposed network (both convolution and de-convolution layers) is trained with numerous CT cases of humanly annotated anatomical structures. All of the 2D CT sections (corresponding to the label maps) along the three body orientations are shuffled, and used to train the FCN. The training process repeats feed-forward computation and back-propagation to minimize the loss function, which is defined as the sum of the pixel-wise losses between the network prediction and the label map annotated by the human experts. The gradients of the loss are propagated from the end to the start of the network, and the method of stochastic gradient descent with momentum is used to refine the parameters of each layer.

The FCN is trained sequentially by adding de-convolution layers [11]. To begin with, a coarse prediction (by a 32-pixel stride) is trained for the modified VGG16 network with one de-convolution layer (called FCN32s). A finer training is then added after adding one further de-convolution layer at the end of the network. This is done by using skips that combine the final prediction layer with a lower layer with a finer stride in the modified VGG16 network. This fine-training is repeated with the growth of the network layers to build FCN16s, 8s, 4s, and 2s which are trained from the predictions of 16, 8, 4, 2 strides on the CT images, respectively. The output of FCN 2s acts as the 2D segmentation result.

2D CT segmentation using trained FCN: The density resolution of the CT images is reduced from 12 to 8 bits using linear interpolation. The trained FCN is then applied to each 2D section independently, and each pixel is labeled automatically. The labels from

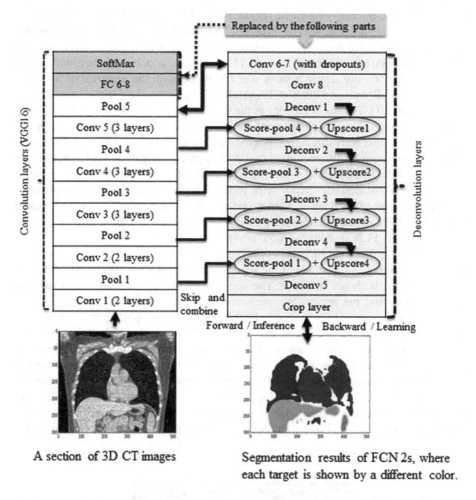

Fig. 2. Semantic image segmentation of 2D CT slice using fully convolutional network (FCN) [11]. Conv: convolution, Deconv: deconvolution, and FC: fully connected.

each 2D section are then projected back to their original 3D locations for the final vote-based labeling, as described above.

3 Experiment and Results

Our experiment used a CT image database that was produced and shared by a research project entitled "Computational Anatomy [13]". This database included 640 3D volumetric CT scans from 200 patients at Tokushima University Hospital. The anatomical ground truth (a maximum of 19 labels that included Heart, right/left Lung, Aorta, Esophagus, Liver, Gallbladder, Stomach and Duodenum (lumen and contents), Spleen, left/right Kidney, Inferior Vein Cava, region of Portal Vein, Splenic Vein, and Superior Mesenteric Vein, Pancreas, Uterus, Prostate, and Bladder) in 240 CT scans was also distributed with the database. Our experimental study used all of the 240 ground-truth CT scans, comprising 89 torso, 17 chest, 114 abdomen, and 20 abdomen-with-pelvis scans. Furthermore, our research work was conducted with the approval of the Institutional Review Boards at Gifu and Tokushima Universities.

We picked 10 CT scans at random as the test samples, using the remaining 230 CT scans for training. As previously mentioned, we took 2D sections along the axial, sagittal, and coronal body directions. For the training samples, we obtained a dataset of 84,823 2D images with different sizes (width: 512 pixels; height: 80–1141 pixels). We trained a single FCN based on the ground-truth labels of the 19 target regions. Stochastic gradient descent (SGD) with momentum was used for the optimization. A mini-batch size of 20 images, learning rate of 10^{-4}, momentum of 0.9, and weight decay of 2^{-4} were used as the training parameters. All the 2D images were used directly as the inputs for FCN training, without any patch sampling.

We tested the proposed FCN network (Fig. 1) using 10 CT cases that were not used in the FCN training. An example of the segmentation result for a 3D CT case covering the human torso is shown in Fig. 3. The accuracy of the segmentation was evaluated per organ type and per image. We measured the intersection over union (IU) (also known as the Jaccard similarity coefficient) between the segmentation result and the ground truth. Because each CT case may contain different anatomical structures—with the information about these unknown before the segmentation—we performed a comprehensive evaluation of multiple segmentation results for all the images in the test dataset by considering the variance of the target numbers and volume. Two measures (voxel accuracy: true positive for multiple label prediction on all voxels in a CT case; frequency-weighted IU: mean value of IUs that normalized by target volumes and numbers in a CT case [11]) were employed for the evaluations. The evaluation results

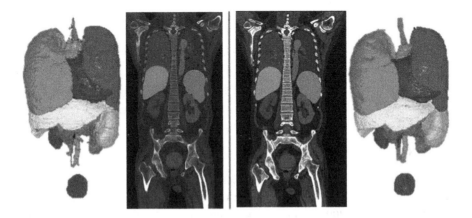

Fig. 3. Left: example of segmentation in 3D CT case, with segmented regions labeled with different colors for one 2D CT slice and 3D visualization based on surface-rendering method. Right: corresponding ground truth segmentation.

for the voxel accuracy, frequency-weighted IU were 0.89 and 0.84, respectively, when averaged over all the segmentation results of the test dataset. These results show that 89 % of the voxels within the anatomical structures (constructed using multiple target regions) were labeled correctly, with a mean overlap ratio of 84 % for 19 target regions in the test dataset. The mean IU values in each organ type are listed in Table 1 for both training and test data.

Table 1. Accuracy evaluations in terms of mean value of IUs per target type between segmentation results of FCN-8s and ground truth in 230 training and 10 test CT scans after voting in 3D [14].

Target name	Mean value of IUs	
	Training samples (230)	Test samples (10)
Right Lung	0.92	0.87
Left Lung	0.91	0.88
Heart	0.87	0.87
Aorta	0.72	0.63
Esophagus	0.18	0.27
Liver	0.91	0.91
Gallbladder	0.58	0.48
Stomach and Duodenum (2nd pos.)	0.48	0.43
Stomach and Duodenum Lumen	0.59	0.61
Contents inside of Stomach and Duodenum	0.21	0.10
Spleen	0.85	0.86
Right Kidney	0.85	0.86
Left Kidney	0.85	0.84
Inferior Vena Cava	0.56	0.51
Portal Vein, Splenic Vein, and Superior Mesenteric Vein	0.32	0.03
Pancreas	0.48	0.45
Uterus	0.23	0.09
Prostate	0.48	0.35
Bladder	0.67	0.72

4   Discussion

We found that the target organs were recognized and extracted correctly in all the test CT images, except for oversights of the portal vein, splenic vein, and superior mesenteric vein in two CT cases. Because our segmentation targets covered a wide range of shapes, volumes, and sizes, either with or without contrast enhancement, and at different locations in the human body, these experimental results demonstrated the potential capability of our approach to recognize whole anatomical structures appearing in CT images. The IUs of the organs with larger volumes (e.g., liver: 0.91, heart: 0.87) were comparable to the accuracies reported from the previous state-of-the-art methods

[2–5]. For some smaller organs (e.g., gallbladder) or line structures (e.g., portal vein, splenic vein, and superior mesenteric vein) that have not been reported in previous work, our segmentation did not show particularly high IUs, but this performance was deemed reasonable because the IU tends to be lower for those organs with smaller volumes. The physical CT image resolution is the major cause of this limited performance, rather than the segmentation method. Our evaluation showed that the average segmentation accuracy of all the targets over all the test CT images was approximately 84 % in terms of the frequency weighted IUs. The segmentation result of each deconvolution layer (FCN 32 s to FCN 2 s) was also investigated. We confirmed the frequency weighted IUs were monotonically increasing (about 0.16, 0.03 and 0.01) from FCN 32s, 16s, 8s and 4s, and no further improvement was observed by FCN 2s. This result showed diminishing returns of gradient descent from the training stage of FCN 8s, which was also mentioned in [11]. From experimental results, we see that our approach can recognize and extract all types of major organs simultaneously, achieving a reasonable accuracy according to the organ volume in the CT images. Furthermore, our approach can deal automatically with segmentation in 2D or 3D CT images with a free scan range (chest, abdominal, whole body region, etc.), which was impossible in previous work [2–5].

Our segmentation process has a high computational efficiency because of its simple structure and GPU-based implementation. The segmentation of one 2D CT slice takes approximately 30 ms (roughly 1 min for a 3D CT scan with 512 slices) when using the Caffe software package [15] and CUDA Library on a GPU (NVIDIA GeForce TITAN-X with 12 GB of memory). The efficiency in terms of system development and improvement is much better than that of previous work that attempted to incorporate human specialist experience into complex algorithms for segmenting different organs. Furthermore, neither the target organ type, number of organs within the image, nor image size limits the CT images that are used for the training process.

For the future work, network performance by using different training parameters as well as cost functions needs to be investigated, especially for de-convolution network. We plan to expand the range of 3D voting process from more than three directions of 2D image sections to improve the segmentation accuracy. Furthermore, bounding box of each organ [16] will be introduced into the network to overcome the insufficient image resolution for segmenting small-size of organ types. A comparison against 3D CNNs will also be investigated.

5   Conclusions

We proposed a novel approach for the automatic segmentation of anatomical structures (multiple organs and interesting regions) in CT images, by majority voting the results from a fully convolutional network. This approach was applied to segment 19 types of targets in 3D CT cases, demonstrating highly promising results. Our work is the first to tackle anatomical segmentation (with a maximum of 19 targets) on scale-free CT scans (both 2D and 3D images) through a deep CNN. Compared with previous work [2–5, 8–10], the novelty and advantages of our study are as follows. (1) Our approach uses an end-to-end, voxel-to-voxel labeling, with a global optimization of parameters, which has the advantage of better performance and flexibility in accommodating the large variety of anatomical structures in different CT cases. (2) It can automatically learn a set of image features to represent all organ types collectively, using an "all-in-one" architecture (a simple structure for both model training and implementation) for image segmentation. This approach leads to more robust image segmentation that is easier to implement and extend. Image segmentation using our approach has more advantages in terms of usability (it can be used to segment any type of organ), adaptability (it can handle 2D or 3D CT images over any scan range), and efficiency (it is much easier to implement and extend) than those of previous work.

Acknowledgments. The authors would like to thank all the members of the Fujita Laboratory in the Graduate School of Medicine, Gifu University for their collaborations. We would like to thank all the members of the Computational Anatomy [13] research project, especially Dr. Ueno of Tokushima University, for providing the CT image database. This research was supported in part by a Grant-in-Aid for Scientific Research on Innovative Areas (Grant No. 26108005), and in part by a Grant-in-Aid for Scientific Research (C26330134), MEXT, Japan.

References

1. Doi, K.: Computer-aided diagnosis in medical imaging: historical review, current status and future potential. Comput. Med. Imaging Graph. **31**, 198–211 (2007)
2. Lay, N., Birkbeck, N., Zhang, J., Zhou, S.K.: Rapid multi-organ segmentation using context integration and discriminative models. In: Gee, J.C., Joshi, S., Pohl, K.M., Wells, W.M., Zöllei, L. (eds.) IPMI 2013. LNCS, vol. 7917, pp. 450–462. Springer, Heidelberg (2013)
3. Wolz, R., Chu, C., Misawa, K., Fujiwara, M., Mori, K., Rueckert, D.: Automated abdominal multi-organ segmentation with subject-specific atlas generation. IEEE Trans. Med. Imaging **32**(9), 1723–1730 (2013)
4. Okada, T., Linguraru, M.G., Hori, M., Summers, R.M., Tomiyama, N., Sato, Y.: Abdominal multi-organ segmentation from CT images using conditional shape-location and unsupervised intensity priors. Med. Image Anal. **26**(1), 1–18 (2015)
5. Bagci, U., Udupa, J.K., Mendhiratta, N., Foster, B., Xu, Z., Yao, J., Chen, X., Mollura, D.J.: Joint segmentation of anatomical and functional images: applications in quantification of lesions from PET, PET-CT, MRI-PET, and MRI-PET-CT images. Med. Image Anal. **17**(8), 929–945 (2013)
6. Shin, H.C., Roth, H.R., Gao, M., Lu, L., Xu, Z., Nogues, I., Yao, J., Mollura, D., Summers, R.M.: Deep convolutional neural networks for computer-aided detection: CNN architectures, dataset characteristics and transfer learning. IEEE Tran. Med. Imaging **35**(5), 1285–1298 (2016)
7. Ciompi, F., de Hoop, B., van Riel, S.J., Chung, K., Scholten, E., Oudkerk, M., de Jong, P., Prokop, M., van Ginneken, B.: Automatic classification of pulmonary peri-fissural nodules in computed tomography using an ensemble of 2D views and a convolutional neural network out-of-the-box. Med. Image Anal. **26**(1), 195–202 (2015)
8. de Brebisson, A., Montana, G.: Deep neural networks for anatomical brain segmentation. In: Proceedings of CVPR, Workshops, pp. 20–28 (2015)
9. Roth, H.R., Farag, A., Lu, L., Turkbey, E.B., Summers, R.M.: Deep convolutional networks for pancreas segmentation in CT imaging. In: Proceedings of SPIE, Medical Imaging 2016: Image Processing, vol. 9413, pp. 94131G-1–94131G-8 (2015)

10. Cha, K.H., Hadjiiski, L., Samala, R.K., Chan, H.P., Caoili, E.M., Cohan, R.H.: Urinary bladder segmentation in CT urography using deep-learning convolutional neural network and level sets. Med. Phys. **43**(4), 1882–1896 (2016)
11. Long, J., Shelhamer, E., Darrell, T.: Fully convolutional networks for semantic segmentation. In: Proceedings of CVPR, pp. 3431–3440 (2015)
12. Simonyan, K., Zisserman, A.: Very deep convolutional networks for large-scale image recognition. In: Proceedings of ICLR. arXiv:1409.1556 (2015)
13. http://www.comp-anatomy.org/wiki/
14. Zhou, X., Ito, T., Takayama, R., Wang, S., Hara, T., Fujita, H.: First trial and evaluation of anatomical structure segmentations in 3D CT images based only on deep learning. In: Medical Image and Information Sciences (2016, in press)
15. http://caffe.berkeleyvision.org
16. Zhou, X., Morita, S., Zhou, X., Chen, H., Hara, T., Yokoyama, R., Kanematsu, M., Hoshi, H., Fujita, H.: Automatic anatomy partitioning of the torso region on CT images by using multiple organ localizations with a group-wise calibration technique. In: Proceedings of SPIE Medical Imaging 2015: Computer-Aided Diagnosis, vol. 9414, pp. 94143K-1–94143K-6 (2015)

Medical Image Description Using
Multi-task-loss CNN

Pavel Kisilev[1(✉)], Eli Sason[1], Ella Barkan[1], and Sharbell Hashoul[1,2]

[1] IBM Haifa Research Lab, Haifa, Israel
pavel.prvt@gmail.com
[2] Carmel Medical Center, Haifa, Israel

Abstract. Automatic detection and classification of lesions in medical images remains one of the most important and challenging problems. In this paper, we present a new multi-task convolutional neural network (CNN) approach for detection and semantic description of lesions in diagnostic images. The proposed CNN-based architecture is trained to generate and rank rectangular regions of interests (ROI's) surrounding suspicious areas. The highest score candidates are fed into the subsequent network layers. These layers are trained to generate semantic description of the remaining ROI's.

During the training stage, our approach uses rectangular ground truth boxes; it does not require accurately delineated lesion contours. It has a clear advantage for supervised training on large datasets. Our system learns discriminative features which are shared in the Detection and the Description stages. This eliminates the need for hand-crafted features, and allows application of the method to new modalities and organs with minimal overhead. The proposed approach generates medical report by estimating standard radiological lexicon descriptors which are a basis for diagnosis. The proposed approach should help radiologists to understand a diagnostic decision of a computer aided diagnosis (CADx) system. We test the proposed method on proprietary and publicly available breast databases, and show that our method outperforms the competing approaches.

Keywords: Deep learning · Mammography · Computer aided diagnosis · Semantic description · Lesion detection · Multi-task loss

1 Introduction

Automatic annotation and description of natural images became recently a very popular topic in computer vision. Various approaches are proposed in a number of papers dealing with the problems of automatic semantic tagging [1], and of automatic description generation of images [2–4]. However, in medical imaging domain, this topic is yet to gain popularity. Obviously, medical image description poses its own set of problems. In particular, specifics of medical images require a pragmatic choice of semantic descriptors. In contrast to natural images, it is important that such semantic description would be standardized. The need for standardized was already recognized in breast imaging in the late 1980s.

© Springer International Publishing AG 2016
G. Carneiro et al. (Eds.): LABELS 2016/DLMIA 2016, LNCS 10008, pp. 121–129, 2016.
DOI: 10.1007/978-3-319-46976-8_13

The American College of Radiology developed the Breast Imaging Reporting and Data System (BI-RADS) [5] that standardizes the assessment and reporting of breast lesions. The BI-RADS system has proved to be efficient in quality assurance. It aided for the comprehension of a non-radiologist report reader, and standardized the communication between clinicians and radiologists. In the past decade, standardization has been implemented in other domains, such as the Pi-RADS in prostate lesions [6], Li-RAD in liver lesions [7]. Other domains (for example, brain tumors or lung diseases) are yet to have fixed standard lexicon, but use similar semi-standardized description systems.

Tumor lesions in different organs and modalities are described by radiologists in similar terms of high level semantic descriptors. The most important semantic descriptors include shape, boundary type, density and other characteristics that are organ or modality specific. Based on these characteristics, a radiologist makes the most vital diagnostic decision about malignancy or benignancy of a tumor. Therefore, automatic classification of lesions requires either explicit or implicit representation of the above semantic descriptors by corresponding image measurements used during the classification process. Typically, Computer Aided Detection (CADe) and Diagnosis (CADx) systems use hand-crafted features such as histograms of intensity values, shape-related features (s.a., aspect ratio), texture descriptors, and others (see [8] for an overview of such systems). Using such features, these systems are able to segment and characterize lesions, and to make a diagnosis (e.g., benign or malignant).

The existing methods can be categorized into two main groups. The first (e.g. [9, 10]) performs independent estimation of semantic descriptors using supervised classification methods. The second (e.g. [11]) is based on unsupervised clustering using k-Nearest Neighbours (KNN) approach. All the above methods assume either given lesion contour or a region of interest (ROI) around the lesion, provided by a radiologist. Recently, a structured learning approach to the problem of semantic description of lesions was proposed in [12]. Hand-crafted features were calculated from semi-automatically segmented lesion contours, and were used to predict semantic descriptors using Structured Support Vector Machine (SSVM) approach.

In this work, we propose a cardinally different approach. Our system is completely based on the Convolutional Neural Network (CNN) which is trained (1) to generate ROI candidates and to rank them, and (2) based on the best candidates, to generate semantic description of lesions inside of the ROIs. Our approach does not require accurately delineated lesions, which is a laborious work usually done by radiologists. We use rectangular ROI's instead, which has a clear advantage for supervised training on large datasets. Our system learns discriminative features shared for both detection and description tasks, eliminating the need for hand-crafted features. The deep network models individual representations and dependencies of the semantic descriptors using novel joint multi-loss training. The main mode of operation of our system is depicted in Fig. 1.

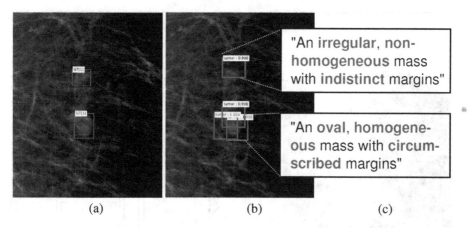

Fig. 1. An example of the output of the proposed multi-task-loss CNN based system. (a) cropped-out mammogram with 2 marked rectangular ground truth areas containing lesions, (b) corresponding top-4 automatically detected bounding box (BB) candidates, (c) automatically generated textual description of lesions in the BB's. The estimated semantic values (in blue) are embedded into predefined sentence templates. The three lower BB's have the same estimated description. (Color figure online)

2 Methodology

We define the problem of ROI detection and of semantic description of a lesion as learning of discriminative features which are partially shared in both detection and description steps. To achieve this, we use CNN-based architecture shown in Fig. 2, and described in details below.

The detection step finds ROI candidates by estimating their bounding box coordinates and the probability of an ROI being a valid lesion. The semantic description step solves a multi-attribute prediction problem; each valid candidate from the detection stage is described by multiple labels (semantic descriptors). In this stage, fully connected layers are trained to map the set of learned convolutional features, to a set of semantic descriptors. We deploy a multi-task loss and jointly train classifiers for all semantic descriptors.

Each ROI is described by a set of J semantic descriptors. The semantic description of the i-th ROI is an assignment: $\mathbf{y}_i = \{y_{i,j}\}, j = 1 \ldots J$ where each j-th semantic descriptor $y_{i,j}$ can have one of the V_j possible discrete values, $Y_j \in \{1, \ldots, V_j\}$, corresponding to the categories in each one of the semantic labels of the radiological lexicon. For example, in mammography, there are $J = 3$ semantic descriptors: *shape*, *margin*, and *density*. For *shape* descriptor, $V_{1(shape)} = 3$ categories: {*oval*, *round*, *irregular*}.

Multi-task-loss CNN for Semantic Description of Medical Images The proposed system architecture is depicted in Fig. 2. Our system is based on the recently proposed Faster R-CNN architecture whose details can be found in [14]. We explain the main differences of our implementation below.

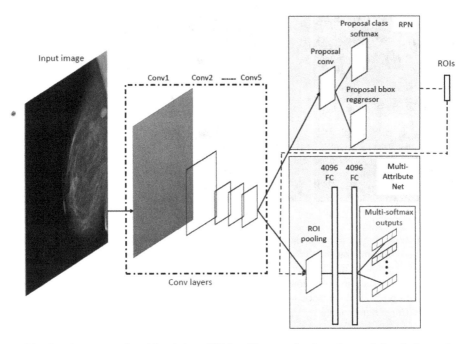

Fig. 2. The proposed multi-task loss CNN architecture for detection and description tasks

The first module (the left rectangle in Fig. 2) is a deep fully convolutional network that produces feature maps from the input image. We use this module as in [14] with a few minor changes. This module consists of 5 fully convolutional layers which are shared between the Detection and the Description stages.

The Region Proposal Network (RPN) module (the upper right rectangle in Fig. 2) generates candidates, and is trained to predict the ROI bounding box (BB) coordinates and its score. The 2 sibling sub-branches of RPN are responsible for the BB coordinates regression and for the 'objectness' score estimation. To accommodate the variety of lesion sizes, we generate BB's at several scales. The above two modules comprise the detection stage of our system.

The second stage of our system (the lower right rectangle in Fig. 2) accepts the candidate ROI's from the first stage as the inputs. In [14], the second stage is a *multi-class* classifier into one of the possible object categories. It uses single softmax loss layer. In contrast to [14], the second stage in our architecture is trained to jointly predict *multiple labels* that represent semantic descriptors. We call this branch the *Multi-Attribute Description Network* (MA-DN). It solves a *multi-class-multi-label* prediction problem. The learning is implemented in a multi-task manner, wherein our network has J sibling output layers as described below.

During the training of the network, we use a mini-batch of positive and negative ROI candidates, taken from 2 images, randomly chosen from the training set. The loss function is defined as the *multi-class-multi-label* loss, and is calculated for each mini-batch as:

$$L(\{p_{ij}\}) = \frac{1}{N}\sum_i\sum_j w_j l(p_{ij}, c_{ij}) \tag{1}$$

Here, i is the index of an ROI, N is the normalization constant according to the mini-batch size ($N \sim 128$ in most of the cases), w_j are the weights of the J terms corresponding to the different semantic descriptors. These weights are used to balance the contributions of different descriptors to the loss, and are chosen empirically in our current implementation.

The log loss for the true class c_{ij} is $l(p_{ij}, c_{ij}) = -\sum_{1...V_j} t_{ij,c_{ij}} \log p_{ij,c_{ij}}$ where t_{ij} is 1 if j-th descriptor of i-th ROI is in the class c_{ij}, and 0 otherwise; $p_{ij,c_{ij}}$ is the predicted probability that the ROI is in the class c_{ij}. The probability p_{ij} for the sample $-i$ and the label j is computed as the softmax over the $V_j + 1$ outputs of the fully connected layers. In order to implement (1), we create branches of fully connected layers for each one of the semantic descriptors, and sum the corresponding log loss terms.

During the joint training of the network branches, the proposed architecture imposes dependencies on the descriptors. In the Experiments section, we show that this architecture improves the accuracy of the descriptor estimation, as compared to the independent training of the separate branches responsible for each one of the descriptors.

Implementation details. The module of the shared convolutional network (the left branch in Fig. 2) processes the whole image with several convolutional (conv) and max pooling layers to produce conv feature maps. This branch follows the AlexNet architecture with five convolutional layers. In the RPN module, we use bounding boxes of the three aspect ratios of 1:1, 1:2 and 2:1, and of the three scales corresponding to the box sides of 32, 96, and 256 pixels. These parameters are chosen based on the statistics of the lesion sizes in the data bases that we use in our experiments.

The MA-DN network (the lower right branch in Fig. 2) accepts as an input the entire image and the RPN-generated bounding boxes (the proposals). The ROI max-pooling layer in the MA-DN branch converts the features inside of any valid ROI into a small feature map with a fixed spatial extent. As a result, each object proposal is represented by a fixed-length feature vector from the feature map of the last fully convolutional layer. Each feature vector is then fed into a sequence of 2 fully connected (fc) layers, each with 4096 neurons that finally branch into J-attribute softmax sibling output layers.

The MA-DN network is trained end-to-end by backpropagation and stochastic gradient descent (SGD) with momentum. Each SGD mini-batch is constructed from 2 images, chosen uniformly at random (we iterate over permutations of the dataset). We use mini-batches of size R = 128, sampling 64 ROI's from each image. During the training of MA-DN, we use object proposals (ROI's) that have intersection over union (IoU) with a ground truth BB of at least 0.5. These ROI's are the examples labelled as the positive class (lesion object). The remaining ROIs are sampled from object proposals that have a maximum IoU with a ground truth BB in the interval [0.05; 0.2]. These are the negative class examples (the background). During the training, we apply data augmentation by shifting the ROI's at random horizontally and vertically by up to 15 pixels. During the testing, we use the BB proposals whose score is greater than 0.85.

Optimization parameters. We use a learning rate of 0.001 for the first 12 K mini-batches, and 0.0001 for the next 16 K mini-batches generated from our datasets. We use a momentum of 0.9 and a weight decay of 0.0005.

We implemented the proposed architecture using the Caffe software framework [15]. Our system is trained on a TitanX GPU with 12 GB memory, and i7 Intel CPU with 64 GB RAM. Training times using around 400 images, each containing 256 ROI's (total about 100 K samples), are as follows. The candidate Detection stage training takes 6 h; the Description stage training takes 4 h.

3 Experiments

Our system is capable of performing end-to-end detection and semantic description of medical findings. However, the main goal of our experiments in this paper is to test thoroughly the proposed description rather than the detection stage. Also, because of the lower performance figures of CADe systems, detection is frequently performed in a semi-automatic manner. In this case, a radiologist marks the suspicious areas around a lesion.

We compare the proposed method, that uses a rectangular ROI's and their corresponding *learned* discriminative CNN-based features, to the methods based on accurately delineated lesion contours and hand-crafted features calculated from them. We also compare the performance of the proposed MA-DN architecture for joint estimation of semantic descriptors to the performance of independently trained classifiers per each descriptor. The independent classifier training was implemented using the same system but with a single semantic descriptor at a time. The results of these comparisons are summarized in Tables 1, 2 and 3, and explained in details below.

Datasets. We apply the proposed method to the breast mammography (MG) and the ultrasound (US) modalities. We used the public DDSM [13] and our proprietary data sets. In the DDSM dataset, we chose mass containing MG images with breast density of BI-RADS 1 and 2. The masses are annotated with semantic descriptors of shape and margin. The final set contains 974 images from 512 (232 benign, and 280 malignant) cases. Our proprietary dataset contains 408 US images from 330 cases, and 646 digital MG images from 281 cases. The proprietary datasets were processed by our trained radiologist who drew accurate lesion boundaries and annotated the lesions with their semantic descriptor values according to the BIRADS.

Experimental methodology. The following three approaches for the lesion description can be considered competing: (1) independent estimation of semantic descriptors (e.g., [10]); we used multiclass SVM classifiers with RBF kernel for each one of descriptors, (2) the KNN based approaches; we implemented the method from [11], and (3) the SSVM based approach of [12] which is easily implemented as well. The objective comparison of various methods for lesion detection and description is difficult. The papers conduct their experiments on different datasets or their subsets. In addition, there are very few publicly available datasets that are sufficiently large for training of deep neural networks. For that reason, we use DDSM, and our proprietary datasets.

Table 1. DDSM dataset: semantic descriptor estimation; mean performance (bold is the best result). The STDs of the metrics are all under 5 % of the mean values.

Semantic descriptor estimation method	Shape			Margin		
	ACC	PPV	TPR	ACC	PPV	TPR
Independent SVM's	0.64	0.64	0.66	0.62	0.63	0.63
k-NN based [11]	0.67	0.67	0.68	0.64	0.65	0.67
SSVM based [12]	0.71	0.71	0.72	0.69	0.68	0.69
Ours, independent	0.78	0.76	0.75	0.74	0.74	0.75
Ours, multi-task	**0.82**	**0.79**	**0.78**	**0.77**	**0.78**	**0.76**

Table 2. Proprietory mammography dataset: semantic descriptor estimation; mean performance (bold is the best result). The STDs of the metrics are all under 5.1 % of the mean values.

Semantic descriptor Estimation method	Shape ACC	Margin ACC	Density ACC
Independent SVM's	0.73	0.72	0.81
k-NN based [11]	0.74	0.76	0.80
SSVM based [12]	0.79	0.78	0.82
Ours, independent	0.84	0.82	0.81
Ours, multi-task	**0.88**	**0.86**	**0.84**

Table 3. Proprietary ultrasound dataset: semantic descriptor estimation; mean performance (bold is the best result). The STDs of the metrics are all under 7.5 % of the mean values.

Semantic descriptor Estimation method	Shape ACC	Orient. ACC	Margin ACC	Echo ACC	Transm. ACC	Boundary ACC
Independent SVM's	0.62	0.98	0.6	0.75	0.79	0.74
k-NN based [11]	0.64	0.92	0.63	0.76	0.78	0.76
SSVM based [12]	0.68	0.94	0.69	0.78	0.81	0.76
Ours, independent	0.77	**0.96**	0.75	0.77	**0.82**	0.78
Ours, multi-task	**0.82**	0.95	**0.81**	**0.78**	**0.82**	**0.8**

All the competing methods for lesion description, apart from ours, require accurate lesion contours. We therefore used a semi-automatic segmentation with a bounding box around a lesion chosen by the radiologist. We then used an active contour algorithm to extract the contours. In DDSM, we used the original annotated contours to define the ROI, and applied the active contour algorithm to refine the ground truth by extracting more accurate contours. We used the contours to compute standard image features usually deployed in detection and segmentation methods (see e.g. in [8, 11]). The groups of features include pixel intensity-, shape- and texture-related descriptors that are combined into a bag of words vector used during the training of classifiers. We used the same set of features in all the experiments. In contrast, our method did not require accurate lesion delineation, and only uses a rectangular ROI.

In all the experiments, we used the following methodology. The set of cases with corresponding images was divided (with stratification) into three equal parts (denoted by segments A, B and C). Segment C was reserved as a testing set. Every algorithm was trained on segment A. The optimal values of parameters, evaluated on the segment B (the validation segment) were picked, and the algorithm was retrained on both segment A and B. Then, the algorithm was tested on segment C. This process was repeated with reversed roles for segments A and B, namely with segment B as the training set and segment A as the validation. This procedure was repeated five times (5 × 2 cross validation), and concluded with 10 trials. For each one of the semantic descriptors, we calculated the means and the standard deviations (STD) of the following performance metrics: (1) the accuracy, ACC = (TP + TN)/M, (2) the positive predictive value, PPV = TP/(TP + FP), and (3) the true positive rate, TPR = TP/(TP + FN). Here M is the total number of samples, TP, TN, FP, and FN are the number of true positives, true negatives, false positives, and false negatives, respectively, and we calculate these in a one-versus-all manner.

In DDSM experiments, we used the following descriptors and their corresponding values: **shape** {*round; oval; irregular*}, **margin** {*circumscribed; indistinct; spiculated; microlobulated; obscured*}. Because of the relatively small number of examples, we used a reduced set of semantic values. In particular, in US experiments, we used 3 classes for margin, shape, and echo, and 2 classes for the rest. In MG experiments, we used 3 classes for shape and margin, and 2 classes for density. We report only the accuracy for these experiments, since these numbers represent well the overall tendency.

As explained above, our main goal in this paper is to test the Description stage. However, we discuss briefly the Detection stage performance as well. In particular, we test the detection rate for the top ROI proposals. Applying the Detection stage of our system to the proprietary breast MG dataset, results in the following figures. The true lesion is detected: in 46 % of the top-1, in 64 % of the top-4, 74 % of the top-10, and 82 % of the top-50 candidates. We obtain similar figures on other datasets.

For the Description stage, the mean figures of the performance metrics for the DDSM dataset are given in Table 1. The STD's of the metrics were under 5 % of the mean values. The mean figures of the performance metrics for the proprietary breast US and MG datasets are summarized in Table 2 and Table 3 respectively. In this case, the STD's of the metrics were all under 5.1 % and 7.5 % of the mean values, respectively.

The proposed method outperforms all the competing methods in the accuracy of semantic description by up to 10 % margin. Furthermore, it is clear from the experimental results, that the proposed MA-DN architecture for joint estimation of semantic values has advantage over the independently trained classifiers per each descriptor.

4   Conclusions

This paper presents a new multi-task-loss CNN based approach for joint automatic detection and semantic description of lesions in diagnostic images. The proposed approach outperforms the competing methods by up to 10 % margin. We attribute this to the ability of deep network to learn good discriminative high level features from data. The learned features are shared in the Detection and the Description stages. The method accepts simple rectangular ground truth boxes, and, therefore, most suitable for supervised training on large datasets. The proposed approach generates standard radiological lexicon description which should help radiologists in understanding of the decision making process of CADx systems. To that end, we plan to concentrate on improving the Detection stage performance, and making the proposed method sufficiently robust to be deployed as an end-to-end detection and description system. We also plan to extend the proposed framework and explore the use of recurrent neural networks in our system.

References

1. Guillaumin, M., Mensink, T., Verbeek, J.J., Schmid, C.: Tagprop: Discriminative metric learning in nearest neighbor models for image auto-annotation. In: ICCV (2009)
2. Farhadi, A., Hejrati, M., Sadeghi, M.A., Young, P., Rashtchian, C., Hockenmaier, J., Forsyth, D.: Every picture tells a story: generating sentences from images. In: Daniilidis, K., Maragos, P., Paragios, N. (eds.) ECCV 2010. LNCS, vol. 6316, pp. 15–29. Springer, Heidelberg (2010). doi:10.1007/978-3-642-15561-1_2
3. V. Ordonez, G. Kulkarni and T. L. Berg. Im2Text: Describing Images Using 1 Million Captioned Photographs. In NIPS 2011, pages 1143–1151
4. Elliott, D., Keller, F.: Image description using visual dependency representations. EMNLP **13**, 1292–1302 (2013)
5. D'Orsi, C.J., Mendelson, E.B., Ikeda, D.M., et al.: Breast imaging reporting and data system: ACR BI-RADS - breast imaging atlas. American College of Radiology, Reston (2003)
6. Weinreb, J., et al.: PI-RADS prostate imaging - reporting and data system: 2015, Version 2. Eur. Urol. **69**(1), 16–40 (2016)
7. Mitchell, D., et al.: Li-RAD in liver lesions. Hepatology **61**(3), 1056–1065 (2015)
8. Oliver, A., Freixenet, J., Martí, J., Pérez, E., Pont, J., Denton, E.R., Zwiggelaar, R.: A review of automatic mass detection and segmentation in mammographic images. Med. Image Anal. **14**(2), 87–110 (2010)
9. Wei, C.-H., Li, Y., Huang, P.J.: Mammogram retrieval through machine learning within BI-RADS standards. J. Biomed. Inform. **44**(4), 607–614 (2011)
10. Rubin, D.L., Burnside, E.S., Shachter, R.: A bayesian network to assist mammography interpretation. In: Brandeau, M.L., Sainfort, F., Pierskalla, W.P. (eds.) Operations Research and Health Care. International Series in Operations Research & Management Science, vol. 70, pp. 695–720. Springer, New York (2004)
11. Narvaez, F., Diaz, G., Romero, E.: Automatic BI-RADS description of mammographic masses. In: Martí, J., Oliver, A., Freixenet, A., Martí, R. (eds.) Digital Mammography. Lecture Notes in Computer Science, vol. 6316, pp. 673–681. Springer, New York (2010)
12. Kisilev, P., Walach, E., Hashoul, S., Barkan, E., Ophir, B., Alpert, S.: Semantic description of medical image findings: structured learning approach. In: BMVC (2015)
13. Heath, M., Bowyer, K., Kopans, D., Moore, R., Philip Kegelmeyer, W.: The digital database for screening mammography. In: Yaffe, M.J. (ed.) Proceedings of the Fifth International Workshop on Digital Mammography, pp. 212–218. Medical Physics Publishing, Madison (2001)
14. Ren, S., He, K., Girshick, R., Sun, J.: Faster R-CNN: Towards real-time object detection with region proposal networks. In: NIPS (2015)
15. Jia, Y., Shelhamer, E., Donahue, J., Karayev, S., Long, J., Girshick, R., Guadarrama, S., Darrell, T.: Caffe: Convolutional architecture for fast feature embedding (2014). arXiv:1408.5093

Fully Automating Graf's Method for DDH Diagnosis Using Deep Convolutional Neural Networks

David Golan[1($\boxtimes$)], Yoni Donner[2], Chris Mansi[3], Jacob Jaremko[4],
Manoj Ramachandran[5], and on behalf of CUDL

[1] Department of Statistics, Stanford University, Stanford, USA
golandavid@gmail.com
[2] Department of Computer Science, Stanford University, Stanford, USA
[3] Graduate School of Business, Stanford University, Stanford, USA
[4] Faculty of Medicine and Dentistry,
Department of Radiology and Diagnostic Imaging,
University of Alberta, Edmonton, Canada
[5] Department of Orthopaedics and Trauma, The Royal London Hospital and Barts
and The London School of Medicine and Dentistry,
Queen Mary University of London, London, UK

Abstract. Developmental dysplasia of the hip (DDH) is a condition affecting up to 1 in 30 infants. DDH is easy to treat if diagnosed early, but undiagnosed DDH can result in life-long hip pain, dysfunction and an increased risk of early onset osteoarthritis, and accounts for around 30 % of all hip replacements in patients under 60. The gold standard for diagnosis in infants is an ultrasound scan, followed by an analysis procedure known as *Graf's method*. The application of Graf's method is notoriously operator-dependent, requiring years of training to reach reasonable and reproducible performance. We describe a novel deep-learning based pipeline that applies Graf's method to ultrasound scans of the hip. We use a convolutional network with an adversarial component to segment the image into relevant landmarks, and define a set of post-processing rules to translate the segmentations into Graf's metrics. Comparing our pipeline to estimates made by experts in DDH diagnosis shows promising results.

1 Introduction

Developmental dysplasia of the hip (DDH) is a neonatal hip developmental condition that is common (affecting up to 1 in 30 infants) and in most cases is relatively easy to treat if identified in a timely manner (e.g. by applying a harness). Treatment at a later age is considerably harder as secondary anatomical

---

The CUDL (Collaborative for Ultrasound Deep Learning) Group is an international multidisciplinary academic collaboration between expert clinicians and computer scientists to apply deep learning networks to ultrasound imaging. For a full list of contributors please see the acknowledgments section. For more information visit www.cudl.ai.

© Springer International Publishing AG 2016
G. Carneiro et al. (Eds.): LABELS 2016/DLMIA 2016, LNCS 10008, pp. 130–141, 2016.
DOI: 10.1007/978-3-319-46976-8_14

changes have occurred and the hip joint becomes irreducible. Undiagnosed DDH impacts quality of life, causing pain and dysfuction, and increasing the risk of early onset osteoarthritis. Indeed, DDH accounts for 30 % of hip replacements in patients under 60 [1]. Due the high cost of undiagnosed DDH compared to the relatively high prevalence and ease of treatment if detected early, some countries sponsor universal screening of any newborn around the age of six weeks (e.g. Germany, Israel).

The gold standard for DDH diagnosis is by an ultrasound scan of the hip joint. The scan involves identifying a plane where key landmarks are visible (Fig. 1), and analysing the relative positions of the landmarks in the image. The most common analysis for DDH ultrasound is the Graf method [2]. A key step of the Graf method involves measuring the α angle – the angle between two imaginary lines corresponding to the ilium and the acetabular roof. A properly located femoral head is located within the acetabulum and contacts the acetabular roof, resulting in an α angle of 60° or more which indicates a normally developing hip joint. Lower α angle values indicate increasingly severe degrees of DDH from minor dysplasia to a completely dislocated hip.

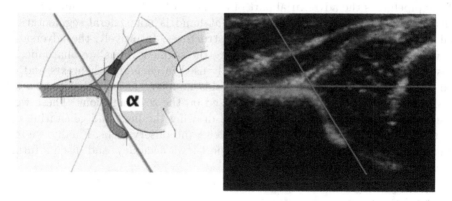

Fig. 1. A cartoon of a newborn's hip joint (left) and an ultrasound image (right) presenting the same anatomy. The ilium and acetabular roof are marked in blue and red, respectively. Graf's method involves drawing a horizontal line corresponding to the ilium (in blue), and a second line corresponding to the acetabular roof (in red). The α angle is the angle between the two lines. (Color figure online)

The application of Graf's method is extremely difficult and operator dependent, for a number of reasons including low image quality, anatomically inadequate images, high variability in the shape of the relevant anatomical features and lack of sufficient training and expertise. Several studies show considerable inter-operator variability, which could change the diagnosis from dysplastic to normal or vice-versa, or change the degree of dysplasia, thus altering the recommended treatment. Importantly, the inter-observer and intra-observer error is lower for normal hips but higher for borderline and abnormal hips [3,4].

Deep learning has been tremendously successful in image processing in general [5,6] and medical imaging analysis in particular [7,8]. Motivated by the success of deep learning in other modalities, we sought to develop an analysis pipeline to automate Graf's method. Both the problem and the solution we suggest have several unique characteristics. First, training data are scarce as images are not typically saved or stored, only reported. Even those images that are saved usually have the markings made by the physician embedded in the image, rendering them of minimal value for training. Second, aiming for a clinical application we were not interested in a black-box classification method where the input is an image and the output is the α angle, but rather in a set of intermediate outputs allowing the visualization and interpretation of the results by a clinician. Third, ultrasound images are notoriously noisy compared to other medical imaging modalities such as CT, X-Ray or MRI.

We designed our pipeline to overcome these issues. To overcome the lack of training data, we first set out to solve a segmentation problem – identifying the ilium and acetabular roof in an image. This allowed us to draw inspiration from other segmentation architectures [9–11] in our network design, and more importantly, to generate training data using crowdsourcing. The second novelty of the pipeline is the adversarial part of the network, which was planned to take advantage of the fact that the problem at hand is not general segmentation, but rather segmentation of well-defined structures. Intuitively, the adversarial network acts as a regularizer, making sure the segmentations are anatomically feasible. Adversarial networks are typically used in generative contexts and we are not aware of studies using them in this manner. The third part is a set of simple heuristics drawing the lines based on the segmentations. These were designed to mimic the expert's process of drawing the lines and generating the α angle, and are based on in-clinic interviews and observations. Finally, we test our pipeline and show that it reaches expert-level accuracy, and discuss future applications of our approach.

2   Methods

2.1   Data

We collected $1,056$ ultrasound scans of infant hips with no annotations. The black frame and text surrounding the images were cropped. We wrote illustrated guidelines explaining how to tag the ilium and the acetabular roof and used a popular crowdsourcing platform – CrowdFlower – to recruit workers to tag the images. Each tagging task was performed by three different workers and the pixel-wise majority vote was taken as the final segmentation. Inspection by experts confirmed that this process produces segmentation results of reasonable quality (see, e.g., Fig. 2).

To validate our method we obtained a set of 100 images where physician annotations were already embedded in the image, for which we could measure the α angles estimated by the expert and compare them to the pipeline's estimates. We note, however, that the embedded annotations (as well as some text,

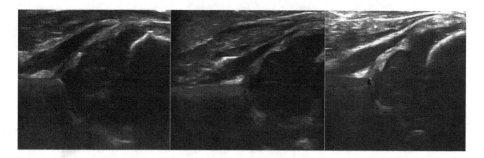

Fig. 2. Examples of bone segmentation by crowdsourcing. The ilium is marked in blue and the acetabular roof in red. Each bone was segmented by three different individuals, and a majority vote over pixels is displayed. (Color figure online)

embedded at the bottom-left corner of the image) may hurt the performance of the network, since it did not observe such inputs at training. We thus refer to this data-set as our "bronze standard".

2.2 Network Architecture

We implemented the segmentation network as a DCNN with multiple down-sampling and upsampling layers for processing the input image at four different scales. During the downwards pass, convolutions are applied with stride-2 resulting in an output half the size of the input. During the upward pass, the output of the previous lower-resolution scale is upsampled using a fractionally-strided convolution and concatenated to the current layer.

The input is a 64×64 grayscale image. A sequence of three 3×3 convolutions is applied at each scale, and the output is upsampled by a fractionally strided 3×3 convolution and joined by filter concatenation to the scale above. Concatenation temporarily increases the number of filters, and the following convolution restores the previous number of filters to keep the complexity constant per scale. Each convolution is followed by batch normalization [12] and ReLU activation. A final convolution with sigmoid activation produces the output. The loss function for the base segmentation network is the mean pixel-wise log-loss. The network architecture is depicted in Fig. 3.

Since the segmentation network processes the image at multiple scales, it captures both local and global context. However, due to the pixel-wise loss function, some global constraints on the output may still not be satisfied, and in practice we have observed that in few cases the outputs included small patches of noise in addition to the correct ilium and acetabular roof. Although these cases were not common, we further improved the base segmentation network to produce outputs that are indistinguishable from actual segmented images to a discriminator network, similar to generative adversarial networks (GAN) [13].

The discriminator network maps $64 \times 64 \times 2$ input images (the two channels correspond to the ilium and acetabular roof) to probabilities. It is trained with

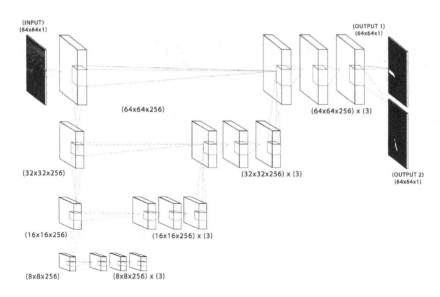

Fig. 3. A diagram of the segmentation DCNN (image dimensions and number of filters not drawn to scale). The input is processed at four scales. At each scale, three 3×3 convolutions with 256 filters are applied, and the output is concatenated to the scale above.

real segmentations as positive examples and outputs of the segmentation network as negative examples. As with GAN, it is trained to minimize the log-loss.

We implemented the discriminator network as a DCNN similar to [14], with a sequence of 3×3 strided convolutions. Unlike [14], we follow each stride-2 convolution with an additional stride-1 convolution. The number of filters is 16 for the first stride-2 convolution and is doubled with every additional downsampling step. After five downsampling steps, the $2 \times 2 \times 256$ layer is flattened, dropout of 0.5 is applied, and a linear layer with sigmoid activation produces the discriminator output probability.

As with GAN, the two networks are trained together, alternating between training steps for the segmentation network and for the discriminator network. The loss function for the discriminator network is the discrimination log-loss $-\mathbf{E}_{(x,y)\in p_{data}(x,y)} \left[\log D\left(y \right) + \log \left(1 - D\left(S\left(x \right) \right) \right) \right]$, and the term $-\lambda \log \left(D\left(S\left(x \right) \right) \right)$ is added to the base segmentation network loss function $-\frac{1}{64^2} \sum_{1 \leq i,j \leq 64} \left(y_{i,j} \log S\left(x \right)_{i,j} + \left(1 - y_{i,j} \right) \log \left(1 - S\left(x \right)_{i,j} \right) \right)$, where $x_{i,j}$ is the pixel at position (i,j) in the input image, $y_{i,j}$ is the true segmentation label for the pixel at position (i,j), S is the segmentation network, D is the discriminator network and λ is a weight balancing the pixel-wise log-loss and the adversarial loss set such that both losses are on roughly the same scale. We note that while adding the adversarial network did not improve the pixel-wise log-loss, it qualitatively improved the segmentations dramatically. The effect of including the adversarial component in the training phase is illustrated in Fig. 4.

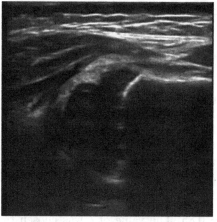 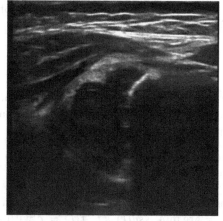

a. Segmentation with adversarial loss.   b. Segmentation without adversarial loss.

Fig. 4. Comparison of segmentations with (left) and without (right) adding the adversarial loss to the overall loss. While including the adversarial loss did not improve the pixel-wise loss, the results were qualitatively improved from an anatomical correctness perspective, which is not directly captured by the pixel-wise loss, as seen in this example.

3 Results

3.1 Training

Implementation was done in TensorFlow [15], using the Adam algorithm [16] for training over 200 epochs with a batch size of 8 images. Training images were augmented with probability 0.5 by rotations drawn uniformly in $[-15, 15]$ degrees and horizontal or vertical stretches by a factor drawn uniformly in $[1, 2]$.

Weight decay was set to 10^{-3} and λ to 10^{-4}. The segmentation network learning rate was 5×10^{-3} initially and multiplied by 0.98 in each training epoch. The discriminator learning rate was set to 0.1 of the segmentation learning rate. Weights were initialized as in [17].

3.2 Post-processing

The outputs of the network were treated as probability maps, one for the ilium and one for the acetabular roof. We denoised the output by first zeroing all entries smaller than the mean activation, and then identifying the largest region of interest using *regionprop* from *skimage* [18], and setting all activations outside of that region to zero. We have found that this simple denoising step is hugely beneficial for downstream analysis. However, more training data might render it unnecessary.

A line $\ell = (a, b)$ describes the set of points (x, y) for which $y = ax + b$. We define the sum of squared distances as

$$ssd(\ell) = \sum_{i,j} d((i,j), \ell)^2 P_{ij}$$

where d denotes the distance from a point to a line, the summation is over all of the pixels of the relevant output image and P_{ij} is the activation probability of the appropriate pixel. We also define

$$f(\ell) = \sum_{i,j} P_{ij} \mathbb{I}\{ia + b < j\}$$

as the fraction of probability map that is found below the line. We then solve $\ell = \arg\min\ ssd(\ell)$ s.t. $f(\ell) = c$ with $c = 0.85$. The value of c was chosen to yield lines that are most visually similar to those typically drawn by doctors by visualizing on a small subset of the training images to avoid overfitting. We note that we have found the α angle to be fairly robust to changes in c, as small changes in c mostly affect the intercept of the line. However, the actual position of the line seemed to be closest to what physicians are expecting with $c = 0.85$. The entire analysis pipeline is illustrated in Fig. 5.

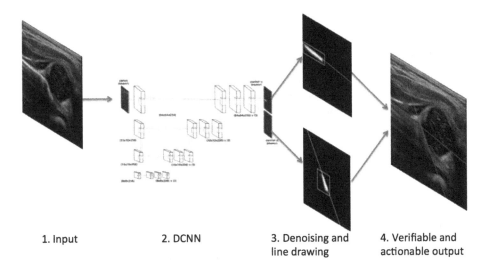

1. Input   2. DCNN   3. Denoising and   4. Verifiable and
                                          line drawing   actionable output

Fig. 5. Analysis pipeline for DDH: (1) A cropped hip ultrasound image is rescaled and (2) fed through our DCNN, resulting in two output images – the segmented ilium and segmented acetabular roof. (3) The output images are then post-processed to reduce noise and lines are drawn as detailed in Subsect. 3.2. (4) Finally, the results are combined to a single image containing the segmentation information, the lines drawn and the computed α angle.

4   Results

We applied our pipeline to our bronze-standard test set. The results demonstrated a correlation of 0.76 between the α angle computed by our pipeline and the human-computed angle, with 77 % of images displaying a discrepancy of less than 5° between the pipeline and the expert. The standard deviation of differences was 4.0°, which is in the range of documented inter-observer variability (3.9° and 3.2° in [19] and [4], respectively. The results are portrayed in Fig. 6.

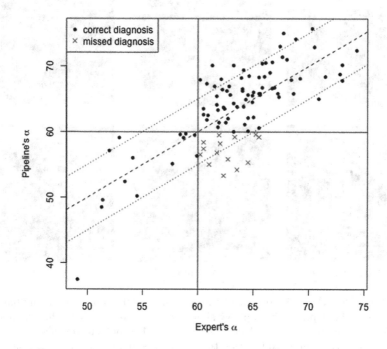

Fig. 6. Comparison of our pipeline's estimates with the expert's. We applied our pipeline to our bronze-standard and plot here the estimated α angle of the pipeline (y-axis) and the estimated α angle of the expert (x-axis). For easy comparison we plot the $y = x$ line (dashed line), and a band of ±5 degrees around it (dotted lines). The estimated αs display a high correlation (0.76) and 77 % fall within a < 5° difference. In terms of hypothetical clinical classification as normal vs. dysplastic, the expert and the pipeline agree in 86 % of cases (marked as black dots), and disagree on 14 % of cases (marked as red crosses). An in-depth examination of the obvious outliers can be found in Fig. 7.

Three images displayed an unreasonable discrepancy of > 10° between the expert and the pipeline (Fig. 7, bottom row). However, inspection of these results by an expert confirmed that the error in these cases is on the expert's side and that the pipeline results are indeed better.

In terms of clinical decision support, great importance is given to the cut-off of 60°, distinguishing normal from dysplastic anatomy. Assuming the expert opinion as ground truth, our pipeline yields no false-negative results, and 14 % false-positive results, similar to the 15 % disagreement between experts documented in [4].

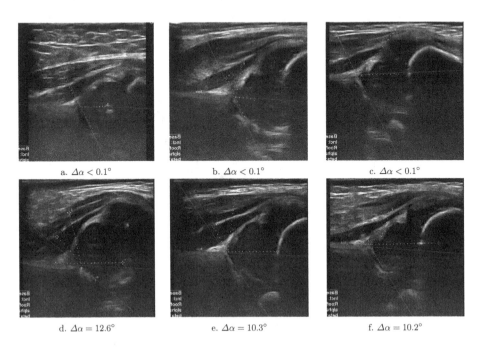

a. $\Delta\alpha < 0.1°$ b. $\Delta\alpha < 0.1°$ c. $\Delta\alpha < 0.1°$

d. $\Delta\alpha = 12.6°$ e. $\Delta\alpha = 10.3°$ f. $\Delta\alpha = 10.2°$

Fig. 7. Examples where the results of the pipeline match (top) or don't match (bottom) those of the expert. The top row shows three examples where the pipeline and the expert's estimate of α are effectively the same. The bottom row shows the three examples where the difference between the α angles estimated, denoted $\Delta\alpha$, is greater than 10°. Network activations for the ilium and acetabular roof and the corresponding lines are highlighted in blue/red respectively. The expert's annotations are the dotted white lines. In some of the images a third white line is visible. This line is used for other routine calculations and can be ignored. (Color figure online)

5   Discussion

In this paper we described a novel pipeline for automatically estimating Graf's alpha angle in ultrasound images of infants' hips based on deep learning. Graf's method is notoriously operator-dependent and requires many years of training to reach a reasonable level of expertise, and automating it would be of great medical and social value. One of the major challenges we faced was the lack of good training data – images with known α angles but with no embedded annotations.

To overcome this challenge, we divided the problem into two parts: segmentation and annotation. This allowed us to harness the power of crowdsourcing to generate good training data for the segmentation problem, while formulating relatively simple rules for performing the annotations on top of the segmentations. We find the results very promising: there is generally a good agreement between the pipeline's estimate and the expert's and in those cases with most disagreement, external expert opinion is in favor of the pipeline's result.

We used two strategies to capture global information. First, our DCNN processes the image at multiple scales. Second, we complement the pixel-wise loss with an adversarial loss to produce outputs that are globally consistent. Adversarial networks have been proposed for unsupervised and semi-supervised learning, but in this work, the adversarial network is used to refine the outputs of fully supervised learning. This approach may be beneficial for other segmentation tasks, and more generally supervised learning tasks where the output has complex structure that may be well-captured by a neural network.

We view our work here as a first step, mostly due to the relatively small amounts of data used as more data is likely to improve the performance of the segmentation. New data should also cover a wider range of ultrasound machines and probe configurations to allow better generalization. One of the considerable advantages of deep learning approaches compared to more "classic" computer vision approaches is it's ability to continue learning as data accumulates. For example, [20] use traditional filters followed by active contours to segment the ilium. We experimented with similar methods and found that they are very sensitive to image quality, and require a considerable amount of fine-tuning.

Another important task is the establishment of a proper gold-standard test set: a large collection of images without annotations, which are then annotated by a number of experts. Ideally follow-up scans should be performed to set the ground-truth in borderline cases. Such data are unfortunately harder to obtain. Once such data are available, current part of the pipeline which are more heuristic (such as setting the value of c) could be automated as well.

Automating DDH diagnosis could have considerable medical and economical implications. Nowadays, many DDH cases go undetected due to lack of universal screening practices in most countries, mostly due to the high cost and low availability of sufficient expertise. Our pipeline provides a step towards universally accessible DDH screening, capturing DDH cases early, when medical intervention is easy and effective. Such universal screening would result in great improvement in the quality of life of millions, as well as a reduction the financial burden caused by early onset osteoarthritis.

Lastly, we believe our approach can be applied to other use-cases beyond DDH, and more importantly, beyond ultrasound, with the ultimate goal of fully automating the analysis of medical imaging data across clinical use-cases and imaging modalities.

Acknowledgments. Members of CUDL who contributed to paper: Jeevesh Kapur, Singapore, Singapore; Jeffrey Young, Stanford, California, US; Meghan Imrie, Stanford, California, US; Claudia Maizen, London, England; Paulien Bjilsma, London,

England; Daniel Reed, London, England; Rosy Jalan, London, England; Ibraheim
El-Daly, London, England; Lukasz Matuszewski, Lublin, Poland; Salih Marangoz,
Istanbul, Turkey; Greg Firth, Johannesburg, South Africa; Leon Izerel, Johannesburg,
South Africa; Ole Rahbek, Aarhus, Denmark; Michel Bach Hellfritzsch, Aarhus, Den-
mark; Christian Wong, Copenhagen, Denmark; Charlotte Strandberg, Gentofte, Den-
mark; Michael Christodolou, Athens, Greece; Abhilash Hareendranathan, Edmonton,
Alberta, Canada; Dornoosh Zonoobi, Edmonton, Alberta, Canada; Nicole Williams,
Adelaide, Australia; Andrew Morris, Adelaide, Australia; Peter Cundy, Adelaide, Aus-
tralia; Rebecca Linke, Adelaide, Australia.

References

1. Furnes, O., Lie, S.A., Espehaug, B., Vollset, S.E., Engesaeter, L.B., Havelin, L.I.:
   Hip disease and the prognosis of total hip replacements. Bone Joint J. **83**(4), 579–
   579 (2001)
2. Graf, R.: The diagnosis of congenital hip-joint dislocation by the ultrasonic com-
   bound treatment. Arch. Orthop. Trauma. Surg. **97**(2), 117–133 (1980)
3. Dias, J.J., Thomas, I.H., Lamont, A.C., Mody, B.S., et al.: The reliability of ultrasonographic assessment of neonatal hips. Bone Joint J. **75**(3), 479–482 (1993)
4. Roovers, E.A., Boere-Boonekamp, M.M., Geertsma, T.S.A., Zielhuis, G.A.,
   Kerkhoff, A.H.M.: Ultrasonographic screening for developmental dysplasia of the
   hip in infants. Bone Joint J. **85**(5), 726–730 (2003)
5. Krizhevsky, A., Sutskever, I., Hinton, G.E.: Imagenet classification with deep convolutional neural networks. In: Advances in Neural Information Processing Systems, pp. 1097–1105 (2012)
6. LeCun, Y., Bengio, Y., Hinton, G.: Deep learning. Nature **521**(7553), 436–444
   (2015)
7. Zhang, W., Li, R., Deng, H., Wang, L., Lin, W., Ji, S., Shen, D.: Deep convolutional
   neural networks for multi-modality isointense infant brain image segmentation.
   NeuroImage **108**, 214–224 (2015)
8. Havaei, M., Davy, A., Warde-Farley, D., Biard, A., Courville, A., Bengio, Y.,
   Pal, C., Jodoin, P.-M., Larochelle, H.: Brain tumor segmentation with deep neural
   networks. Med. Image Anal. (2016)
9. Long, J., Shelhamer, E., Darrell, T.: Fully convolutional networks for semantic
   segmentation. In: Proceedings of the IEEE Conference on Computer Vision and
   Pattern Recognition, pp. 3431–3440 (2015)
10. Hariharan, B., Arbeláez, P., Girshick, R., Malik, J.: Hypercolumns for object seg-
    mentation and fine-grained localization. In: Proceedings of the IEEE Conference
    on Computer Vision and Pattern Recognition, pp. 447–456 (2015)
11. Newell, A., Yang, K., Deng, J.: Stacked hourglass networks for human pose esti-
    mation. arXiv preprint arXiv:1603.06937 (2016)
12. Ioffe, S., Szegedy, C., Normalization, B.: Accelerating Deep Network Training by
    Reducing Internal Covariate Shift. arXiv:1502.03167, pp. 1–11 (2015)
13. Goodfellow, I., Pouget-Abadie, J., Mirza, M.: Generative Adversarial Networks,
    arXiv preprint, pp. 1–9 (2014)
14. Radford, A., Metz, L., Chintala, S.: Unsupervised Representation Learning with
    Deep Convolutional Generative Adversarial Networks. arXiv, pp. 1–15 (2015)
15. Abadi, M., Agarwal, A., Barham, P., Brevdo, E., Chen, Z., Citro, C., Corrado, G.S.,
    Davis, A., Dean, J., Devin, M., et al.: TensorFlow: large-scale machine learning on
    heterogeneous distributed systems. arXiv preprint arXiv:1603.04467 (2016)

16. Kingma, D.P., Ba, J.L.: Adam: a method for stochastic optimization. In: International Conference on Learning Representations, pp. 1–13 (2015)
17. He, K., Zhang, X., Ren, S., Sun, J.: Delving Deep into Rectifiers: Surpassing Human-Level Performance on ImageNet Classification. arXiv preprint, pp. 1–11 (2015)
18. Van der Walt, S., Schönberger, J.L., Nunez-Iglesias, J., Boulogne, F., Warner, J.D., Yager, N., Gouillart, E., Yu, T.: Scikit-image: image processing in Python. PeerJ **2**, e453 (2014)
19. Zieger, M.: Ultrasound of the infant hip. Part 2. Validity of the method. Pediatr. Radiol. **16**(6), 488–492 (1986)
20. Cevik, K.K., Kocer, H.E., Andac, S.: Segmentation of the ilium and femur regions from ultrasound images for diagnosis of developmental dysplasia of the hip. J. Med. Imaging Health Inf. **6**(2), 449–457 (2016)

Multi-dimensional Gated Recurrent Units for the Segmentation of Biomedical 3D-Data

Simon Andermatt$^{(\boxtimes)}$, Simon Pezold, and Philippe Cattin

Department of Biomedical Engineering, University of Basel, Allschwil, Switzerland
simon.andermatt@unibas.ch

Abstract. We present a supervised deep learning method to automatically segment 3D volumes of biomedical image data. The presented method takes advantage of a neural network with the main layers consisting of multi-dimensional gated recurrent units. We apply an on-the-fly data augmentation technique which allows for accurate estimations without the need for either a huge amount of training data or advanced data pre- or postprocessing. We show that our method performs amongst the leading techniques on a popular brain segmentation challenge dataset in terms of speed, accuracy and memory efficiency. We describe in detail advantages over a similar method which uses the well-established long short-term memory.

Keywords: Deep learning · GRU · Multi-dimensional RNN · Segmentation

1 Introduction

With the rapid advancements of imaging technologies, their ubiquitous availability and dropping prices, vast amounts of data are collected. This is particularly true for medical imaging. Accurate segmentation and delineation of e.g. pathologies in this medical data, however, pose real challenges as this is still mainly a manual process. In late phase drug studies with thousands of patients, multiple 3d datasets with different MR sequences are often collected per patient. If quantitative analysis of the immense amount of data is required, the time that has to be spent on the data by trained experts is enormous. A successful automated segmentation technique would decrease manual work to a minimum, cutting the costs and time spent on developing new treatments.

Automatic segmentation of biomedical volumetric data is, however, a challenging problem due to its high dimensionality, imaging noise, artifacts and other factors. Recent advances in the field of deep learning, especially the enabling effect of modern GPUs along with the advent of general purpose GPU computing, led to a revival of convolutional neural networks [9]. These feed-forward networks show great promise, but need a large number of layers to solve a difficult task accurately. A recurrent neural network (RNN), in contrast, can become arbitrarily deep due to its additional temporal dimension. Each timestep computed in an RNN corresponds roughly to one layer in a feed-forward network,

© Springer International Publishing AG 2016
G. Carneiro et al. (Eds.): LABELS 2016/DLMIA 2016, LNCS 10008, pp. 142–151, 2016.
DOI: 10.1007/978-3-319-46976-8_15

with the weights in one RNN being the same for each timestep. This property allows defining substantially more complexity very elegantly without the need for a huge number of layers or parameters.

The multi-dimensional Long Short-Term Memory (MD-LSTM) proposed by Stollenga et al. [13], called *PyraMiD-LSTM*, applied these insights to the Long Short-Term Memory (LSTM) [6]. It defines two LSTMs for each spatial dimension, using said spatial dimension as temporal dimension. The first one processes the data along that dimension, the second one in the opposite direction. In order to make full use of the spatial information, not only the direct predecessor along the temporal direction is taken into account, but also its local neighborhood. This can be neatly expressed using convolutions.

A relatively new RNN called Gated Recurrent Unit (GRU) [2] grew popular in recent years and became a strong competitor for the LSTM. It can be seen as a simplified version of the LSTM, which uses an update gate instead of a forget and input gate and combines the hidden and cell state [11]. It has been shown that it performs comparably to the LSTM in the task of sequence modeling [3]. Another study suggests that GRU and LSTM report similar performance on selected tasks [5]. An empirical search among more than 10 000 RNN architectures showed that on the selected tasks, although not the best performing RNN on every task, the GRU outperformed the standard LSTM architecture [8]. A larger time dimension in an RNN can mean that larger time dependencies can be represented. The lower memory requirement of the GRU means that larger volumes can be fed into the network and larger networks can be designed for the same volume size.

For all these reasons, a modification of the GRU to be able to process volumetric data seems compelling. We propose the multi-dimensional GRU (MD-GRU), which is capable of accurate segmentation of 3d data. We hint at the theoretical memory savings compared to the MD-LSTM and show that the performance of MD-GRU is comparable if not superior. Furthermore, we show that its convergence rate, computation time and combination of fewer gates favor the MD-GRU. We apply our method on a popular brain segmentation challenge dataset, achieving a score among the top 3 best performing methods.

2   Methods

2.1   Data

We used the publicly available MrBrainS [10] challenge dataset, which was one of the datasets used to evaluate the PyraMiD-LSTM. The MrBrainS challenge data consists of 5 labeled samples and 15 testing samples, where each sample has a T1 weighted, T1 inversion recovery and a FLAIR scan. The additional high-resolution T1 scan was not used, as the labeling was performed on the low resolution data. The training data contained two different label maps, one for training and one for testing. The training map consists of classes for cortical gray matter (GM), basal ganglia, white matter (WM), WM lesions, cerebrospinal fluid (CSF), ventricles, cerebellum, brainstem and background. The testing map only

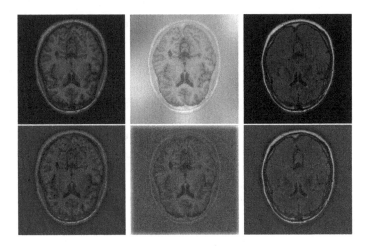

Fig. 1. Slice 19 of the 5th training sample. *Top row (left to right):* T1, T1_IR and T2_FLAIR. *Bottom row:* respective highpass filtered versions.

defines classes for GM, WM and CSF, the respective classes of the training map are merged. Brainstem and cerebellum are not included in the evaluation and do therefore not appear labeled in the testing map.

2.2 Convolutional Gated Recurrent Unit

The standard GRU as proposed in [2] is defined as

$$r^j = \sigma([W_r x]^j + [U_r h_{t-1}]^j), \tag{1}$$

$$z^j = \sigma([W_z x]^j + [U_z h_{t-1}]^j), \tag{2}$$

$$\tilde{h}_t^j = \phi([W x]^j + [U(r \odot h_{t-1})]^j), \tag{3}$$

$$h_t^j = z^j \odot h_{t-1}^j + (1 - z^j) \odot \tilde{h}_t^j, \tag{4}$$

where x is the input data, r^j is the reset gate, z^j is the update gate of the hidden unit j and the activation is performed in h^j. The operator $\odot$ represents an elementwise multiplication. The functions $\sigma(\cdot)$ and $\phi(\cdot)$ stand for the logistic function and the hyperbolic tangent. W and U are the weight matrices for the current input and last step's output data respectively. Along the lines of Stollenga et al. [13], we adapt these equations to be able to process 3D volumes and introduce our convolutional GRU (C-GRU):

$$r^j = \sigma\left(\sum_i^I (x^i * w_r^{i,j}) + \sum_k^J (h_{t-1}^k * u_r^{k,j}) + b_r^j\right), \tag{5}$$

$$z^j = \sigma\left(\sum_i^I (x^i * w_z^{i,j}) + \sum_k^J (h_{t-1}^k * u_z^{k,j}) + b_z^j\right), \tag{6}$$

$$\tilde{h}_t^j = \phi \left(\sum_i^I (x^i * w^{i,j}) + r^j \odot \sum_k^J (h_{t-1}^k * u^{k,j}) + b^j \right), \qquad (7)$$

$$h_t^j = z^j \odot h_{t-1}^j + (1 - z^j) \odot \tilde{h}_t^j, \qquad (8)$$

where $*$ represents a convolution. Compared to the vanilla GRU, we introduced slight changes. We decided to use a bias b on each gate. We factored r^j out of the convolution operation between u and h_{t-1}. This change was motivated by the fact that an additional convolution would require r to have twice the support it needs now because of the chained convolution. Moreover, we reorder the data for each C-RNN such that the two spatial dimensions are closest to memory, and the temporal dimension is ordered according to the temporal direction, as explained in the next paragraph. We motivated that decision with faster possible processing speeds on the GPU, since all convolutions now require data that lies close in memory. The computations of one C-GRU are visualized as a computational graph in Fig. 2a.

The MD-GRU consists of two times D C-GRUs, where D is the dimensionality of the image data and we need one C-GRU for each of the two directions. We set the input data of channel i as $x^i \in \mathbb{R}^{S_1 \times \cdots \times S_D}$. For each spatial dimension d, we create the copies $x^{i,d,-1}, x^{i,d,+1} \in \mathbb{R}^{S_d \times S_1 \times \cdots \times S_D}$ of x and apply the following data transformations:

$$x^{i,d,+1}(s_d, s_1, \ldots, s_D) = x^i(s_1, \ldots, s_d, \ldots, s_D), \qquad (9)$$

$$x^{i,d,-1}(S_d - s_d, s_1, \ldots, s_D) = x^i(s_1, \ldots, s_d, \ldots, s_D), \qquad (10)$$

where s_d is the index of the assigned dimension of the C-GRU and S_d is the size of dimension d. The inverse operation is applied to $h^{j,d,+1}, h^{j,d,-1} \in \mathbb{R}^{S_d \times S_1 \times \cdots \times S_D}$ to gather the final output h^j:

$$h^j(s_1, \ldots, s_D) = \sum_{d=1}^{D} \left(h^{j,d,+1}(s_d, s_1, \ldots, s_D) + h^{j,d,-1}(S_d - s_d, s_1, \ldots, s_D) \right).$$

$$(11)$$

Figure 2b details this process for the MD-GRU. We apply the same technique for our implementation of the MD-LSTM.

2.3 Experiments

Network. We model our network similar to [13]. We include three multi-dimensional RNN (MD-RNN) layers of 16, 32 and 64 channels which are connected with pixelwise fully connected hidden layers of 25 and 45 channels respectively, each followed by a hyperbolic tangent activation function. The last MD-RNN is attached to a pixelwise fully connected layer with c channels, the same number as classes in the data. We estimate the probabilities for each class using a softmax in the last layer and consequently choose the multinomial logistic loss for the training of our network. Figure 2c shows our network setup for the case of MD-GRU.

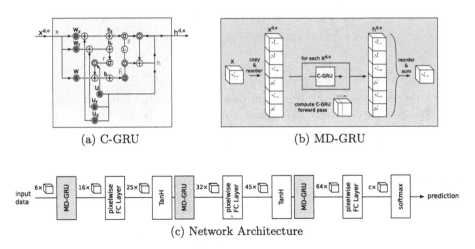

(a) C-GRU   (b) MD-GRU

(c) Network Architecture

Fig. 2. (a) Directed graph denoting the computations in one C-GRU. The variables $x^{d,o}$, $h^{d,o}$ with $o \in \{-1,+1\}$ represent the input and output data across all I and J channels respectively. The $\circledast$ operator denotes here the sum per channel j over the convolutions with each channel i or k, as used in Eqs. (5)–(7). (b) Proposed arrangement of 6 C-GRUs in a MD-GRU for three-dimensional data. (c) Setup of our network.

Setting. All experiments were calculated on an NVIDIA GTX Titan X GPU with 12 GB global memory. Our implementation of MD-LSTM and MD-GRU relied on the fast convolution routines provided by NVIDIA's cuDNN [1]. For other layers, the already available implementations of the CAFFE[1] framework [7] were used.

Preprocessing. For all volumes, unsharp masking was done using a Gaussian smoothed image ($\sigma = 5$ voxels) which was then subtracted from the original images to produce highpass filtered volumes. The original images and the high-pass filtered images were normalized to $\sigma = 1$ and $\mu = 0$, assuming normally distributed values. In this way we followed a procedure similar to [13], but omitted the histogram equalization. Figure 1 shows the original and preprocessed data for training sample 5 at slice 19.

Data Augmentation. In the training stage, at each iteration, a random location in the training data was selected and a deformation field was generated and applied to the subvolumes, which were then fed into the network. We used a procedure similar to [12], but made the grid size dependent on the data. We did not use random deformations in the feasibility study mentioned in Sect. 3.1. For the testing phase, no deformations were applied.

---

[1] Version 1.0.0-rc3, commit 9c46289.

Training. In three training steps we iteratively increase the subvolume size from $64 \times 64 \times 8$ voxels to $128 \times 128 \times 12$ and finally to $200 \times 200 \times 15$, keeping the third dimension smaller to account for the anisotropic MR volume resolution. We relied on AdaDelta [15] to omit the manual tuning of a learning rate. For the challenge, we additionally used DropConnect [14] of 0.5 on the input connections of each C-GRU to prevent overfitting. Training took around two days.

Testing. In the testing phase, we divided the volume into a grid of equally sized subvolumes of $120 \times 120 \times 8$, which were padded by 50, 50 and 4 voxels respectively on all sides of the volume. The padding was later used to stitch the results together using a Gaussian ($\mu = 0$, $\sigma = (10, 10, 0.8)$) to produce interpolation weights, since the borders contain starting artifacts from the individual RNNs and do not contain adequate results. Since we trained for nine classes, but only four classes were needed for the final evaluation, we simply combined the binary labels for the CSF with the ventricles, the cortical GM with the basal ganglia and the WM with the WM lesions. Everything else was considered background. Testing one volume of the MRBrainS data required 32 iterations, which needed around two minutes.

3   Results

3.1   Feasibility Study

To point out differences between the MD-GRU and the MD-LSTM, we ran the same setup with the multi-dimensional RNN layers either being an MD-GRU or an MD-LSTM. We used the first four volumes in the training set of the MrBrainS challenge and trained both networks for 3 000 iterations on the largest possible resolution which was feasible for both (limited to $192 \times 192 \times 14$ by our MD-LSTM implementation). On average, one training iteration for MD-GRU and MD-LSTM took 9.1 and 12.8 s, respectively. The Dice coefficients for CSF, GM, WM and ICV between the computed segmentation of the 5th training volume and the provided reference segmentation are shown in Table 1 for both the MD-GRU and MD-LSTM. Slice 19 of the computed segmentations and the reference segmentation are displayed in Fig. 3 together with a plot of a running average of 100 iterations of the loss function for each iteration of the training procedure.

Table 1. Feasibility study. Dice coefficients in percent for gray and white matter (GM/WM), cerebrospinal fluid (CSF) and intracranial volume (ICV).

	GM	WM	CSF	ICV
MD-LSTM	**88.09**	90.08	82.62	97.56
MD-GRU	87.88	**90.15**	**83.19**	**97.73**

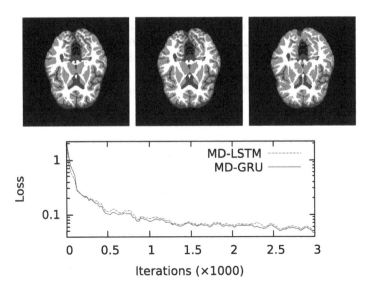

Fig. 3. Feasibility study. *Top row:* slice 19 of the 5th training volume used for the evaluation. The images from left to right represent the results of the MD-LSTM, the MD-GRU and the manual labeling. *Bottom row:* convergence rates for the feasibility study of both MD-GRU and MD-LSTM.

3.2   MD-GRU on MRBrainS

In our attempt to beat the highscore of the MRBrainS challenge, we used our described data augmentation method. Each subvolume was deformed randomly throughout all three training phases. We used all provided low resolution volumes and their highpass filtered versions. Table 2 lists our performance according to the Dice coefficients, 95th-percentile of the Hausdorff distance and average volume difference of the GM, WM, CSF and ICV. Nine measures were relevant

Table 2. MrBrainS challenge. Results of the six best performing methods for GM, WM, CSF and ICV of all three used metrics (Dice, 95th-percentile of the Hausdorff distance (HD) and average volume difference (AVD)). A bold number means best out of these six. The results reflect the state on August 12, 2016.

Team name	Rank	GM			WM			CSF			ICV		
		Dice	HD	AVD	Dice	HD	AVD	Dice	HD	AVD	Dice	HD	AVD
CU_DL2	1	**86.15**	**1.45**	6.60	**89.46**	**1.94**	6.05	**84.25**	2.19	7.69	98.10	2.75	1.54
CU_DL	2	86.12	1.47	6.42	89.39	**1.94**	**5.84**	83.96	2.28	7.44	97.99	3.16	1.83
MD-GRU [proposed]	3	85.40	1.55	**6.09**	88.98	2.02	7.69	84.13	2.17	7.44	**98.15**	**2.37**	0.86
PyraMiD-LSTM2	4	84.89	1.67	6.35	88.53	2.07	5.93	83.05	2.30	7.17	98.04	2.86	**0.69**
FBI/LMB Freiburg [4]	5	85.44	1.58	6.60	88.86	1.95	6.47	83.47	2.22	8.63	97.98	2.51	1.06
IDSIA [13]	6	84.82	1.70	6.77	88.33	2.08	7.05	83.72	**2.14**	**7.09**	**98.15**	2.44	0.95

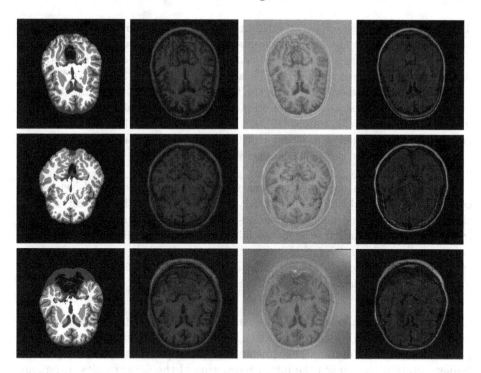

Fig. 4. MrBrainS challenge. *Rows (top to bottom):* 5th, 10th and 15th test sample. *Columns (left to right):* slice 19 of our segmentation results, T1, T1_IR and T2_FLAIR.

for the final evaluation: Dice, modified Hausdorff distance and average volume distance in each of the categories GM, WM and CSF. The sum of the ranks in these nine categories is used as the performance score and determines the final rank. Figure 4 shows the computed segmentation at slice 19 of samples 5, 10 and 15 of the test data.

4   Discussion

The feasibility study has shown that MD-GRU has great potential for the segmentation of volumetric images, since it achieved comparable results to the MD-LSTM in less time with the same settings.

Using deformation as a data augmentation strategy and DropConnect for regularization in the challenge, we ranked 3rd out of 37. Unfortunately, none of the results in the top five of the challenge highscore are published so far. The 4th and 6th entries are both incarnations of the already discussed MD-LSTM, where only the latter was described in [13] and the former likely contains unpublished improvements to their method. In contrast to [13], we did not omit the original T1_IR images. Yet some obvious misclassifications could be traced back to strong bias field artifacts in the T1_IR images. Given the small training size, using the

T1_IR images leads to apparent fitting to the bias field. Furthermore, we were not able to replicate the training volume size of Stollenga et al. [13] due to a higher memory requirement of our implementation, since we decided to copy the input and output data for each RNN layer, as detailed in Sect. 2.2. This has to be kept in mind when comparing the two approaches. Relationships between areas that are located at a certain distance in the data could therefore not be modeled in our network, where [13] was able to use the full spatial context in two dimensions as well as a larger third dimension. In their last training step more than half of the data was covered while we could only fit a bit more than a fifth in our memory.

The contribution on rank five was computed using the 3D U-Net [4]. It consists of a hierarchical convolutional neural network with shortcut connections, which is trained using various on-the-fly data augmentation techniques, including the deformation strategy used in this paper. The challenge results and corresponding adaptations of the algorithm to fit the challenge data are, however, not yet published. We believe that data augmentation is key for successful applications to problems with such a small training size.

Conclusion. With the MD-GRU, we combined the enormous expressive power of RNNs with a highly beneficial data augmentation strategy, resulting in a powerful supervised automatic segmentation technique. With a memory-savvy implementation that omits the initial reordering of the data, results surpassing the state of the art should be possible with MD-GRU.

References

1. Chetlur, S., Woolley, C., Vandermersch, P., Cohen, J., Tran, J., Catanzaro, B., Shelhamer, E.: cuDNN: Efficient Primitives for Deep Learning. arXiv:1410.0759 [cs], October 2014
2. Cho, K., van Merrienboer, B., Gulcehre, C., Bahdanau, D., Bougares, F., Schwenk, H., Bengio, Y.: Learning Phrase Representations Using RNN Encoder-Decoder for Statistical Machine Translation. arXiv:1406.1078 [cs, stat], June 2014
3. Chung, J., Gulcehre, C., Cho, K., Bengio, Y.: Empirical Evaluation of Gated Recurrent Neural Networks on Sequence Modeling. arXiv:1412.3555 [cs], December 2014
4. Çiçek, Ö., Abdulkadir, A., Lienkamp, S.S., Brox, T., Ronneberger, O.: 3D U-Net: Learning Dense Volumetric Segmentation from Sparse Annotation. arXiv:1606.06650 [cs], June 2016
5. Greff, K., Srivastava, R.K., Koutník, J., Steunebrink, B.R., Schmidhuber, J.: LSTM: A Search Space Odyssey. arXiv:1503.04069 [cs], March 2015
6. Hochreiter, S., Schmidhuber, J.: Long short-term memory. Neural Comput. **9**(8), 1735–1780 (1997)
7. Jia, Y., Shelhamer, E., Donahue, J., Karayev, S., Long, J., Girshick, R., Guadarrama, S., Darrell, T.: Caffe: Convolutional Architecture for Fast Feature Embedding. arXiv preprint arXiv:1408.5093 (2014)
8. Jozefowicz, R., Zaremba, W., Sutskever, I.: An empirical exploration of recurrent network architectures. In: Proceedings of The 32nd International Conference on Machine Learning, pp. 2342–2350 (2015)

9. Krizhevsky, A., Sutskever, I., Hinton, G.E.: ImageNet classification with deep convolutional neural networks. In: Pereira, F., Burges, C.J.C., Bottou, L., Weinberger, K.Q. (eds.) Advances in Neural Information Processing Systems 25, pp. 1097–1105. Curran Associates Inc, Red Hook (2012)
10. Mendrik, A.M., Vincken, K.L., Kuijf, H.J., et al.: MRBrainS challenge: online evaluation framework for brain image segmentation in 3T MRI scans. Comput. Intell. Neurosci. **2015**, 16 (2015). doi:10.1155/2015/813696. Article ID 813696
11. Olah, C.: Understanding LSTM Networks, August 2015. http://colah.github.io/posts/2015-08-Understanding-LSTMs/
12. Ronneberger, O., Fischer, P., Brox, T.: U-Net: convolutional networks for biomedical image segmentation. In: Navab, N., Hornegger, J., Wells, W.M., Frangi, A.F. (eds.) MICCAI 2015. LNCS, vol. 9351, pp. 234–241. Springer, Heidelberg (2015)
13. Stollenga, M.F., Byeon, W., Liwicki, M., Schmidhuber, J.: Parallel multi-dimensional LSTM, with application to fast biomedical volumetric image segmentation. In: Cortes, C., Lawrence, N.D., Lee, D.D., Sugiyama, M., Garnett, R. (eds.) Advances in Neural Information Processing Systems 28, pp. 2998–3006. Curran Associates Inc., Red Hook (2015)
14. Wan, L., Zeiler, M., Zhang, S., Cun, Y.L., Fergus, R.: Regularization of neural networks using dropconnect. In: Dasgupta, S., McAllester, D. (eds.) Proceedings of the 30th International Conference on Machine Learning (ICML-13), JMLR Workshop and Conference Proceedings, vol. 28, pp. 1058–1066, May 2013
15. Zeiler, M.D.: ADADELTA: An Adaptive Learning Rate Method. arXiv:1212.5701 [cs], December 2012

Learning Thermal Process Representations for Intraoperative Analysis of Cortical Perfusion During Ischemic Strokes

Nico Hoffmann[1,2(✉)], Edmund Koch[1], Gerald Steiner[1], Uwe Petersohn[2], and Matthias Kirsch[3]

[1] Clinical Sensing and Monitoring, Technische Universität Dresden, 01307 Dresden, Germany
nico.hoffmann@tu-dresden.de
[2] Applied Knowledge Representation and Reasoning, Technische Universität Dresden, 01062 Dresden, Germany
[3] Department of Neurosurgery, University Hospital Carl Gustav Carus, 01307 Dresden, Germany

Abstract. Thermal imaging is a non-invasive and marker-free approach for intraoperative measurements of small temperature variations. In this work, we demonstrate the abilities of active dynamic thermal imaging for analysis of tissue perfusion state in case of cerebral ischemia. For this purpose, a NaCl irrigation is applied to the exposed cortex during hemicraniectomy. The caused temperature changes are measured by a thermal imaging system whilst tissue heating is modeled by a double exponential function. Modeled temperature decay constants allow us to characterize tissue perfusion with respect to its dynamic thermal properties. As intraoperative imaging prevents the usage of computational intense parameter optimization schemes we discuss a deep learning framework that approximates these constants given a simple temperature sequence. The framework is compared to common Levenberg-Marquardt based parameter optimization approaches. The proposed deep parameter approximation framework shows good performance compared to numerical optimization with random initialization. We further validated the approximated parameters by an intraoperative case suffering acute cerebral ischemia. The results indicate that even approximated temperature decay constants allow us to quantify cortical perfusion. Latter yield a standardized representation of cortical thermodynamic properties and might guide further research regarding specific intraoperative therapies and characterization of pathologies with atypical cortical perfusion.

Keywords: Neurosurgery · Intraoperative thermal imaging · Deep learning · Parameter approximation

1 Introduction

Thermal imaging is a contactless, marker-free, white-light independent and non-invasive method for online measurement of temperature variations up to $30\,\mu\mathrm{K}$.

© Springer International Publishing AG 2016
G. Carneiro et al. (Eds.): LABELS 2016/DLMIA 2016, LNCS 10008, pp. 152–160, 2016.
DOI: 10.1007/978-3-319-46976-8_16

Current uncooled devices use infrared microbolometer focal plane array detectors measuring a field of view of 16×12 cm with an underlying spatial resolution of $250 \, \mu m$ per pixel at a framerate of 50 Hz. The detected infrared radiation arriving at the microbolometer array is processed and stored as two-dimensional image.

In brain tissue, temperature variations are primarily caused by heat transfers originating from cerebral perfusion. Note, that the local cerebral blood flow correlates with cell metabolism and can be used as marker for tissue state and neural activity. Intraoperative thermal neuroimaging now allows online inference of diagnostic information about perfusion- and neural activity related disorders. [1] demonstrated an approach to distinguish cancerous from healthy tissue based on thermal imaging. [2] evaluated the cortical blood flow by analysing the spatial distribution of a cold bolus applied through a central line with multivariate analysis tools.

In the remaining, the thermal behavior in case of ischemic strokes is analyzed. Latter denote the shortage of substrates of delimited areas of the brain by blockage of vessels (embolism or thrombosis). Severe strokes lead to a swelling of brain tissue, which raises intracranial pressure (ICP) leading to bad or fatal prognosis if not treated appropriately. Hemicraniectomy can be considered as last resort to decrease ICP. We extend the approach of Steiner et al. [2] by combining deep learning and active dynamic thermal imaging during decompressive hemicraniectomy to characterize the perfusion state of cortical tissue. The proposed method integrates seamlessly into typical intraoperative workflows and is not limited to perfused areas in contrast to the Cold Bolus approach of Steiner et al. We also extend prior findings of Gorbach et al. [3] by a sound mathematical model with efficient approximation of tissue thermodynamics yielding standardized parameters of cortical perfusion.

2   Intraoperative Reasoning About Cortical Perfusion

Gorbach et al. [3] proposed irrigating the surface of cortical tissue for some time to propagate heat through several tissue layers. In contrast, we employ available intraoperative tools to prevent the need for additional sterile tools. The surgeon typically has a tool (e.g. syringe) to purge sterile sodium chloride (NaCl) onto tissue. Hereby, it is possible to selectively apply NaCl to a delimited area of the exposed cortex for a specific duration. This irrigation induces a steep drop in temperature followed by a temperature increase caused by heat transfers. In human tissue, this heating correlates with thermodynamic properties of the underlying tissue, thermal conductivity and tissue perfusion state. By modeling this behavior and estimating respective parameters, it is possible to characterize the imaged tissue.

2.1   Modelling Tissue Perfusion

In 1948, Pennes [4] proposed the biologically inspired "Bioheat equation". He proposed the following model to describe internal as well as external influences to the heat distribution in living tissue:

$$c_p\rho\frac{\delta T(x,y,z)}{\delta t} = \kappa\nabla^2 T(x,y,z,t) + q_b + q_m + q_{ex} \tag{1}$$

with the specific heat c_p, material density ρ, temperature distribution $T(x,y,z)$ at time t $T(x,y,z,t)$ and thermal inductivity κ. He further added biological parameters describing the heat power density of q_b blood flow, q_m metabolism and external power density q_{ex}.

Several authors have shown the discretization of Penne's equation (see for example Gutierrez et al. [5]). In our case, we are facing several a priori unknown parameters whose estimation schemes would introduce significant computational complexity and potentially inaccurate estimates. To counter these challenges, we propose to employ Nowakowski's approach to approximate tissue's thermal behavior by a double exponential function [6] at time t

$$T(t,\theta) = T_{equ} + \Delta T_1 exp(-t\gamma_1) + \Delta T_2 exp(-t\gamma_2) \tag{2}$$

$\theta_i = (\Delta T_1, \Delta T_2, \gamma_1, \gamma_2, T_{equ})$ denotes the set of all model parameters with T_{equ} resembling the tissue's equilibrium temperature, ΔT_1 and ΔT_2 being the scaling coefficients of both exponential functions. Decay constants γ_1 and γ_2 (unit s^{-1}) denote the amplitude of the tissue's temperature change rate.

By applying a cold liquid to the exposed cortex, we expect at least two orthogonal components that explain subsequent heating. One component represents the temperature changes of the applied cool fluid. The other component describes the temperature change of the affected underlying tissue. Latter gets dominant after the fluid drained from the surface. Since the cortex can be regarded as convex shape with high curvature, it is reasonable to expect the fluid to drain continuously and fast. We therefore expect γ_2 of the fluid to be larger than γ_1 of the imaged tissue allowing a reliable distinction and therefore estimation of both.

2.2   Levenberg-Marquardt Algorithm

Non-linear least squares is a standard approach for solving Eq. 2. Given n data samples y_i and time points t_i $(1 \le i \le n)$ the problem formulation reads

$$\widetilde{\theta} \in \underset{\theta}{argmin} \sum_{i=1}^{n} ||y_i - T(t_i,\theta)||_2^2 := \sum_{i=1}^{n} ||f_i||_2^2 \tag{3}$$

Minimizing this equation yields an estimate of thermal perfusion parameters $\widetilde{\theta}$. As the optimization problem is non-linear, iterative optimization schemes are required for minimization. The (damped) Levenberg-Marquardt algorithm (LMA) depicts a fast iterative scheme to estimate $\widetilde{\theta}$ by only relying on the model's Jacobian $J = [J_1^T \ldots J_n^T]^T$. Given sample i, row vector $J_i = \delta f_i/\delta\theta$ denotes the gradient of f_i with respect to θ

$$J_i = [-t_i\Delta T_1 exp(t_i\gamma_1) \ -t_i\Delta T_2 exp(t_i\gamma_2) \ -exp(t_i\gamma_1) \ -exp(t_i\gamma_2) \ -1]$$

In each iteration, θ is replaced by $\theta + \nu$ whereas ν is determined by solving

$$(J^T J + \lambda I)\nu = J^T(y - T(\theta))$$

with identity matrix I, some (non-negative) damping factor λ, $y = [y_1 \ldots y_n]^T$ and $T(\theta) = [T(t_1, \theta) \ldots T(t_n, \theta)]^T$. Depending on the target function and initial values LMA can achieve quadratic convergence [7]. A detailed discussion of LMA can be found elsewhere (see for example [7,8]).

2.3 Approximating Thermal Process Parameters by Deep Neural Networks

As we have to estimate θ for each pixel of our thermal video sequence even efficient numerical optimization schemes can be time consuming or require a vast amount of computational resources. In order to tackle both challenges, we trained a deep parameter approximation network (DPA) that learns the underlying manifold so that it approximates θ given a length k thermal sequence $(T(t_1), T(t_2), \ldots, T(t_k))$. The network is described by some $\eta : \mathbb{R}^k \to \mathbb{R}^5$. In order to catch non-linear dependencies a regularized (using dropout layers [9]) multi-layer neural network topology is employed. S-shaped rectified linear activation layer [10] further allow to catch non-convex effects. The whole topology of the proposed network is shown in Fig. 1 and is trained by adaptive moment estimation [11]. As we are approximating the parameter space of an a priori known model, supervised training data is generated by sampling Eq. 2. This yields a training set $\mathcal{X} = (T_j, \theta_j)$ of m samples with $T_j \in \mathbb{R}^k$, $\theta_j \in \mathbb{R}^5$ and $1 \leq j \leq m$.

3   Results and Discussion

We performed several experiments to evaluate the performance of the proposed irrigation analysis framework. All intraoperative procedures were approved by the Human Ethics Committee of the Technische Universität Dresden (no. EK 323122008). Informed consent was obtained postoperatively in accordance with the approved scheme. In the following, we evaluate the detector's performance in experimental test and training datasets. Afterwards, the approach is used to analyze exemplary intraoperative data. All computations were done on a workstation with dual Intel Xeon E5-2630, 128 GB Ram and Nvidia Geforce GTX Titan Black graphics card.

3.1   Deep Parameter Approximation

DPA training data was generated by sampling 1 million normal distributed instances $(\theta^*) \sim N(\mu, \Sigma)$ (see Eq. 2) with $\mu = (-0.5, -1, -6, -6, 28)^T$ and 5×5 diagonal matrix $\Sigma = diag(0.5, 0.5, 6, 6, 4)$. Thermal time series can now be generated by $T^* = T(t_k, \theta^*)$ with $0 \leq t_k \leq 4$ and $1 \leq i \leq 400$. In order to quantify the performance of the proposed optimization schemes with respect to groundtruth parameter θ^* and synthetic temperature series $T^* = (T_1^*, \ldots, T_k^*)^*$ 10000 samples were drawn from the same distribution. The baseline method was chosen to be a damped Levenberg-Marquardt optimizing scheme given three parameter

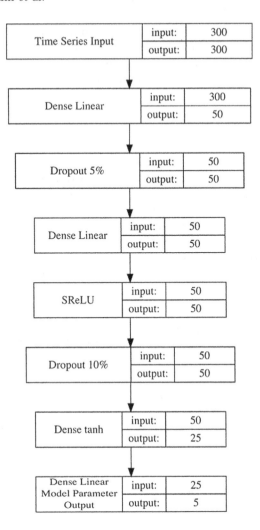

Time Series Input	input:	300
	output:	300

Dense Linear	input:	300
	output:	50

Dropout 5%	input:	50
	output:	50

Dense Linear	input:	50
	output:	50

SReLU	input:	50
	output:	50

Dropout 10%	input:	50
	output:	50

Dense tanh	input:	50
	output:	25

Dense Linear Model Parameter Output	input:	25
	output:	5

Fig. 1. This figure shows the deep neural network used to approximate thermal perfusion parameters of Eq. 2.

initialization strategies: uninformed guess (RAND) of θ_0 is acquired by sampling $\theta_0^{\text{RAND}} \sim N([0\ 0\ 0\ 0\ 28]^T, \Sigma)$ whereas near-optimal initializations (NO) are realized by sampling $\theta_0^{\text{NO}} \sim N(\theta^*, 0.1\Sigma)$. The latter is expected to yield best performance as it is initialized near to the optimal solution. Both strategies employ $\Sigma = I_5$ with I_5 being a 5×5 identity matrix. The last strategy initializes LMA by the output of the deep parameter approximation network given T^* denoted by LMA-DPA: $\theta_0^{\text{DPA}} = \eta(T^*)$. Latter should be close to the optimal solution for what reason we expect better performance than by random initialization.

Table 1. This table shows the achieved performance of the proposed deep parameter approximation (DPA) scheme compared to traditional Levenberg-Marquardt based numerical optimization given three different initialization schemes.

Method	Iterations	Runtime [s]	ϵ	ϵ_γ
DPA	1	0.00001	1.384 ± 0.742	0.098 ± 0.061
LMA-NO	31.64 ± 96.7	0.006	0.63 ± 3.13	0.001 ± 0.006
LMA-DPA	37 ± 81	0.005	$\mathbf{0.026 \pm 0.181}$	$\mathbf{0.0001 \pm 0.0006}$
LMA-RAND	130 ± 147	0.014	2.913 ± 5.325	0.282 ± 0.292

The accuracy of the parameter estimates $\widetilde{\theta} = [\widetilde{\gamma_1} \ \widetilde{\gamma_2} \ \widetilde{\Delta T_1} \ \widetilde{\Delta T_2} \ \widetilde{T_{equ}}]$ is quantified by two measures $\epsilon = ||\widetilde{\theta} - \theta^*||_2^2$ and $\epsilon_\gamma = ||[\gamma_1^* \ \gamma_2^*]^T - [\widetilde{\gamma_1} \ \widetilde{\gamma_2}]^T||_2^2$. Latter is particularly interesting as the temperature decay constants correlate with cortical perfusion and denote the most important parameters for subsequent analysis. Runtime denotes the time required to optimize a single temperature sequence of length k. The results are shown in Table 1. The results suggest that DPA approximates the model parameters more accurately than Levenberg-Marquardt optimization with random initialization and significantly reduced overall runtime. When used as initialization for LMA it is interesting to note that the approximated parameters seem to lie close to the actual parameters as LMA-DPA achieves better performance than LMA-NO with less variation. The standard deviation of the resulting number of iterations as well as accuracy $\epsilon, \epsilon_\gamma$ further suggests that the convergence behaviour of employed optimization scheme strongly correlates with the initial parameter estimate θ_0. One reason for this behaviour is the non-convex nature of the stated optimization problem (Eq. 3). This puts further emphasisis on parameter initialization especially when subsequent analysis requires accurate parameter estimates. As we have shown, deep parameter approximation networks might be one approach to this challenge.

3.2   Case Study

The examined case suffered an acute ischemic stroke of middle cerebral artery requiring a decompressive hemicraniectomy to decrease intracerebral pressure. Accompanying and without influencing the surgical intervention we performed thermographic measurements of the exposed cortex and recorded intraoperative irrigations of cold NaCl. Latter causes a steep temperature drop and subsequent heating. These irrigations are common in neurosurgery in order to prevent cortical drying. We further segmented the infarct demarcation in postoperative computed tomography (CT) scans and mapped thermal image sequences onto the cortex for easier orientation (Fig. 2b). Heating parameters were approximated by the discussed DPA approach being applied to the heating sequence caused by the cortical irrigation. Figure 2c visualizes the approximated values of γ_1. Low values of γ_1 indicate reduced perfusion and metabolism which also explains the clear correlation with the infarct demarcation in postoperative CT (see Fig. 2a).

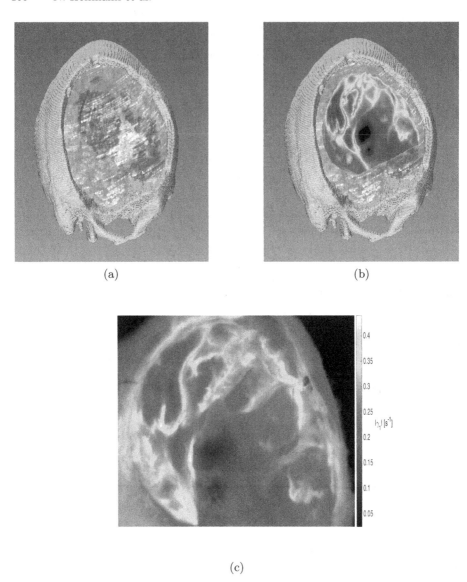

(a)   (b)

(c)

Fig. 2. (A) visualizes the infarct demarcation as green-blue object in a post-operative CT recording with the convex shape being the trepanation. (B) depicts the temperature distribution at equilibrium temperature after the cortical irrigation. Blue visualizes temperatures at 22 °C and red resembles temperatures at 32 °C. (C) shows the spatial distribution of γ_1. Black represents ischemic/low perfusion state whilst the brighter colors denote stronger perfusion. Note that op towel got hit by cold NaCl irrigation as well causing some heating off the trepanation. The estimated underperfused tissue state correlates with post-operative infarct demarcation. Compared to equilibrium temperature, thermal decay constant γ_1 allows to infer standardized and more detailed information regarding tissue perfusion. The transition between healthy and ischemic tissue (orange to red colors) might be subject for further inspections and therapies. (Color figure online)

4   Conclusion

Thermography is an emerging whitelight-independent, non-invasive method to measure the temperature distribution of surfaces. By application of temperature gradients, this method is extended to active dynamic thermography. In medical domain this enables analysis of abnormal tissue and vascular pathologies by dynamic thermal properties.

We employ active dynamic thermography to analyze the perfusion of the exposed human cortex during neurosurgical interventions in case of ischemic strokes. Our approach requires the application of a temperature gradient to the exposed cerebral cortex in order to quantify cortical perfusion. These gradients are induced by applying a cold NaCl irrigation to the exposed cerebral cortex. Subsequent tissue heating is modeled by a double exponential function and its parameter's are approximated efficiently by a novel deep parameter learning framework. The parameters include thermal decay constants that quantify the rate of tissue heating. We demonstrated that these decay constants correlate with tissue perfusion state and allow to draw conclusions regarding infarct demarcations as imaged by pre/post-operative CT measurements. This enables the surgeon to inspect the progression of cerebral ischemia and allows inferring further diagnostic information. In order to improve clinical significance of our results and enhance the accuracy of our deep parameter approximation network further research on larger cohorts is required. A more advanced parameter approximation network might allow to reliably estimate the parameters of Penne's bioheat equation and therefore infer fine-grain information about tissue composition. We further expect that other pathologies can be characterized by their dynamic thermal behavior as well especially if they correlate with atypical metabolism or perfusion.

Acknowledgment. The authors would also like to thank all other organizations and individuals that supported this research project.

References

1. Gorbach, A.M., Heiss, J.D., Kopylev, L., Oldfield, E.H.: Intraoperative infrared imaging of brain tumors. J. Neurosurg. **101**(6), 960–969 (2004)
2. Steiner, G., Sobottka, S.B., Koch, E., Schackert, G., Kirsch, M.: Intraoperative imaging of cortical cerebral perfusion by time-resolved thermography and multivariate data analysis. J. Biomed. Opt. **16**(1), 016001–016006 (2011)
3. Gorbach, A., Heiss, J.D., Kopylev, L., Oldfield, E.H.: Intraoperative infrared imaging of brain tumors. J. Neurosurg. **101**, 960 (2004)
4. Pennes, H.H.: Analysis of tissue and arterial blood temperatures in the resting human forearm. J. Appl. Physiol. **1**, 93–122 (1948)
5. Gutierrez, G., Giordano, M.: Study of the bioheat equation using Monte Carlo simulations for local magnetic hyperthermia. In: Proceedings of the ASME International Mechanical Engineering Congress and Exposition (2008)

6. Nowakowski, A.: Quantitative active dynamic thermal IR-imaging and thermal tomography in medical diagnostics. In: Medical Infrared Imaging. Taylor and Francis (2013)

7. Yamashita, N., Fukushima, M.: On the rate of convergence of the Levenberg-Marquardt method. In: Alefeld, G., Chen, X., et al. (eds.) Topics in Numerical Analysis. Computing Supplementa, pp. 239–249. Springer, Vienna (2001)

8. Moré, J.J.: The Levenberg-Marquardt algorithm: implementation and theory. Numerical Analysis. Lecture Notes in Mathematics, vol. 630, pp. 105–116. Springer, Heidelberg (1978)

9. Srivastava, N., Hinton, G., Krizhevsky, A., Sutskever, I., Salakhutdinov, R.: Dropout: a simple way to prevent neural networks from overfitting. J. Mach. Learn. Res. **15**, 1929–1958 (2014)

10. Jin, X., Xu, C., Feng, J., Wei, Y., Xiong, J., Yan, S.: Deep learning with s-shaped rectified linear activation units. CoRR, vol. abs/1512.07030 (2015)

11. Kingma, D.P., Ba, J.: Adam: a method for stochastic optimization. CoRR, vol. abs/1412.6980 (2014)

Automatic Slice Identification in 3D Medical Images with a ConvNet Regressor

Bob D. de Vos[1]($\boxtimes$), Max A. Viergever[1], Pim A. de Jong[2], and Ivana Išgum[1]

[1] Image Sciences Institute, University Medical Center Utrecht,
Utrecht, The Netherlands
bddevos@gmail.com
[2] Department of Radiology, University Medical Center Utrecht,
Utrecht, The Netherlands

Abstract. Identification of anatomical regions of interest is a prerequisite in many medical image analysis tasks. We propose a method that automatically identifies a slice of interest (SOI) in 3D images with a convolutional neural network (ConvNet) regressor.

In 150 chest CT scans two reference slices were manually identified: one containing the aortic root and another superior to the aortic arch. In two independent experiments, the ConvNet regressor was trained with 100 CTs to determine the distance between each slice and the SOI in a CT. To identify the SOI, a first order polynomial was fitted through the obtained distances.

In 50 test scans, the mean distances between the reference and the automatically identified slices were 5.7 mm (4.0 slices) for the aortic root and 5.6 mm (3.7 slices) for the aortic arch.

The method shows similar results for both tasks and could be used for automatic slice identification.

Keywords: Slice identification · Localization · Detection · Convolutional neural network · Regression · Deep learning

1 Introduction

Manual and automatic localization of organs, anatomical structures, or points, is a prerequisite for many tasks in medical image analysis. Hence, several automatic methods for localization of organs have been described in literature (e.g. [4,11]). These methods typically indicate a region around the organ of interest and enable dedicated analysis of this region only. Similarly, several methods have been proposed that describe automatic localization of anatomical landmark points (e.g. [5,9]). Moreover, clinical work often requires localization of specific anatomical regions that are visualized in a specific image slice. For example specific slices are chosen to analyze body composition in population studies to e.g. quantify sarcopenia, myopenia, or visceral obesity [10]. This requires an expert to scroll through a 3D medical image to identify the slice of interest before analysis. Such cases would benefit from automatic slice identification.

© Springer International Publishing AG 2016
G. Carneiro et al. (Eds.): LABELS 2016/DLMIA 2016, LNCS 10008, pp. 161–169, 2016.
DOI: 10.1007/978-3-319-46976-8_17

In this work we propose a method to automatically identify a single slice of interest (SOI) in a 3D medical image with a convolutional neural network (ConvNet) regressor. The ConvNet regressor is trained to compute a distance between every slice of a given image and the SOI. To obtain a smooth result, a first order polynomial is fitted through the obtained distances. The slice with zero distance indicates the SOI. Negative distances indicate slices located inferior to the SOI and positive distances indicate slices located superior to the SOI.

In this work the method was evaluated in two independent experiments in a set of 150 chest CT scans. In the first experiment the method was evaluated on identification of the axial slice that visualizes the aortic root, and in the second experiment on identification of the axial slice superior to the aortic arch.

2   Data

In this work 150 low-dose chest CT scans were randomly selected from a set of scans acquired at baseline in the National Lung Screening Trial (NLST) [1]. The scans were made during inspiratory breath-hold in supine position with the arms elevated above the head and without contrast enhancement. Scans were acquired on multiple scanners from four CT scanner vendors (General Electrics, Philips, Siemens, and Toshiba) and were reconstructed with soft or sharp reconstruction kernels and with varying image resolution (see Table 1). No ECG synchronization and no contrast enhancement were applied.

Table 1. Characteristics of the chest CT scans. Note the variability in resolution and number of slices per scan.

Number of scans	150
In plane voxel size (mm)	0.50–0.86
Slice increment (mm)	1.00–2.50
In plane matrix size	512×512
Number of slices	108–363

To define the reference, in each scan two slices of interest were manually identified (Fig. 1): the slice containing the aortic root, and the first slice superior to the aortic arch. The aortic root is a landmark that separates the heart from the aortic arch and can be used to e.g. locate the coronary ostia. The slice above the aortic arch is typically used as a landmark for body composition analysis.

3   Method

To automatically identify a SOI, a ConvNet regressor is trained with a set of CT scans. From every scan, all slices are extracted and provided to the ConvNet with its distance to the SOI. To identify a SOI in a test scan, all slices from the scan are extracted and evaluated by the ConvNet that outputs the relative

-2   -1   0   +1   +2

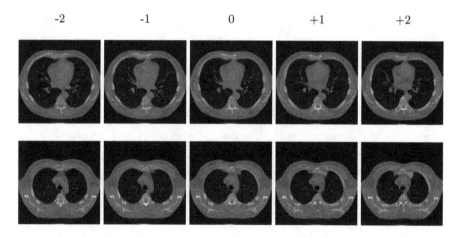

Fig. 1. Examples of CT slices adjacent to the slice of interest in localization of the aortic root (top) and slice superior to the aortic arch (bottom). For both examples, four consecutive slices are shown. The first two columns show slices two and one inferior to the slice of interest, respectively. The middle column shows the slice of interest. The last two columns show one and two slices superior to the slice of interest, respectively. Note the similarity in consecutive slices; this illustrates the difficulty of identifying a single slice of interest.

distance to the SOI. The SOI receives zero distance, slices inferior have a negative distance, and slices superior to the SOI have a positive distance. To ensure a smooth result, a first order polynomial is fitted through the ConvNet outputs (Fig. 2).

The employed ConvNet regressor consists of five convolutional layers and two fully connected layers, and a single node as output. It uses (2×2) strided convolutions to reduce feature-map sizes, batch normalization [6] in each layer to speed up training, and it uses exponential linear units [3] for activation (except for the output layer). The output layer provides the distance (in mm) to the SOI without providing image resolution to the network. See Fig. 3 for the complete architecture.

The CT scans used in this study were randomly divided into a training set of 75 scans (14,707 slices) and a validation set of 25 scans (3,784 slices). An independent set of 50 scans (10,100 slices) was used to test the method and it was not used during development of the method.

Before analysis, slices were downsampled by a factor of four with linear interpolation. Resampling the slices to a lower resolution reduced the number of necessary parameters of the ConvNet, but it still allowed to distinguish anatomy in the slices. In addition, during training, slices were randomly cropped to 112×112 pixels and randomly rotated between $-10°$ and $10°$ to allow the ConvNet to learn plausible variations of the positions of a subject in the scanner. During validation and testing the slices were evenly cropped around all borders, but not rotated.

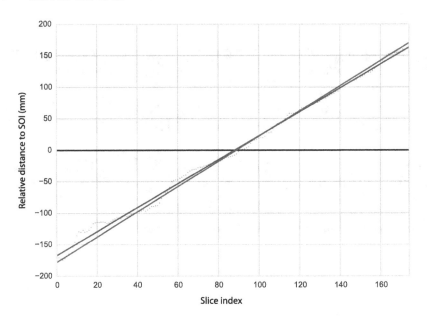

Fig. 2. Result of automatic slice identification. The plot shows slice indices on the x-axis and distances to the target slice in mm on the y-axis. The reference distance to the target slice is plotted in green. The target slice index is located at the intersection of the green line with the x-axis. The predicted distances are indicated as blue dots, with the fitted polynomial as a blue line. Note that negative distances indicate slice positions inferior to the target slice, and positive distances indicate positions superior to the target slice. (Color figure online)

During training, the ConvNet regressor was randomly presented axial slices in mini-batches of 100 slices in 100 epochs. Per epoch, all slices of the training set were presented once to the ConvNet. The distance of the extracted slice to the target slice was given as the target regression value. Adam [7] was used with a learning rate of 0.001 to minimize the mean squared distance to the target regression value. After each epoch the mean squared distance was evaluated on the validation set and the best performing model was chosen.

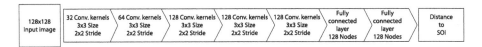

Fig. 3. Architecture of the convolutional neural network regressor. The network expects input image slices of 128×128 pixels. It consists of five layers with strided convolutions, two layers that are fully connected, and a single output node. In each layer batch normalization and exponential linear units are used, except in the output layer. The output layer provides the relative distance to the slice of interest (SOI) in mm.

4   Results

Table 2 lists the obtained results of the method on the independent test set of 50 scans. The results show that for both tasks the automatic methods find slices that are on average less than 4 slices from the SOI. For both tasks, the method tended to automatically select slices slightly inferior to the reference slice. This bias is also shown in Fig. 4, which shows boxplots of all automatic results. Using distance (in mm) as an evaluation criterion, the results of identification of the slice that visualizes the aortic root show a narrower distribution than localization of the slice superior to the aortic arch, but it also has two outliers. When using number of slices as evaluation criterion, the distribution of the results is similar for both tasks. This difference in the distributions is caused by the difference in image resolution, caused by variation in slice increment among the analyzed images.

Table 2. Mean distances and standard deviations (std) between the automatically identified slices and the reference slices. Distances are given in millimeters and number of slices. The first and second rows show the mean of the relative distances of the estimated slice to the slice of interest (SOI), with negative numbers indicating estimations inferior to the SOI, and positive numbers indicating estimations superior to the SOI. The third and fourth rows show the mean of absolute distances of the estimated slices to the SOI.

	Aortic root	Aortic arch sup
Distance in mm (std)	−1.51 (8.00)	−1.78 (7.03)
Distance in slices (std)	−0.82 (6.26)	−1.37 (5.20)
Absolute distance in mm (std)	5.74 (5.65)	5.59 (4.55)
Absolute distance in slices (std)	4.02 (4.83)	3.72 (3.85)

In 12 % of the scans the method identified the correct slice, the method was one slice off in 19 %, and two slices off in 16 %. Furthermore, in the case of larger errors the method still produced sensible results: see Fig. 5 showing the four largest errors of the method. All these errors were caused by the offset of the fitted polynomial with respect to the reference.

5   Discussion

The results show that automatic slice identification is feasible with the proposed method in chest CT.

The chest CTs used in this study show large variability with respect to image acquisition (e.g. CT scanner and patient positioning) and reconstruction (e.g. reconstruction kernel and image resolution). In addition, the scans are part of a screening study and were therefore acquired with low radiation dose and without

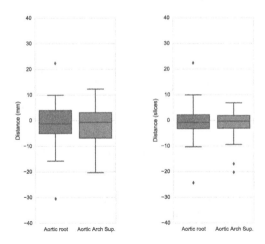

Fig. 4. Boxplots of the distances in mm (left) and in number of slices (right) between the automatically identified slices and the reference slices of interest. Negative distances indicate that the predicted slice is inferior to the reference slice. Positive distances indicate that the predicted slice is located superior to the reference slice.

contrast enhancement. Hence, the scans contained high noise levels and low soft tissue contrast. Furthermore, no ECG-synchronization was applied, so scans contained cardiac motion artifacts, especially in the slices that visualize the aortic root. Nevertheless, the results are comparable between the two tasks and showed that in 47 % of the scans the distance to the target slice was within 2 slices. The tasks were not very stringently defined, and given the variation in anatomy among subjects and slice thickness, the obtained results are likely similar to the interobserver variability (see Fig. 1). In this study, only a single observer defined the reference standard. In the future work, we aim to establish agreement among observers.

Our ConvNet follows the architecture of popular networks like AlexNet [8] and VGG-net [2]; it has an increasing number of kernels and two fully connected layers. Different architecture could also be used, but likely performance would not change dramatically if the same training set would be employed. Furthermore, in our experiments a relatively small set of 75 CT scans, each scan containing about 150 slices was used for training. ConvNets are known for achieving excellent results when trained with a large set of images. Possibly, performance could be further improved by increasing the training set size that would cover a range of anatomical variations and variotions in image acquisition. Also, in future work, we will investigate whether performance could reach an expert level when trained with a substantially larger data set.

Even though Fig. 5 shows the largest errors, it illustrates the most common errors in the experiments. Either the fitted polynomial runs parallel to the reference, which indicates a correct estimation of the subject's length, or the fitted polynomial has a different slope, which indicates incorrect estimation of the

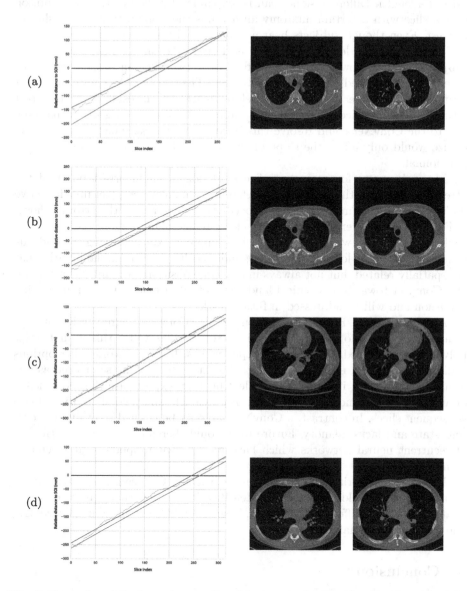

Fig. 5. Examples of the largest errors found in automatic slice identification. The left column shows predicted (blue) and reference distances (green). The middle column shows the reference slices of interest (SOIs). The right column shows the automatically selected slices. The two largest errors in detecting the slices of interest that visualize the aortic root are shown in (a) (−30.44 mm) and (b) (2.40 mm). The two largest errors in selecting the slice superior to the aortic arch are shown in (c) (−20.29 mm) and (d) (−16.92 mm). Except for the results in (a), the fitted slopes run parallel to the reference slope. Both errors (b) and (d) occured in the same scan. (Color figure online)

subject's length. Different slopes can be explained by the incorrect assumption that a slice with a certain anatomy always has the same distance to a slice of interest. Even though subjects bear an anatomical resemblance, they are often of different size and length. The here used chest CTs are acquired so that the subject's chest is shown in the full field of view, regardless of patient size. Also, slice increment varied among the used scans. These may have caused incorrect estimation of a subject's size and therefore length, which results in an incorrect estimation of distance to the slice of interest. Adding voxel sizes as parameters to the ConvNet could resolve this issue. Nevertheless, incorrect estimation of size would only affect the slope of the polynomial and not the offset of the polynomial.

The only cause for erroneous slice detection is an incorrect offset of the fitted polynomial with respect to the reference. An incorrect offset may have two underlying causes. First, the fitting procedure could generate the error as shown in Fig. 5d, where determined distances closer to the SOI are more precise, which could be resolved by weighing distant slices differently during fitting. Second, the ConvNet could have learned to also respond on other anatomical landmarks that are spatially related, but not always in the same position. Guiding the attention of a ConvNet towards anatomical landmarks of interest would be an interesting extension and will be addressed in future work.

As illustrated in Fig. 5a, the output of the ConvNet regressor is not necessarily strictly monotonically increasing. To compensate for this, a first order polynomial was fitted through the output values. In future work other options could be considered, especially those taking into account the sequential aspect of image slices. E.g., in manual slice identification, experts use their knowledge of anatomy and memorize information of previously analyzed slices to evaluate subsequent slices. In contrast, a ConvNet can only be trained to evaluate a current state and lacks memory. Future work could therefore benefit from the use of recurrent neural networks which have an inherent property that resembles memory.

Finally, the algorithm has been tested in chest CT scans only. We expect that the method could be applied for identification of slices that contain different anatomies or have different orientation, in scans of different anatomical coverage, and in different modalities.

6   Conclusion

Automatic identification of slices of interest in 3D medical images can be achieved with a convolutional neural network regressor. For each slice extracted from an image the regressor determines the distance to the slice of interest. The proposed method might be used for slice identification in medical image analysis.

Acknowledgments. This study was funded by the Netherlands Organization for Scientific Research (NWO)/Foundation for Technology Sciences (STW); Project 12726.

The authors thank the National Cancer Institute for access to NCI's data collected by the National Lung Screening Trial. The statements contained herein are solely those of the authors and do not represent or imply concurrence or endorsement by NCI.

The authors gratefully acknowledge the support of NVIDIA Corporation with the donation of the Tesla K40 GPU used for this research.

References

1. The National Lung Screening Trial: Overview and study design. Radiology **258**(1),243–253 (2011)
2. Chatfield, K., Simonyan, K., Vedaldi, A., Zisserman, A.: Return of the devil in the details: delving deep into convolutional nets. arXiv preprint arXiv:1405.3531 (2014)
3. Clevert, D.A., Unterthiner, T., Hochreiter, S.: Fast and Accurate Deep Network Learning by Exponential Linear Units (ELUs). arXiv:1511.07289 [cs], November 2015
4. Criminisi, A., Robertson, D., Konukoglu, E., Shotton, J., Pathak, S., White, S., Siddiqui, K.: Regression forests for efficient anatomy detection and localization in computed tomography scans. Med. Image Anal. **17**(8), 1293–1303 (2013)
5. Han, D., Gao, Y., Wu, G., Yap, P.T., Shen, D.: Robust anatomical landmark detection with application to MR brain image registration. Comput. Med. Imaging Graph. **46**, 277–290 (2015). Part 3
6. Ioffe, S., Szegedy, C.: Batch normalization: accelerating deep network training by reducing internal covariate shift. JMLR **37** (2015)
7. Kingma, D., Ba, J.: Adam: A Method for Stochastic Optimization. arXiv:1412.6980 [cs], December 2014
8. Krizhevsky, A., Sutskever, I., Hinton, G.E.: Imagenet classification with deep convolutional neural networks. In: Advances in Neural Information Processing Systems, pp. 1097–1105 (2012)
9. Liu, D., Zhou, S.K.: Anatomical landmark detection using nearest neighbor matching and submodular optimization. In: Ayache, N., Delingette, H., Golland, P., Mori, K. (eds.) MICCAI 2012, Part III. LNCS, vol. 7512, pp. 393–401. Springer, Heidelberg (2012)
10. Malietzis, G., Aziz, O., Bagnall, N., Johns, N., Fearon, K., Jenkins, J.: The role of body composition evaluation by computerized tomography in determining colorectal cancer treatment outcomes: a systematic review. Eur. J. Surg. Oncol. (EJSO) **41**(2), 186–196 (2015)
11. Zheng, Y., Georgescu, B., Comaniciu, D.: Marginal space learning for efficient detection of 2D/3D anatomical structures in medical images. In: Prince, J.L., Pham, D.L., Myers, K.J. (eds.) IPMI 2009. LNCS, vol. 5636, pp. 411–422. Springer, Heidelberg (2009)

Estimating CT Image from MRI Data Using 3D Fully Convolutional Networks

Dong Nie[1,2], Xiaohuan Cao[1,3], Yaozong Gao[1,2],
Li Wang[1], and Dinggang Shen[1(✉)]

[1] Department of Radiology and BRIC,
University of North Carolina at Chapel Hill, Chapel Hill, USA
dgshen@med.unc.edu
[2] Department of Computer Science,
University of North Carolina at Chapel Hill, Chapel Hill, USA
[3] School of Automation, Northwestern Polytechnical University, Xian, China

Abstract. Computed tomography (CT) is critical for various clinical applications, e.g., radiotherapy treatment planning and also PET attenuation correction. However, CT exposes radiation during CT imaging, which may cause side effects to patients. Compared to CT, magnetic resonance imaging (MRI) is much safer and does not involve any radiation. Therefore, recently researchers are greatly motivated to estimate CT image from its corresponding MR image of the same subject for the case of radiotherapy planning. In this paper, we propose a 3D deep learning based method to address this challenging problem. Specifically, a 3D fully convolutional neural network (FCN) is adopted to learn an end-to-end nonlinear mapping from MR image to CT image. Compared to the conventional convolutional neural network (CNN), FCN generates structured output and can better preserve the neighborhood information in the predicted CT image. We have validated our method in a real pelvic CT/MRI dataset. Experimental results show that our method is accurate and robust for predicting CT image from MRI image, and also outperforms three state-of-the-art methods under comparison. In addition, the parameters, such as network depth and activation function, are extensively studied to give an insight for deep learning based regression tasks in our application.

1 Introduction

Computed tomography (CT) imaging is widely used for both diagnostic and therapeutic purposes in various clinical applications. In the cancer radiation therapy, CT image provides Hounsfield units, which is essential for dose calculation in treatment planning. Besides, CT image is also of great importance for attenuation correction of positron emission tomography (PET) in the popular PET-CT scanner [8].

However, patients are exposed to radiation during CT imaging, which can damage normal body cells and further increase potential risks of cancer. Brenner and Hall [1] reported that 0.4 % of cancers were due to CT scanning performed

© Springer International Publishing AG 2016
G. Carneiro et al. (Eds.): LABELS 2016/DLMIA 2016, LNCS 10008, pp. 170–178, 2016.
DOI: 10.1007/978-3-319-46976-8_18

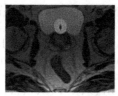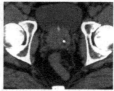

Fig. 1. A pair of corresponding pelvic MR (left) and CT (right) images from the same subject.

in the past, and this rate will increase to as high as 1.5 to 2 % in the future. Therefore, the use of CT scan should be with great caution. Magnetic resonance imaging (MRI) is a safe imaging protocol. It also provides more anatomical details than CT for diagnostic purpose, but unfortunately cannot be used for either dose calculation or attenuation correction. To reduce unnecessary imaging dose for patients, it is clinically desired to estimate CT image from MR image in many applications.

It is technically difficult to directly estimate CT image from MR image. As shown in Fig. 1, CT and MR images have very different appearances. For example, in CT image, the intensity difference between the prostate and bladder is much smaller than that in MR image. Besides, MR image contains richer texture information than CT image. Therefore, it is challenging to directly estimate a mapping from MRI intensity to CT intensity.

Recently, many researches focus on estimating one modal image from another modality image, e.g., estimating CT image using MRI data. (a) The first category is atlas-based method. These methods first register an atlas (with the attenuation map) to the new subject MR image, and then warp the corresponding attenuation map of atlas to the new MR image as its estimated attenuation map of atlas to the new MR image as its estimated attenuation map [2,3]. However, the performance of these atlas-based methods highly depends on the registration accuracy. (b) The second category is learning-based method, in which non-linear model is learnt from MRI to CT image. Huynh et al. [5] presented an approach to predict CT image from MRI using structured random forest. Such methods often have to first represent the input MR image by features and then map features to output CT image. Thus, the performance of these methods is bound to the quality of feature extraction.

On the other hand, recently the convolutional neural network (CNN) [9] becomes popular in both computer vision and medical imaging fields. As a multi-layer and fully trainable model, CNN is able to capture the complex non-linear mapping from the input space to the output space. For the case of 2D image, 2D CNN has been widely used in many applications. However, it is unreasonable to directly apply 2D CNN to process 3D medical images because 2D CNN considers the image appearance slice by slice, thus potentially causing discontinuous prediction results across slices. To address this issue, 3D CNNs have been proposed. Ji et al. [6] presented a 3D CNN model for action recognition in an uncontrolled environment. Tran et al. [13] used 3D CNN to effectively learn spatio-temporal features on a large-scale video dataset. Li et al. [11] applied deep learning models to estimate the missing PET image from the MR image of the same subject.

In this paper, we propose to learn the non-linear mapping from MR to CT images through a 3D fully convolutional neural network (FCN), which is a variation of the conventional CNN. Compared to CNN, FCN generates the structured output, which can better preserve the neighborhood information in the predicted CT image [12]. Specifically, an input MR image is first partitioned into overlapping patches. For each patch, FCN is used to predict the corresponding CT patch. Finally, all predicted CT patches are merged into a single CT image by averaging the intensities of overlapping CT regions. The proposed method is evaluated on a real pelvic CT/MR dataset. Experimental results demonstrate that our method can effectively predict CT image from MR image, and also outperforms three state-of-the-art methods under the comparison. Besides, extensive experiments have been conducted to validate the choice of several key parameters in the FCN, such as network depth and activation function. These parameter evaluation results provide good insight for other regression applications using deep learning.

2   Methods

Deep learning model can learn a hierarchy of features, i.e., high-level features built upon low-level features. CNN [4,9] is one popular type of deep learning models, in which trainable filters and local neighborhood pooling operations are applied in an alternating sequence starting with the raw input images. When trained with appropriate regularization, CNN can achieve superior performance on visual object recognition and image classification tasks [10]. However, most of CNNs are designed for 2D natural images. They are not well suited for medical image analysis, since most of medical images are 3D volumetric images, such as MRI, CT and PET. Compared to 2D CNN, 3D CNN can better model the 3D spatial information due to the use of 3D convolution operations. 3D convolution preserves the spatial neighborhood of 3D image. As a result, 3D CNN can solve the discontinuity problem across slices, which are suffered by 2D CNN. Mathematically, the 3D convolution operation is given by Eq. 1

$$a_{ij}(x,y,z) = f\left(\sum_{c=1}^{C}\sum_{p=0}^{P_i-1}\sum_{q=0}^{Q_i-1}\sum_{r=0}^{R_i-1} W_{ijc}(x,y,z)a_{(i-1)c}(x+p,y+q,z+r)\right)$$

(1)

where x, y, z denotes the 3D voxel position. W is a 3D filter. a is a 3D feature map from the previous $(i-1)$-th layer. Initially, a is the input MRI patch. c and C is the index and number of feature maps in the previous layer. i and j are the layer index and filter index, respectively. P_i, Q_i and R_i are the dimensions of the i-th filter in 3D space, respectively. f is an activation function that encodes the non-linearity in the CNN.

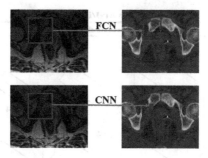

Fig. 2. Illustration of difference between FCN and CNN. The left column shows MR slices, and the right one shows corresponding CT slices.

Structured CNN - FCN: The output of conventional CNN is a single target value, which is unable to preserve neighborhood information in the output space. In this paper, we propose to use FCN to produce the structured output. Instead of predicting the CT intensity voxel by voxel, we use FCN to estimate the CT image in a patch-by-patch manner, as shown in Fig. 2. Compared to using CNN for voxel-wise CT prediction, using FCN for patch-wise CT prediction has several obvious advantages. First, the neighborhood information can be preserved in each predicted CT patch. Second, the prediction efficiency can be greatly improved since a entire CT patch can be predicted by a single pass of forward propagation in the neural network.

In the following paragraphs, we will describe the network architecture of FCN used in the MRI-to-CT prediction. Compared to the conventional CNN, the pooling layers are not used in this application. This is because the pooling layers often reduce the spatial resolution of feature maps. Although this property is desirable for tasks, such as image classification, since the pooling over local neighborhood could enhance invariance to certain image distortions, it is not desired in the task of image prediction, where subtle image distortions need to be precisely captured in the prediction process.

3D FCN for Estimating CT Images from MRI Data: Based on the 3D convolution described above, a variety of FCN architectures can be devised. In the following, we describe a 3D FCN architecture, as shown in Fig. 3, for estimating CT patch from MR patch. The training data for this CNN model consists of patches extracted from subjects with both MR and CT images. The size of input MRI patch is $32 \times 32 \times 16$ and the size of output CT patch is $24 \times 24 \times 12$. The input and output patches are in correspondence, which means that they share the same center position in their aligned image space. To generate training samples for FCN, we randomly extracted a large number of patches from 3D MRI volume as inputs, and the corresponding CT image patches as outputs. Patches that cross the boundaries or locate completely in the background were removed. The total number of patches extracted from each volume was 6000, which was sufficient to cover majority of the 3D image volume.

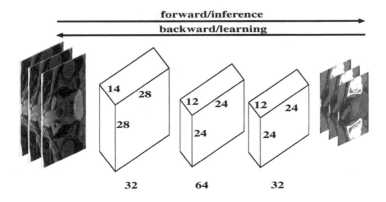

Fig. 3. The 3D FCN architecture for estimating CT image from MRI image.

In the FCN architecture, we first apply 3-D convolution with a filter size of $7 \times 7 \times 3$ on the input MRI patch to construct 32 feature maps in the first hidden layer. One voxel is padded along the first two dimensions. In the second layer, the outputs of the first layer are fed into another convolutional layer with 64 filters of size $5 \times 5 \times 3$. The third convolutional layer contains 32 feature maps. Each of the feature maps is connected to all the input feature maps through filters of size $3 \times 3 \times 3$. The output layer contains only one feature map generated by 1 filter of size $3 \times 3 \times 3$, and it corresponds to the predicted CT image patch. To keep the same image size, one voxel is padded along three dimensions in the last two layers. In all layers, we set stride as one voxel. The latent nonlinear relationship between MR and CT images is encoded by the large number of parameters in the network.

Caffe [7] is modified to implement the architecture shown in Fig. 3. The network parameters of FCN are updated by back-propagation using stochastic gradient descent algorithm. To train the network, the model hyper-parameters need to be appropriately determined. Specifically, the network weights are initialized by xavier algorithm [4], which can automatically determine the scale of initialization based on the number of input and output neurons. For the network bias, we initialize it to be 0. The initial learning rate and weight decay parameter are determined by conducting a coarse line search, followed by decreasing the learning rate during training. In particular, we have approximately 200,000 training patches. A Titan X GPU is utilized to train the network.

3   Experiments and Results

Data Acquisition and Preprocessing: Our pelvic dataset consists of 22 subjects, each with MR and CT images. The spacings of CT and MR images are $1.172 \times 1.172 \times 1$ mm^3 and $1 \times 1 \times 1$ mm^3, respectively. In the training stage, CT image is manually aligned to its corresponding MR image to build voxel-wise correspondences. After alignment, CT and MR images of the same subjects have the same image size and spacing. Since only pelvic regions are concerned in this study, we further crop the aligned CT and MR images to reduce the computational burden. Finally, each preprocessed image has a size of $153 \times 193 \times 50$ and a spacing of $1 \times 1 \times 1$ mm^3. A typical example of preprocessed CT and MR images is given in Fig. 1.

Parameter Selection of FCN: We evaluate the proposed method on 22 subjects in a leave-one-out cross validation. In our implementation, we adopt FCN to learn the nonlinear mapping from MR image to CT image. There are several factors that could affect the learning process, such as activation function, network depth, the number of filters in each layer and so on. In this paper, we evaluate the effect of different network depths and activation functions in learning this nonlinear mapping. In particular, three popular nonlinear functions are explored, which are the rectified linear units (Relu), sigmoid and tanh functions, respectively. The performance of FCN under different activation functions is shown in Fig. 4. In addition, we also analyze the impact of FCN under different network depths in Fig. 4. The experimental results show that with the Relu activation function, the performance of FCN gradually increases as the increase of network depth. However, for both sigmoid and tanh activation function, PSNR decreases with a deeper network. The best results are obtained with a shallow network (2-layer/3-layer). A simple interpretation is that sigmoid/tanh may suffer from gradient vanishing problem in a deep network although layer-wise training is used, while the Relu does not suffer such problem. The bad performance of Relu is due to the limited nonlinearity of Relu compared to two other activation functions. By increasing the network depth, the nonlinearity can be effectively increased, which renders the improved performance of Relu as the depth increases.

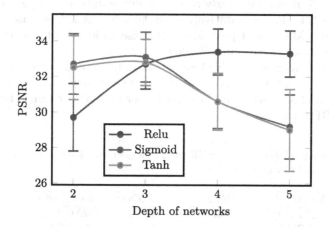

Fig. 4. Sensitivity analysis of 3 activation functions with respect to network depth.

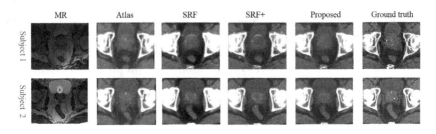

Fig. 5. Visual comparison of original MR images, the estimated CT images by our method and the ground truth CT images on 2 subjects.

Experimental Results: To demonstrate the advantage of the proposed method in terms of prediction accuracy, we compare our method with three widely used approaches:

- Atlas-based method (**Atlas**): Here, the MR image of each atlas is first aligned [15] onto the target MR image, and the resulting deformation field is used to warp the CT image of each atlas. The final prediction is obtained by averaging all warped CT images of all atlases.
- Structured Random forest based method (**SRF**): Structured random forest [5] was used to learn a nonlinear mapping between MR image and its corresponding CT image.
- Structured random forest and auto-context model (**SRF+**) based method: Besides the structured random forest, auto-context model (ACM) [14] is further used to iteratively refine the prediction of CT images.

The prediction results by different methods on two typical MR images are shown in Fig. 5. It can be clearly seen that our results are consistent with the ground-truth CT. To quantitatively evaluate our method, we use both mean absolute error (MAE) and peak signal-to-noise ratio (PSNR) to measure the prediction accuracy, as shown in Table 1.

Quantitative results in Table 1 show that our method outperforms other 3 methods in terms of both MAE and PSNR. Specifically, our method gives an average PSNR of 33.4, which is obviously better than 32.1 obtained by the state-of-the-art SRF+ method.

Table 1. Average of MAE and PSNR on 22 subjects by 4 different methods: Atlas, SRF, SRF+, and FCN (Proposed).

MAE	Mean(std.)	Med.	**PSNR**	Mean(std.)	Med.
Atlas	66.1(6.9)	66.7	Atlas	29.0(2.1)	29.6
SRF	51.2(3.8)	51.5	SRF	31.7(0.9)	31.8
SRF+	48.1(4.6)	48.3	SRF+	32.1(0.9)	31.8
FCN	**42.4(5.1)**	**42.6**	FCN	**33.4(1.1)**	**33.2**

4   Conclusions

We have developed a 3D FCN model for estimating CT images from MRI images by directly taking MR image patches as input and CT patches as output. The nonlinear relationship between two imaging modalities is captured by a large number of trainable mapping and parameters in the network. We have applied this model to predict CT images from their corresponding MR images. Experiments demonstrate that our proposed method can significantly outperform the three state-of-the-art methods. We also conduct a simple exploration for the important factors in the deep learning regression, which gives an insight of parameter selection in other related regression tasks. Although we considered the FCN model for CT image prediction, this model can also be applied to other related tasks. In our future works, we will explore ways of expediting the computation and designing more effective deep learning models to improve the prediction speed and accuracy.

References

1. Brenner, D.J., Hall, E.J.: Computed tomography an increasing source of radiation exposure. N. Engl. J. Med. **357**(22), 2277–2284 (2007)
2. Burgos, N., et al.: Robust CT synthesis for radiotherapy planning: application to the head and neck region. In: Navab, N., Hornegger, J., Wells, W.M., Frangi, A.F. (eds.) MICCAI 2015. LNCS, vol. 9350, pp. 476–484. Springer, Heidelberg (2015)
3. Catana, C., et al.: Toward implementing an MRI-based PET attenuation-correction method for neurologic studies on the MR-PET brain prototype. J. Nucl. Med. **51**(9), 1431–1438 (2010)
4. Glorot, X., Bengio, Y.: Understanding the difficulty of training deep feedforward neural networks. In: International Conference on Artificial Intelligence and Statistics, pp. 249–256 (2010)
5. Huynh, T., et al.: Estimating CT image from MRI data using structured random forest and auto-context model (2015)
6. Ji, S., et al.: 3D convolutional neural networks for human action recognition. IEEE Trans. Pattern Anal. Mach. Intell. **35**(1), 221–231 (2013)
7. Jia, Y., et al.: Caffe: convolutional architecture for fast feature embedding. In: Proceedings of the ACM International Conference on Multimedia, pp. 675–678. ACM (2014)
8. Kinahan, P.E., et al.: Attenuation correction for a combined 3D PET/CT scanner. Med. Phys. **25**(10), 2046–2053 (1998)
9. LeCun, Y., et al.: Deep learning. Nature **521**(7553), 436–444 (2015)
10. LeCun, Y., et al.: Gradient-based learning applied to document recognition. Proc. IEEE **86**(11), 2278–2324 (1998)
11. Li, R., Zhang, W., Suk, H.-I., Wang, L., Li, J., Shen, D., Ji, S.: Deep learning based imaging data completion for improved brain disease diagnosis. In: Golland, P., Hata, N., Barillot, C., Hornegger, J., Howe, R. (eds.) MICCAI 2014, Part III. LNCS, vol. 8675, pp. 305–312. Springer, Heidelberg (2014)
12. Nie, D., Wang, L., Gao, Y., Sken, D.: Fully convolutional networks for multi-modality isointense infant brain image segmentation. In: IEEE 13th International Symposium on Biomedical Imaging (ISBI), pp. 1342–1345. IEEE (2016)

13. Tran, D., et al.: Learning spatiotemporal features with 3D convolutional networks. arXiv preprint arXiv:1412.0767 (2014)
14. Zhuowen, T., et al.: Auto-context and its application to high-level vision tasks and 3D brain image segmentation. IEEE Trans. Pattern Anal. Mach. Intell. **32**(10), 1744–1757 (2010)
15. Vercauteren, T., et al.: Diffeomorphic demons: efficient non-parametric image registration. NeuroImage **45**(1), S61–S72 (2009)

The Importance of Skip Connections in Biomedical Image Segmentation

Michal Drozdzal[1,2]([✉]), Eugene Vorontsov[1,2]([✉]), Gabriel Chartrand[1,3], Samuel Kadoury[2,4], and Chris Pal[2,5]

[1] Imagia Inc., Montréal, Canada
{michal,eugene,gabriel}@imagia.com
[2] École Polytechnique de Montréal, Montréal, Canada
{samuel.kadoury,christopher.pal}@polymtl.ca
[3] Université de Montréal, Montréal, Canada
[4] CHUM Research Center, Montréal, Canada
[5] Montreal Institute for Learning Algorithms, Montréal, Canada

Abstract. In this paper, we study the influence of both long and short skip connections on Fully Convolutional Networks (FCN) for biomedical image segmentation. In standard FCNs, only long skip connections are used to skip features from the contracting path to the expanding path in order to recover spatial information lost during downsampling. We extend FCNs by adding short skip connections, that are similar to the ones introduced in residual networks, in order to build very deep FCNs (of hundreds of layers). A review of the gradient flow confirms that for a very deep FCN it is beneficial to have both long and short skip connections. Finally, we show that a very deep FCN can achieve near-to-state-of-the-art results on the EM dataset without any further post-processing.

Keywords: Semantic segmentation · FCN · ResNet · Skip connections

1 Introduction

Semantic segmentation is an active area of research in medical image analysis. With the introduction of Convolutional Neural Networks (CNN), significant improvements in performance have been achieved in many standard datasets. For example, for the EM ISBI 2012 dataset [2], BRATS [13] or MS lesions [18], the top entries are built on CNNs [3,4,7,15].

All these methods are based on Fully Convolutional Networks (FCN) [12]. While CNNs are typically realized by a contracting path built from convolutional, pooling and fully connected layers, FCN adds an expanding path built with deconvolutional or unpooling layers. The expanding path recovers spatial information by merging features skipped from the various resolution levels on the contracting path.

M. Drozdzal and E. Vorontsov—Equal contribution.

© Springer International Publishing AG 2016
G. Carneiro et al. (Eds.): LABELS 2016/DLMIA 2016, LNCS 10008, pp. 179–187, 2016.
DOI: 10.1007/978-3-319-46976-8_19

Variants of these skip connections are proposed in the literature. In [12], upsampled feature maps are summed with feature maps skipped from the contractive path while [15] concatenate them and add convolutions and non-linearities between each upsampling step. These skip connections have been shown to help recover the full spatial resolution at the network output, making fully convolutional methods suitable for semantic segmentation. We refer to these skip connections as long skip connections.

Recently, significant network depth has been shown to be helpful for image classification [8,9,14,20]. The recent results suggest that depth can act as a regularizer [8]. However, network depth is limited by the issue of vanishing gradients when backpropagating the signal across many layers. In [20], this problem is addressed with additional levels of supervision, while in [8,9] skip connections are added around non-linearities, thus creating shortcuts through which the gradient can flow uninterrupted allowing parameters to be updated deep in the network. Moreover, [19] have shown that these skip connections allow for faster convergence during training. We refer to these skip connections as short skip connections.

In this paper, we explore deep, fully convolutional networks for semantic segmentation. We expand FCN by adding short skip connections that allow us to build very deep FCNs. With this setup, we perform an analysis of short and long skip connections on a standard biomedical dataset (EM ISBI 2012 challenge data). We observe that short skip connections speed up the convergence of the learning process; moreover, we show that a very deep architecture with a relatively small number of parameters can reach near-state-of-the-art performance on this dataset. Thus, the contributions of the paper can be summarized as follows:

- We extend Residual Networks to fully convolutional networks for semantic image segmentation (see Sect. 2).
- We show that a very deep network without any post-processing achieves performance comparable to the state of the art on EM data (see Sect. 3.1).
- We show that long and short skip connections are beneficial for convergence of very deep networks (see Sect. 3.2)

2   Residual Network for Semantic Image Segmentation

Our approach extends Residual Networks [8] to segmentation tasks by adding an expanding (upsampling) path (Fig. 1(a)). We perform spatial reduction along the contracting path (left) and expansion along the expanding path (right). As in [12,15], spatial information lost along the contracting path is recovered in the expanding path by skipping equal resolution features from the former to the latter. Similarly to the short skip connections in Residual Networks, we choose to sum the features on the expanding path with those skipped over the long skip connections.

We consider three types of blocks, each containing at least one convolution and activation function: bottleneck, basic block, simple block (Fig. 1(b)–(d)). Each block is capable of performing batch normalization on its inputs as well as spatial downsampling at the input (marked blue; used for the contracting path) and spatial upsampling at the output (marked yellow; for the expanding path). The bottleneck and basic block are based on those introduced in [8] which include short skip connections to skip the block input to its output with minimal modification, encouraging the path through the non-linearities to learn a residual representation of the input data. To minimize the modification of the input, we apply no transformations along the short skip connections, except when the number of filters or the spatial resolution needs to be adjusted to match the block output. We use 1×1 convolutions to adjust the number of filters but for spatial adjustment we rely on simple decimation or simple repetition of rows and columns of the input so as not to increase the number of parameters. We add an optional dropout layer to all blocks along the residual path.

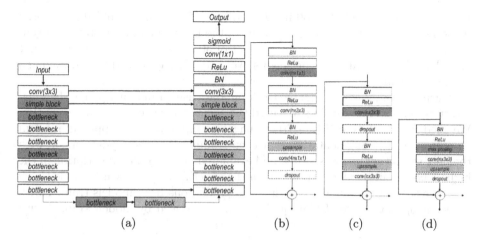

Fig. 1. An example of residual network for image segmentation. (a) Residual Network with long skip connections built from bottleneck blocks, (b) bottleneck block, (c) basic block and (d) simple block. Blue color indicates the blocks where an downsampling is optionally performed, yellow color depicts the (optional) upsampling blocks, dashed arrow in figures (b), (c) and (d) indicates possible long skip connections. Note that all blocks (b), (c) and (d) can have a dropout layer (depicted with dashed line rectangle). (Color figure online)

We experimented with both binary cross-entropy and dice loss functions. Let $o_i \in [0, 1]$ be the ith output of the last network layer passed through a sigmoid non-linearity and let $y_i \in \{0, 1\}$ be the corresponding label. The binary cross-entropy is then defined as follows:

$$L_{bce} = \sum_i y_i \log o_i + (1 - y_i) \log (1 - o_i) \tag{1}$$

The dice loss is:

$$L_{Dice} = -\frac{2 \sum_i o_i y_i}{\sum_i o_i + \sum_i y_i} \tag{2}$$

182   M. Drozdzal et al.

We implemented the model in Keras [5] using the Theano backend [1] and trained it using RMSprop [21] (learning rate 0.001) with weight decay set to 0.001. We also experimented with various levels of dropout.

3   Experiments

In this section, we test the model on electron microscopy (EM) data [2] (Sect. 3.1) and perform an analysis on the importance of the long and short skip connections (Sect. 3.2).

3.1   Segmenting EM Data

EM training data consist of 30 images (512 × 512 pixels) assembled from serial section transmission electron microscopy of the Drosophila first instar larva ventral nerve cord. The test set is another set of 30 images for which labels are not provided. Throughout the experiments, we used 25 images for training, leaving 5 images for validation.

During training, we augmented the input data using random flipping, sheering, rotations, and spline warping. We used the same spline warping strategy as [15]. We used full resolution (512 × 512) images as input without applying random cropping for data augmentation. For each training run, the model version with the best validation loss was stored and evaluated. The detailed description of the highest performing architecture used in the experiments is shown in Table 1.

Interestingly, we found that while the predictions from models trained with cross-entropy loss were of high quality, those produced by models trained with

Table 1. Detailed model architecture used in the experiments. Repetition number indicates the number of times the block is repeated.

Layer name	Block type	Output resolution	Output width	Repetition number
Down 1	conv 3 × 3	512 × 512	32	1
Down 2	simple block	256 × 256	32	1
Down 3	bottleneck	128 × 128	128	3
Down 4	bottleneck	64 × 64	256	8
Down 5	bottleneck	32 × 32	512	10
Across	bottleneck	32 × 32	1024	3
Up 1	bottleneck	64 × 64	512	10
Up 2	bottleneck	128 × 128	256	8
Up 3	bottleneck	256 × 256	128	3
Up 4	simple block	512 × 512	32	1
Up 5	conv 3 × 3	512 × 512	32	1
Classifier	conv 1 × 1	512 × 512	1	1

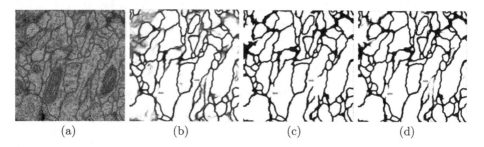

(a)   (b)   (c)   (d)

Fig. 2. Qualitative results on the test set. (a) original image, (b) prediction for a model trained with binary cross-entropy, (c) prediction of the model trained with dice loss and (d) model trained with dice loss with 0.2 dropout at the test time.

Table 2. Comparison to published entries for EM dataset. For full ranking of all submitted methods please refer to challenge web page: http://brainiac2.mit.edu/ isbi_challenge/leaders-board-new. We note the number of parameter, the use of post-processing, and the use of model averaging only for FCNs.

Method	V_{rand}	V_{info}	FCN	Post-processing	Average over	Parameters (M)
CUMedVision [4]	0.977	0.989	YES	YES	6	8
Unet [15]	0.973	0.987	YES	NO	7	33
IDSIA [6]	0.970	0.985	NO	-	-	-
motif [23]	0.972	0.985	NO	-	-	-
SCI [11]	0.971	0.982	NO	-	-	-
optree-idsia [22]	0.970	0.985	NO	-	-	-
PyraMiD-LSTM [17]	0.968	0.983	NO	-	-	-
Ours (L_{Dice})	0.969	0.986	YES	NO	Dropout	11
Ours (L_{bce})	0.957	0.980	YES	NO	1	11

the Dice loss appeared visually cleaner since they were almost binary; borders that would appear fuzzy in the former (see Fig. 2(b)) would be left as gaps in the latter (Fig. 2(c)). However, we found that the border continuity can be improved for models with the Dice loss by implicit model averaging over output samples drawn at test time, using dropout [10] (Fig. 2(d)). This yields better performance on the validation and test metrics than the output of models trained with binary cross-entropy (see Table 2).

Two metrics used in this dataset are: Maximal foreground-restricted Rand score after thinning (V_{rand}) and maximal foreground-restricted information theoretic score after thinning (V_{info}). For a detailed description of the metrics, please refer to [2].

Our results are comparable to other published results that establish the state of the art for the EM dataset (Table 2). Note that we did not do any post-processing of the resulting segmentations. We match the performance of UNet, for which predictions are averaged over seven rotations of the input images, while using less

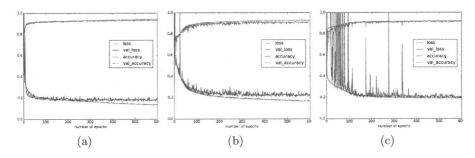

Fig. 3. Training and validation losses and accuracies for different network setups: (a) model 1: long and short skip connections enabled, (b) model 2: only short skip connections enabled and (c) model 3: only long skip connections enabled.

Table 3. Best validation loss and its corresponding training loss for each model.

Method	Training loss	Validation loss
Long and short skip connections	0.163	0.162
Only short skip connections	0.188	0.202
Only long skip connection	0.205	0.188

parameters and without sophisticated class weighting. Note that among other FCN available on the leader board, CUMedVision is using post-processing in order to boost performance.

3.2 On the Importance of Skip Connections

The focus in the paper is to evaluate the utility of long and short skip connections for training fully convolutional networks for image segmentation. In this section, we investigate the learning behavior of the model with short and with long skip connections, paying specific attention to parameter updates at each layer of the network. We first explored variants of our best performing deep architecture (from Table 1), using binary cross-entropy loss. Maintaining the same hyperparameters, we trained (Model 1) with long and short skip connections, (Model 2) with only short skip connections and (Model 3) with only long skip connections. Training curves are presented in Fig. 3 and the final loss and accuracy values on the training and the validation data are presented in Table 3.

We note that for our deep architecture, the variant with both long and short skip connections is not only the one that performs best but also converges faster than without short skip connections. This increase in convergence speed is consistent with the literature [19]. Not surprisingly, the combination of both long and short skip connections performed better than having only one type of skip connection, both in terms of performance and convergence speed. At this depth, a network could not be trained without any skip connections. Finally, short skip connections appear to stabilize updates (note the smoothness of the validation loss plots in Figs. 3(a) and (b) as compared to Fig. 3(c)).

We expect that layers closer to the center of the model can not be effectively updated due to the vanishing gradient problem which is alleviated by short skip connections. This identity shortcut effectively introduces shorter paths through fewer non-linearities to the deep layers of our models. We validate this empirically on a range of models of varying depth by visualizing the mean model parameter updates at each layer for each epoch (see sample results in Fig. 4). To simplify the analysis and visualization, we used simple blocks instead of bottleneck blocks.

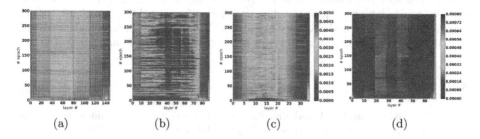

(a)   (b)   (c)   (d)

Fig. 4. Weight updates in different network setups: (a) the best performing model with long and short skip connections enabled, (b) only long skip connections enabled with 9 repetitions of simple block, (c) only long skip connections enabled with 3 repetitions of simple block and (d) only long skip connections enabled with 7 repetitions of simple block, without batch normalization. Note that due to a reduction in the learning rate for Figure (d), the scale is different compared to Figures (a), (b) and (c).

Parameter updates appear to be well distributed when short skip connections are present (Fig. 4(a)). When the short skip connections are removed, we find that for deep models, the deep parts of the network (at the center, Fig. 4(b)) get few updates, as expected. When long skip connections are retained, at least the shallow parts of the model can be updated (see both sides of Fig. 4(b)) as these connections provide shortcuts for gradient flow. Interestingly, we observed that model performance actually drops when using short skip connections in those models that are shallow enough for all layers to be well updated (eg. Figure 4(c)). Moreover, batch normalization was observed to increase the maximal updatable depth of the network. Networks without batch normalization had diminishing updates toward the center of the network and with long skip connections were less stable, requiring a lower learning rate (eg. Figure 4(d)).

It is also interesting to observe that the bulk of updates in all tested model variations (also visible in those shown in Fig. 4) were always initially near or at the classification layer. This follows the findings of [16], where it is shown that even randomly initialized weights can confer a surprisingly large portion of a model's performance after training only the classifier.

4   Conclusions

In this paper, we studied the influence of skip connections on FCN for biomedical image segmentation. We showed that a very deep network can achieve results near the state of the art on the EM dataset without any further post-processing. We confirm that although long skip connections provide a shortcut for gradient flow in shallow layers, they do not alleviate the vanishing gradient problem in deep networks. Consequently, we apply short skip connections to FCNs and confirm that this increases convergence speed and allows training of very deep networks.

Acknowledgements. We would like to thank all the developers of Theano and Keras for providing such powerful frameworks. We gratefully acknowledge NVIDIA for GPU donation to our lab at École Polytechnique. The authors would like to thank Lisa di Jorio, Adriana Romero and Nicolas Chapados for insightful discussions. This work was partially funded by Imagia Inc., MITACS (grant number IT05356) and MEDTEQ.

References

1. Al-Rfou, R., Alain, G., Almahairi, A., et al.: Theano: a python framework for fast computation of mathematical expressions. CoRR abs/1605.02688 (2016)
2. Arganda-Carreras, I., Turaga, S.C., Berger, D.R., et al.: Crowdsourcing the creation of image segmentation algorithms for connectomics. Front. Neuroanat. **9**, 142 (2015). doi:10.3389/fnana.2015.00142
3. Brosch, T., Tang, L.Y.W., Yoo, Y., et al.: Deep 3D convolutional encoder networks with shortcuts for multiscale feature integration applied to multiple sclerosis lesion segmentation. IEEE TMI **35**(5), 1229–1239 (2016)
4. Chen, H., Qi, X., Cheng, J., Heng, P.A.: Deep contextual networks for neuronal structure segmentation. In: Proceedings of the 13th AAAI Conference on Artificial Intelligence, 12–17 February 2016, Phoenix, Arizona, USA, pp. 1167–1173 (2016)
5. Chollet, F.: Keras (2015). https://github.com/fchollet/keras
6. Ciresan, D., Giusti, A., Gambardella, L.M., Schmidhuber, J.: Deep neural networks segment neuronal membranes in electron microscopy images. In: NIPS, vol. 25, pp. 2843–2851. Curran Associates, Inc. (2012)
7. Havaei, M., Davy, A., Warde-Farley, D., et al.: Brain tumor segmentation with deep neural networks. CoRR abs/1505.03540 (2015)
8. He, K., Zhang, X., Ren, S., Sun, J.: Deep residual learning for image recognition. CoRR abs/1512.03385 (2015)
9. He, K., Zhang, X., Ren, S., Sun, J.: Identity mappings in deep residual networks. CoRR abs/1603.05027 (2016)
10. Kendall, A., Badrinarayanan, V., Cipolla, R.: Bayesian segNet: model uncertainty in deep convolutional encoder-decoder architectures for scene understanding. CoRR abs/1511.02680 (2015)
11. Liu, T., Jones, C., Seyedhosseini, M., Tasdizen, T.: A modular hierarchical approach to 3D electron microscopy image segmentation. J. Neurosci. Methods **226**, 88–102 (2014)
12. Long, J., Shelhamer, E., Darrell, T.: Fully convolutional networks for semantic segmentation. In: CVPR, November 2015 (to appear)

13. Menze, B.H., Jakab, A., Bauer, S., et al.: The multimodal brain tumor image segmentation benchmark (BRATS). IEEE Trans. Med. Imaging **34**(10), 1993–2024 (2015). doi:10.1109/TMI.2014.2377694
14. Romero, A., Ballas, N., Kahou, S.E., Chassang, A., Gatta, C., Bengio, Y.: FitNets: hints for thin deep nets. CoRR abs/1412.6550 (2014)
15. Ronneberger, O., Fischer, P., Brox, T.: U-net: convolutional networks for biomedical image segmentation. CoRR abs/1505.04597 (2015)
16. Saxe, A., Koh, P.W., Chen, Z., Bhand, M., Suresh, B., Ng, A.Y.: On random weights and unsupervised feature learning. In: Getoor, L., Scheffer, T. (eds.) Proceedings of the 28th International Conference on Machine Learning (ICML-11), pp. 1089–1096. ACM, New York (2011)
17. Stollenga, M.F., Byeon, W., Liwicki, M., Schmidhuber, J.: Parallel multidimensional LSTM, with application to fast biomedical volumetric image segmentation. CoRR abs/1506.07452 (2015)
18. Styner, M., Lee, J., Chin, B., et al.: 3D segmentation in the clinic: a grand challenge II: MS lesion segmentation, November 2008
19. Szegedy, C., Ioffe, S., Vanhoucke, V.: Inception-v4, inception-resnet and the impact of residual connections on learning. CoRR abs/1602.07261 (2016)
20. Szegedy, C., Liu, W., Jia, Y., Sermanet, P., Reed, S.E., Anguelov, D., Erhan, D., Vanhoucke, V., Rabinovich, A.: Going deeper with convolutions. CoRR abs/1409.4842 (2014)
21. Tieleman, T., Hinton, G.: Lecture 6.5—RmsProp: divide the gradient by a running average of its recent magnitude. COURSERA: Neural Netw. Mach. Learn. (2012)
22. Uzunbaş, M.G., Chen, C., Metaxsas, D.: Optree: a learning-based adaptive watershed algorithm for neuron segmentation. In: Golland, P., Hata, N., Barillot, C., Hornegger, J., Howe, R. (eds.) MICCAI 2014, Part I. LNCS, vol. 8673, pp. 97–105. Springer International Publishing, Cham (2014)
23. Wu, X.: An iterative convolutional neural network algorithm improves electron microscopy image segmentation. CoRR abs/1506.05849 (2015)

Understanding the Mechanisms of Deep Transfer Learning for Medical Images

Hariharan Ravishankar, Prasad Sudhakar[✉],
Rahul Venkataramani, Sheshadri Thiruvenkadam, Pavan Annangi,
Narayanan Babu, and Vivek Vaidya

GE Global Research, Bangalore, India
prasad.sudhakar@ge.com

Abstract. The ability to automatically learn task specific feature representations has led to a huge success of deep learning methods. When large training data is scarce, such as in medical imaging problems, transfer learning has been very effective. In this paper, we systematically investigate the process of transferring a Convolutional Neural Network, trained on ImageNet images to perform image classification, to kidney detection problem in ultrasound images. We study how the detection performance depends on the extent of transfer. We show that a transferred and tuned CNN can outperform a state-of-the-art feature engineered pipeline and a hybridization of these two techniques achieves 20 % higher performance. We also investigate how the evolution of intermediate response images from our network. Finally, we compare these responses to state-of-the-art image processing filters in order to gain greater insight into how transfer learning is able to effectively manage widely varying imaging regimes.

1 Introduction

Automated organ localization and segmentation from ultrasound images is a challenging problem because of specular noise, low soft tissue contrast and wide variability of data from patient to patient. In such difficult problem settings, data driven machine learning methods, and especially deep learning methods in recent times, have found quite a bit of success. Usually, a large amount of labeled data is needed to train machine learning models and a careful feature engineering is required for each problem. The question of how much data is needed for satisfactory performance of these methods is still unanswered, with some recent works in this direction [7]. However, *transfer learning* has been successfully employed in data scarce situations, with model knowledge being effectively transferred across (possibly unrelated) tasks/domains. It is fascinating that a model, learnt for an unrelated problem setting can actually solve a problem at hand with minimal retraining. In this paper, we have attempted to demonstrate and understand the effectiveness and mechanism of transfer learning a CNN, originally learnt on camera images for image recognition, to solve the problem of automated kidney localization from ultrasound B-mode images.

G. Carneiro et al. (Eds.): LABELS 2016/DLMIA 2016, LNCS 10008, pp. 188–196, 2016.
DOI: 10.1007/978-3-319-46976-8_20

Kidney detection is challenging due to wide variability in its shape, size and orientation. Depending upon the acquisition scan plane, inconsistency in appearance of internal regions (renal sinus) and presence of adjacent structures like diaphragm, liver boundaries, etc. pose additional challenges. This is also a clinically relevant problem as kidney morphology measurements are essential in assessing renal abnormalities [13], planning and monitoring radiation therapy, and renal transplant.

There have been semi-automated and automated kidney detection approaches reported in literature. In [22], a texture model is built by an expectation maximization algorithm using features inferred from a bank of Gabor filters, followed by iterative segmentation to combine texture measures into parametric shape model. In [16], Markov random fields and active contour methods have been used to detect kidney boundaries in 3D ultrasound images. Recently, machine learning approaches [1,17] based on kidney texture analysis have proven successful for segmentation of kidney regions from 2-D and 3-D ultrasound images.

2   State of the Art

CNNs [15] provide effective models for vision learning tasks by incorporating spatial context and weight sharing between pixels. A typical deep CNN for a learning task has, as input, N channel image patches P_k of size $n_1 \times n_2$, where $P_k : \{1, 2, \cdots, n_1\} \times \{1, 2, \cdots, n_2\} \to D \subset \mathbb{R}$, $k = 1, 2, \cdots, N$. The output is M feature maps, $G_j \in \mathbb{R}^{m_1 \times m_2}$, $j = 1, 2, \cdots, M$, defined as convolutions using MN filters v_k^j, $(j = 1, 2, \cdots, M)$, $(k = 1, 2, \cdots, N)$ of size $S = s_1 \times s_2$, and M scalars b^j, $j = 1, 2, \cdots, M$. We then have:

$$G_j = \mathcal{S}_\downarrow \left(\sigma \left(\sum_k P_k * v_k^j + b^j \right) \right), j = 1, 2, \cdots, M. \qquad (1)$$

Here, $*$ denotes convolution, σ is a non-linear function (sigmoid or a linear cutoff (ReLU)). $\mathcal{S}_\downarrow$ is a down sampling operator. The number of feature maps, filter size, and size of the feature maps are hyperparameters in the above expression, with a total of $M(NS + 1)$ parameters that one has to optimize for a learning task. A deep CNN architecture is multi-layered, with the above expression being hierarchically stitched together, given the number of input/output maps, sizes of filters and maps for each layer, resulting in a huge number of parameters to be optimized. When data is scarce, the learning problem is under-determined and therefore transferring CNN parameters from a pre-learned model helps.

For medical image problems, transfer learning is additionally attractive due to the heterogeneity of data types (modalities, anatomies, etc.) and clinical challenges. In [4], the authors perform breast image classification using a CNN model trained on ImageNet. Shie et al. [18] employ the CaffeNet, trained on ImageNet, to extract features and classify Otitis Media images. In [6], a pre-trained CNN is used to extract features on ultrasound images to localize a certain standard plane that is important for diagnosis.

Studies on transferability of features across CNNs include [23] and more specifically [19,21] for medical images. While our work demonstrates yet another success of transfer learning for medical imaging and the tuning aspects of transfer learning, we

1. Reason out the effectiveness of transfer learning by methodically comparing the response maps from various layers of transfer learnt network with traditional image processing filters.
2. Investigate the effect of level of tuning on performance. We demonstrate that full network adaptation leads to learning problem specific features and also establishes the superiority over off-the-shelf image processing filters.
3. Re-establish the relevance and complementary advantages of state-of-the-art, hand-crafted features and merits of hybridisation approaches with CNNs, to help us achieve next level performance improvement [24].

3   Methods

From a set of training images, we build classifiers to differentiate between kidney and non-kidney regions. On a test image, the maximum likelihood detection problem of finding the best kidney region of interest (ROI) S^* from a set of candidate ROIs $\{S\}$ is split into two steps, similar to [3,17]. The entire set $\{S\}$ is passed through our classifier models and the candidates with positive class labels (Y) are retained (Eq. (2)). The ROI with highest likelihood (L) from the set $\{S^+\}$ is selected as the detected kidney region (Eq. (3))

$$\{Y, L\} = MLClassifier(S) \text{ and } \{S^+ \in S \mid Y = 1\}, \tag{2}$$

$$S^* = \arg\max(L^+), \text{ where } \{L^+ = L(S^+)\}. \tag{3}$$

We propose to employ CNNs as feature extractors similar to [10] to facilitate comparisons with traditional texture features. We also propose to use a well-known machine learning classifier, to evaluate performance of different feature sets, thereby eliminating the effects of having soft-max layer for CNNs and a different classifier on traditional features as our likelihood functions.

3.1   Dataset and Training

We considered a total of 90 long axis kidney images acquired on GE Healthcare LOGIQ E9 scanner, split into two equal and distinct sets, for training and validation. The images contained kidney of different sizes with lengths varying between 7.5 cm and 14 cm and widths varying between 3.5 cm and 7 cm, demonstrating wide variability in the dataset. The orientation of the kidneys varied between $-25°$ and $+15°$. The images were acquired at varying depths of ultrasound acquisition ranging between 9 cm and 16 cm. Accurate rectangular ground truth kidney ROIs were manually marked by a clinical expert.

To build our binary classification models from training images, we swept the field of view (FOV) to generate many overlapping patches of varying sizes

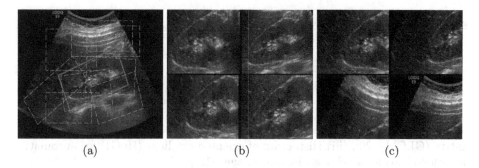

Fig. 1. (a) Sample generation (b) Positive patches (c) Negative patches

(see Fig. 1) that satisfied clinical guidelines on average adult kidney dimensions and aspect ratio [8]. We downsampled these ROIs to a common size and were further binned into two classes based on their overlap with ground truth annotations. We used Dice similarity coefficient (DSC) as the metric and a threshold of 0.8 (based on visual and clinical feedback) was used to generate positive and negative class samples. This was followed by feature extraction and model building.

3.2   Transfer Learned Features

Our study on transfer learning was based on adapting the popular CaffeNet [11] architecture built on ImageNet database to ultrasound kidney detection, whose simplified schematic is in Fig. 2. We extracted features after the 'fc7' layer from all the updated nets, resulting in 4096 features. The features extracted were:

1. **Full Network adaptation (CaffeNet_FA)** - Initialized with weights from CaffeNet parameters, the entire network weights were updated by training on kidney image samples from Sect. 3.1. The experiment settings were: stochastic gradient descent update with a batch size of 100, momentum of 0.5 and weight decay of 5×10^{-4}.
2. **Partial Network adaptation (CaffeNet_PA)** - To understand the performance difference based on level of tuning, we froze the weights of 'conv1' and 'conv2' layers, while updating the weights of other layers. The reasoning behind freezing the first two layers was to evaluate how sharable were the low-level features and also to help us in interpret-ability (Sect. 5). The experiment settings were same as those for full network adaptation.
3. **Zero Network adaptation (CaffeNet_NA)** - Finally, we also extracted features from the original CaffeNet model without modifying the weights.

3.3   Traditional Texture Features

Some of the well-studied texture features used for ultrasound images include (i) Haar features [3] for fetal anatomy studies, (ii) Gray Level Co-Occurrence

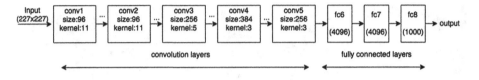

Fig. 2. Simple schematic of CaffeNet architecture [40]

Matrix (GLCM) [20], (iii) Histogram of oriented gradient (HoG) (for automatic view classification of echocardiogram images [12]).

Haar features have been reported to have the best performance for kidney detection n [17]. For our study, we extracted Haar features similar to [3], yielding a total of ∼2000 features.

3.4   Gradient Boosting Machine (GBM)

Ensemble classifiers have been shown to be successful in ultrasound organ detection problems. In [3], authors have used probabilistic boosting tree classifier for fetal anatomy detection. In [17], it has been noted that gradient boosting machine (GBM) have outperformed adaboost classfiers. In an empirical comparison study of supervised learning algorithms [5] comparing random forests and boosted decision trees, calibrated boosted trees had the best overall performance with random forests being close second. Motivated by these successes, we have chosen to use Gradient boosting tree as our classifier model. We build GBM classifiers for all the feature sets explained in Sects. 3.2 and 3.3 using GBM implementation inspired by [2], with parameters: shrinkage factor and sampling factor set to 0.5, maximum tree depth = 2 and number of iterations = 200.

3.5   Hybrid Approach

Investigation of the failure modes of baseline method (Haar + GBM) and CaffeNet_FA revealed that they had failed on different images (Sect. 4). To exploit the complementary advantages, we propose a simple scheme of averaging the spatial likelihood maps from GBMs of these two approaches and employing it in (2), which yields dramatic improvement.

4   Results

To quantitatively evaluate the performance on 45 validation images, we used two metrics: (1) Number of localization failures - the number of images for which the dice similarity coefficient between detected kidney ROI and ground truth annotation was < 0.80. (2) Detection accuracy - average dice overlap across 45 images between detection results and ground truth, which. From Table 1, we see that CaffeNet features without any adaptation outperformed baseline by 2 % in average detection accuracy with same number of failures. This improvement is consistent with other results reported in literature [18], where CaffeNet features outperform state-of-the-art pipeline. However, by allowing these network weights to get adapted to the kidney data, we achieved a performance boost of 4% over the baseline method, with number of failure cases reducing to 10 from 12. Interestingly, tuning with the first two convolutional layers frozen yielded intermediate performance, suggesting that multiple levels of feature adaptation are important to the problem.

Table 1. Performance comparison on unseen 45 validation images

Method	Haar features	CaffeNet_NA	CaffeNet_PA	CaffeNet_FA	Haar + CaffeNet_FA
Average dice overlap	0.793	0.825	0.831	0.842	**0.857**
# of failures	12/45	12/45	11/45	10/45	**3/45**

Figure 3(a) and (b) shows a case in which the baseline method was affected by the presence of diaphragm, kidney and liver boundaries creating a texture similar to renal-sinus portion, while CaffeNet had excellent localization. Figure 3(c) and (d) illustrate a case where CaffeNet resulted in over-segmentation containing the diaphragm, clearly illustrating that in limited data problems careful feature-engineering incorporating domain knowledge still carries a lot of relevance. Finally, we achieved a best performance of 86% average detection accuracy using the hybrid approach (Sect. 3.5). More importantly, the number of failures of the hybrid approach was 3/45, which is 20% better than either of the methods.

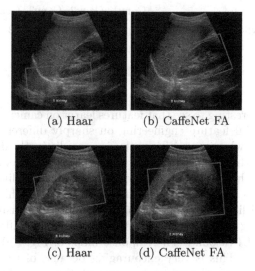

(a) Haar   (b) CaffeNet FA

(c) Haar   (d) CaffeNet FA

Fig. 3. Visual comparison of baseline method with CaffeNet transfer

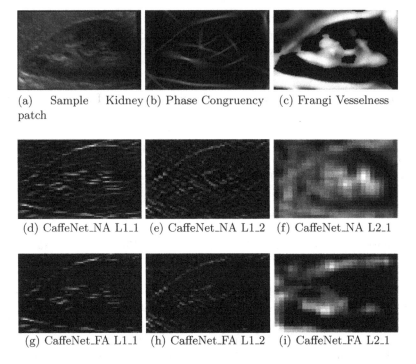

(a) Sample Kidney (b) Phase Congruency   (c) Frangi Vesselness
patch

(d) CaffeNet_NA L1_1 (e) CaffeNet_NA L1_2 (f) CaffeNet_NA L2_1

(g) CaffeNet_FA L1_1 (h) CaffeNet_FA L1_2 (i) CaffeNet_FA L2_1

Fig. 4. Filter responses for learned &hand-engineered features for a sample patch (CaffeNet_FA(NA) LX_Y denotes response image from Y^{th} filter of layer X)

Table 2. No. of filters in each layer that changed by more than 40 % in ℓ_2 norm

	Layer				
	Conv1	Conv2	Conv3	Conv4	Conv5
# of filters with ≥ 40 % change	0	5	125	22	62

5 Discussion

It is indeed very interesting to see that features learnt on camera images were able to outperform careful feature engineering on sharply different detection problems, in modalities whose acquisition physics are distinctly different. Figure 4 compares some of the response images generated from layers 1 and 2 of the learned network with traditional image processing outputs like Phase Congruency [14] and Frangi vesselness filter [9] for an example patch.

Here, we would like to highlight two main points: (1) Visually, we find the output has intriguing similarities with the outputs of hand crafted feature extractors optimized for Ultrasound. The response maps of Fig. 4(g) and (i) are similar to 4(b) and (c). This is very encouraging because of the fact that CNNs learns features that are equivalent to some of these widely used non-linear feature extractors. (2) The second important observation here is the reduction in speckle noise on CaffeNet_FAL1_1, compared to CaffeNet_PAL1_1. By carefully tuning CaffetNet features on ultrasound data, the model was able to learn the underlying noise characteristics, while preserving edges, and this resulted in a much improved response map as shown in Fig. 4(g) and (i).

Further, we quantitatively analyzed changes (% in ℓ_2 norm) in filter weights in each layer to identify significant trends. Table 2 shows a large number of filters have significantly changed in the 3rd layer, with filters in the 1st and 2nd layer showing minimal change. This is possibly due to the lower level features being fairly the same for both natural and ultrasound images. We also noted that the use of ReLU as the activation function also avoided the vanishing gradient problem, resulting in this skew in distribution of weight changes across layers. The response images past layer 2 proved to be difficult to interpret, and may require more intensive techniques. Our quantitative results and the literature in the field show that a great deal of the power of deep networks lies in these layers, and so we feel this is an important area for our future investigation.

In a clinical context, the interpretability of models is crucial and we feel this insight into why the deep CNN was able to outperform hand-crafted features is as important as the results demonstrated in Sect. 4. We also see this as opening up new ways of understanding and utilizing deep networks for medical problems.

References

1. Ardon, R., Cuingnet, R., Bacchuwar, K., Auvray, V.: Fast kidney detection and segmentation with learned kernel convolution and model deformation in 3D ultrasound images. In: Proceedings of ISBI, pp. 268–271 (2015)
2. Becker, C., Rigamonti, R., Lepetit, V., Fua, P.: Supervised feature learning for curvilinear structure segmentation. In: Mori, K., Sakuma, I., Sato, Y., Barillot, C., Navab, N. (eds.) MICCAI 2013, Part I. LNCS, vol. 8149, pp. 526–533. Springer, Heidelberg (2013)
3. Carneiro, G., Georgescu, B., Good, S., Comaniciu, D.: Detection and measurement of fetal anatomies from ultrasound images using a constrained probabilistic boosting tree. IEEE Trans. Med. Imaging 27(9), 1342–1355 (2008)
4. Carneiro, G., Nascimento, J., Bradley, A.P.: Unregistered multiview mammogramanalysis with pre-trained deep learning models. In: Navab, N., Hornegger, J., Wells, W.M., Frangi, A.F. (eds.) MICCAI 2015. LNCS, vol. 9351, pp. 652–660. Springer, Heidelberg (2015)
5. Caruana, R., Niculescu-Mizil, A.: An empirical comparison of supervised learning algorithms. In: Proceedings of ICML, pp. 161–168 (2006)
6. Chen, H., Ni, D., Qin, J., Li, S., Yang, X., Wang, T., Heng, P.A.: Standard plane localization in fetal ultrasound via domain transferred deep neural networks. IEEE J. Biomed. Health Inform. 19(5), 1627–1636 (2015)
7. Cho, J., Lee, K., Shin, E., Choy, G., Do, S.: How much data is needed to train a medical image deep learning system to achieve necessary high accuracy? In: ICLR (2016)
8. Emamian, S.A., Nielsen, M.B., Pedersen, J.F., Ytte, L.: Kidney dimensions at sonography: correlation with age, sex, and habitus in 665 adult volunteers. Am. J. Roentgenol. 160(1), 83–86 (1993)

9. Frangi, A.F., Niessen, W.J., Vincken, K.L., Viergever, M.A.: Multiscale vessel enhancement filtering. In: Wells, W.M., Colchester, A.C.F., Delp, S.L. (eds.) MICCAI 1998. LNCS, vol. 1496, pp. 130–137. Springer, Heidelberg (1998)
10. Girshick, R., Donahue, J., Darrell, T., Malik, J.: Rich feature hierarchies for accurate object detection and semantic segmentation (2014)
11. Jia, Y., Shelhamer, E., Donahue, J., Karayev, S., Long, J., Girshick, R., Guadarrama, S., Darrell, T.: Caffe: Convolutional architecture for fast feature embedding. In: Proceedings of the ACM International Conference on Multimedia, pp. 675–678 (2014)
12. Keramidas, E.G., Iakovidis, D.K., Maroulis, D.E., Karkanis, S.A.: Efficient and effective ultrasound image analysis scheme for thyroid nodule detection. In: Kamel, M.S., Campilho, A. (eds.) ICIAR 2007. LNCS, vol. 4633, pp. 1052–1060. Springer, Heidelberg (2007)
13. Kop, A.M., Hegadi, R.: Kidney segmentation from ultrasound images using gradient vector force. IJCA 2, 104–109 (2010). Special Issue on RTIPPR
14. Kovesi, P.: Phase congruency detects corners and edges. In: Proceedings of the Australian Pattern Recognition Society Conference: DICTA, pp. 309–318 (2003)
15. Krizhevsky, A., Sutskever, I., Hinton, G.E.: Imagenet classification with deep convolutional neural networks. In: Proceedings of Advances in Neural Information Processing Systems NIPS, pp. 1106–1114 (2012)
16. Martin-Fernandez, M., Alberola-Lopez, C.: An approach for contour detection of human kidneys from ultrasound images using Markov random fields and active contours. Med. Image Anal. 9(1), 1–23 (2005)
17. Ravishankar, H., Annangi, P.: Automated kidney morphology measurements from ultrasound images using texture and edge analysis. In: SPIE Medical Imaging (2016)
18. Shie, C.K., Chuang, C.H., Chou, C.N., Wu, M.H., Chang, E.Y.: Transfer representation learning for medical image analysis. In: EMBC, pp. 711–714 (2015)
19. Shin, H., Roth, H.R., Gao, M., Lu, L., Xu, Z., Nogues, I., Yao, J., Mollura, D.J., Summers, R.M.: Deep convolutional neural networks for computer-aided detection: CNN architectures, dataset characteristics and transfer learning. IEEE Trans. Med. Imaging 35(5), 1285–1298 (2016)
20. Sohail, A.S.M., Rahman, M.M., Bhattacharya, P., Krishnamurthy, S., Mudur, S.P.: Retrieval and classification of ultrasound images of ovarian cysts combining texture features and histogram moments. In: Proceedings of ISBI, pp. 288–291, April 2010
21. Tajbakhsh, N., Shin, J.Y., Gurudu, S.R., Hurst, R.T., Kendall, C.B., Gotway, M.B., Liang, J.: Convolutional neural networks for medical image analysis: full training or fine tuning? IEEE Trans. Med. Imaging 35(5), 1299–1312 (2016)
22. Xie, J., Jiang, Y., Tsui, H.T.: Segmentation of kidney from ultrasound images based on texture and shape priors. IEEE Trans. Med. Imaging 24(1), 45–57 (2005)
23. Yosinski, J., Clune, J., Bengio, Y., Lipson, H.: How transferable are features in deep neural networks? In: Proceedings Advances in Neural Information Processing Systems NIPS, pp. 3320–3328 (2014)
24. Zheng, Y., Liu, D., Georgescu, B., Nguyen, H., Comaniciu, D.: 3D deep learning for efficient and robust landmark detection in volumetric data. In: Navab, N., Hornegger, J., Wells, W.M., Frangi, A.F. (eds.) MICCAI 2015. LNCS, vol. 9349, pp. 565–572. Springer, Heidelberg (2015). doi:10.1007/978-3-319-24553-9_69

A Region Based Convolutional Network for Tumor Detection and Classification in Breast Mammography

Ayelet Akselrod-Ballin$^{(\boxtimes)}$, Leonid Karlinsky, Sharon Alpert,
Sharbell Hasoul, Rami Ben-Ari, and Ella Barkan

IBM Research - Haifa, Haifa, Israel
ayeletb@il.ibm.com

Abstract. This paper addresses the problem of detection and classification of tumors in breast mammograms. We introduce a novel system that integrates several modules including a breast segmentation module and a fibroglandular tissue segmentation module into a modified cascaded region-based convolutional network. The method is evaluated on a large multi-center clinical dataset and compared to ground truth annotated by expert radiologists. Preliminary experimental results show the high accuracy and efficiency obtained by the suggested network structure. As the volume and complexity of data in healthcare continues to accelerate generalizing such an approach may have a profound impact on patient care in many applications.

1 Introduction

Breast cancer is the second leading cause of death for women [1]. Despite the advances in imaging technology, Mammography (MG), X-ray imaging of the breast, remains the primary modality for screening and diagnosis of breast cancer. In current practice, screening for early detection is performed for asymptomatic individuals, where an expert radiologist examines the images and performs detection and classification of potential abnormalities. Nevertheless, MG analysis is challenging, due to the subtle fine-grained (FG) visual categories and large variability of appearance in abnormalities (e.g. different sizes, shapes, boundaries, and intensities) [2], making abnormalities difficult to detect and classify, even by an expert radiologist. The problem is further complicated by the non-rigidity of the breast, and the varying viewing conditions, leading to significant intra-expert and inter-expert variability. Still, due to the accelerated advances in technology, the information overload, the limited amount of expert time, and diagnosis errors, it is essential to augment the radiologist with decision supporting computational tools utilizing image processing and machine learning (ML) technology.

The objective of this paper is to introduce a novel algorithm for detection and classification of abnormalities based on a powerful region-based convolutional networks approach. Classification is performed according to the Breast Imaging-Reporting

---

A. Akselrod-Ballin and L. Karlinsky—contributed equally to this work.

© Springer International Publishing AG 2016
G. Carneiro et al. (Eds.): LABELS 2016/DLMIA 2016, LNCS 10008, pp. 197–205, 2016.
DOI: 10.1007/978-3-319-46976-8_21

and Data System (BI-RADS) score [3]. The BI-RADS score ranges from 0 to 6 and is defined as (0 more information is needed,1 negative, 2 benign finding, 3 probably benign <2 % likelihood of cancer, 4 suspicious abnormality, 5 highly suggestive of malignancy, and 6 proven malignancy). This study dealt only with scores 1 to 5 based on radiological features and without correlation with clinical information. We demonstrate our results on tumor detection and classification where due to the small amount of training data in some of the score classes, we include the three major clinical classes of normal {1}, benign {2} and malignant {3, 4, 5}. Figure 1, demonstrates examples of tumors with different BI-RADS score.

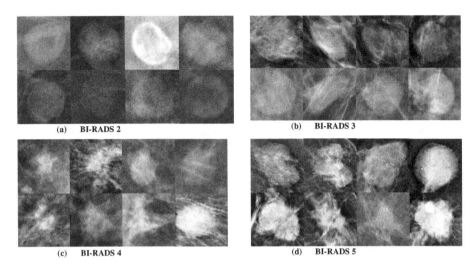

(a)   BI-RADS 2

(b)   BI-RADS 3

(c)   BI-RADS 4

(d)   BI-RADS 5

Fig. 1. Examples of tumors with different BI-RADS score.

Deep Neural Networks (DNN) have shown outstanding performance in image recognition tasks such as classification and detection and have been applied success-fully in many fields [4]. Recently deep learning methods have also been utilized in medical imaging tasks where an additional difficulty stems from the limited number large labeled datasets, which are required for efficient training and avoiding parameter over fitting. Nevertheless, several deep learning algorithms for breast mammography lesion and calcification classification have been reported, for detailed report see [5, 6].

Prominent work in the field, include [7], where a multi-view convolutional neural network (CNN) based approach was developed. First a separate CNN model was trained for each unregistered view and each segmentation map fine tuning from an Imagenet pre-trained model. Then, using the features obtained the authors trained another CNN classifier that estimated the BI-RADS score. Arevalo et al. [8] used convolutional architectures within a supervised learning framework taking advantage of expert knowledge represented by previously manually segmented lesions by radi-ologists in both mammographic views. Most of the previous work has focused on binary classification of micro-calcification (MC) or tumors which is different than performing detection localization and classification of abnormalities. The study of [9] is closely related to our Region-Based CNN (R-CNN) work. The authors present a system consisting of four modules, the first is a multi-scale deep belief nets (DBN) with a Gaussian mixture model (GMM) classifier for region proposal generation, the second is a cascade of R-CNNs, the thirds is a cascade of two random forests and finally, a post processing step merges regions with a high overlap ratio.

A variety of methods have been reported in the computer vision literature for region proposals. Classically, R-CNN [10], solves the detection problem by two modules, the first generates generic region proposals (image regions likely to contain objects) using low level cues such as color and texture, while the second computes CNN features and classifies them into object categories. Fast R-CNN [11] modified some of the drawbacks of R-CNN, by replacing the extraction of region proposal images by direct pooling of region features within a single CNN operating on the entire image and also introducing a regression stage for region box refinement. Recently, Faster R-CNN [12], introduced end-to-end joint training of both the region proposal module and the region classification module, both represented by CNNs with significant weight sharing. This also led to much higher detection speeds and higher detection quality than the original R-CNN [10]. The advantage of joint end-to-end training is that it allows avoiding sequentially-trained tasks and also that it may improve results since the shared representation allows the tasks to influence each other.

Our contribution is twofold: First the best of our knowledge this is the first work to utilizing state-of-the-art Faster-R-CNN in a full efficient pipeline for tumor detection and classification tasks in mammography images. Second we modify the original CNN architecture used in Faster-R-CNN in order to adapt the deep learning process to the specific problem domain, training and testing on a large multi-center dataset for both detection and classification tasks.

2   Methods

The system takes as input a Mammography (MG) image of $\sim$4k $\times$ 3k pixel and begins by segmenting the breast tissue automatically, removing the background and pectoral muscle and cropping image accordingly. In the second step a priori anatomical image is generated detecting the Fibro-glandular tissue based on a fuzzy logic approach [13]. The third step divides the images based on a grid representation to multiple overlapping sub images (parts) which are then used to train and test a modified Faster-RCNN [12]. The fourth step integrates the results obtained from the parts onto the entire image. Finally the output produces the detection and classification results represented by bounding-boxes with a confidence/probability score where pixels that were not detected are defined as normal breast tissue class. Figure 2 shows the outline of the system.

2.1   Breast Anatomical Segmentation and Candidate Extraction

To obtain accurate detection of tumors it is essential to perform segmentation of the breast and the pectoral muscle. Additionally, we generate an anatomical prior identifying the fibroglandular tissue to be used for reduction of FP. The fibroglandular segmentation is based on the approach described in [13]. Due to the lack of space we refer the reader to the paper for details.

As a result of GPU memory limitations a grid was defined on the image, dividing the image to overlapping parts of fixed size 800 × 800. The use of overlapping parts can also be seen as a data augmentation technique as each lesion appears in several overlapping parts. This allows us to create several samples from each lesion appearing in the original data.

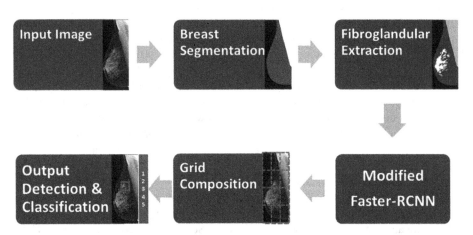

Fig. 2. (a) System outline. Given an MG Input (1) Breast tissue segmentation removal of background and pectoral muscle (2) Fibro-glandular tissue extraction. (3) The image is divided to multiple overlapping subparts utilized in the Faster-RCNN training and testing. (4) Composition: the bounding boxes detected are projected on image grid. The process ends with tumor detection and the corresponding BI-RADS classification.

2.2   Modified Faster-R-CNN

The system is composed of two main components: (1) a region proposal network (RPN), a deep fully convolutional network that is trained to detect windows on the input image that are likely to contain objects of interest regardless of their class. The RPN simultaneously predicts objects bounds and objectness scores at each position on a wide range of scales and aspect ratios, following which top scoring 500 predictions are kept. (2) Fast R-CNN detection network that is trained to classify candidate object windows returned by the RPN, each window is classified into one of the classes of interest or rejected as a false alarm. Both RPN and Fast-RCNN share a large common set of bottom layers allowing computation re-use and hence a significant speed-up at test time.

Faster-R-CNN training is a four-step alternating algorithm consisting of the following steps: (1) Train RPN, initialized with an ImageNet pre-trained model. (2) Train a separate classification network using the proposals generated in step 1. As proposed in [11], the network operates on the entire image and uses pooling from the proposal regions in order to generate deep features for classification. (3) Use the network from stage 2 to initialize the RPN but freeze the parameters of the shared bottom layers and only fine-tune the top RPN layers (non-shared). (4) Keep the shared layers frozen and repeat stage 2 using the proposals generated in step 3. We have modified the original Faster-RCNN net of [12] to include information from the finer bottom levels during classification (Fast-RCNN) stage. This allows to consider low level (higher resolution) information such as color and texture during the classification stage and improves the classification results. When considering visually similar objects such as malignant lesions and patches of suspicious normal tissue, intricate visual details need to be taken into account in order to make the distinction. In other words, the problem addressed in this paper is inherently fine grained and significantly different than the one of classifying visually dis-similar objects as in many visual challenges such as PASCLA-VOC used for testing in [12]. Therefore, features from lower levels of the CNN need to be taken into the account when making the decision as they are the only ones looking on the considered region proposals in the high enough resolution. Figure 3, provides a schematic view of the modification in the network.

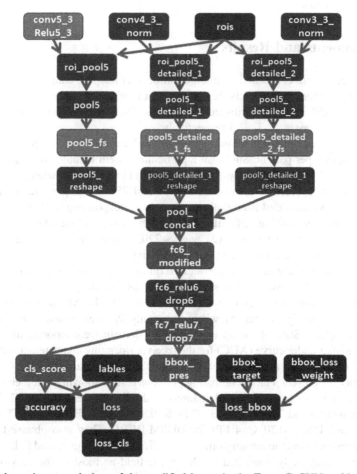

Fig. 3. Schematic zoomed view of the modified layers in the Faster R-CNN architecture. The boxes connected to conv4_3 and conv3_3 represent additional layers in the modified network.

Given a training set of images and RoIs $\{I_i, r_{1i}, c_{1i}, r_{2i}, c_{2i}\}$, where each RoI is defined by a four-tuple that specifies its top-left corner (r; c) and bottom right corner and the class and a test set of images $\{I_j\}$. The output includes all the objects in the test set and their bounding boxes represented in a six-tuple ($\{I_j, r_{1j}, c_{1j}, r_{2j}, c_{2j}\}$, class, and score). Namely, given a test input the system will automatically detect and classify into one of three classes including normal tissue (BI-RADS 1), benign (BI-RADS 2), and malignant tumors (BI-RADS 3, 4, 5).

Our implementation is based on the Faster R-CNN architecture [12] using VGG-16 architecture [14] and caffe implementation [15]. The system was trained on a single TitanX GPU with 12 GB on chip memory, and i7 Intel CPU with 64 GB RAM. Training times required ~ 36 h, while testing takes 0.2 s per image. During training 2000 top-scoring boxes are sampled from the RPN, during testing top scoring 500 boxes are sampled using standard non-maximal suppression (NMS) based on box overlap. We used the SGD solver with learning rate of 0.001, batch size 2, momentum 0.99, and 60 epochs.

3   Experiments and Results

The experiments were conducted on a large multicenter hospital data set annotated and examined by expert radiologists (the fourth author). The data sets consists of approximately 850 images distributed in terms of BI-RADS to 400, 200, 150, 100 corresponding to classes 2, 3, 4, 5 respectively.

The dataset was split into training (80 %), and testing (20 %) sets following a stratified sampling per patient. Such that a particular patient belongs to only one of the subsets. The total number of patients in experiment (1) was ~ 300, where training and testing of the model were performed with 4000 and 750 image parts respectively. In experiment (2), we excluded from both sets images corresponding to BI-RADS {3}, to demonstrate the recognition difficulties which the intermediate class brings. The number of patients in experiment (2) was ~ 220, where training and testing were performed with 3000 and 700 image parts respectively.

Results in the field are commonly evaluated on the DDSM-BCRP [16] and INBreast [17] datasets. The INBreast comprises a set of 115 cases containing 410 images, where only 116 images contain benign or malignant masses. The DDSM-BCRP dataset contains 79 images of malignant masses, where commonly 39 cases are used for training and 40 cases for testing. State of the art results in this domain were reported in [7] which produced an Area under curve (AUC) for the receiver operating characteristics (ROC) of $0.91 \pm .05$ on INBreast and $0.97 \pm .0.03$ on DDSM. [8] obtained an AUC score of 0.826. Finally [9] present a table comparing previous results showing that their approach produces the best results to date in both datasets: with TPR $0.96 \pm .0.03$ @ 1.2 FPI (false positive per image) and TPR = $0.87 \pm .0.14$ @ 0.8 FPI for INBreast; and TPR = 0.75 @ 4.8 FPI and TPR = 0.70 @ 4 FPI for DDSM-BCRP. They also obtained the best results reported in respect to running time of 20 s. Table 1 and Figs. 4 and 5. It is difficult to compare to previously published results in the field as most of the previous work focused on binary classification of masses. Also previous work mainly report on DDSM and INBreast which are limited in size. Our method is evaluated on a large multi-center data set, while most methods report results on smaller data sets of tumors. Also we evaluate both the detection, localization and classification of tumors and report the AUC of precision recall, commonly used in computer vision literature [4, 10]. Nevertheless, examining only classification results, the methodology can be considered as promising in terms of accuracy and extremely efficient in terms of time (Table 1) and Figs. 4 and 5.

Table 1. Results of two experiments for Detection and Classification of tumors.

Experiment	Detection AUC (average precision)	Classification accuracy	#images	Running time
(1) benign BI-RADS- 2 & malignant {345}	0.6	0.78	850	0.2 s
(2) benign BI-RADS- 2 & malignant {45}	0.72	0.77	850	0.2 s

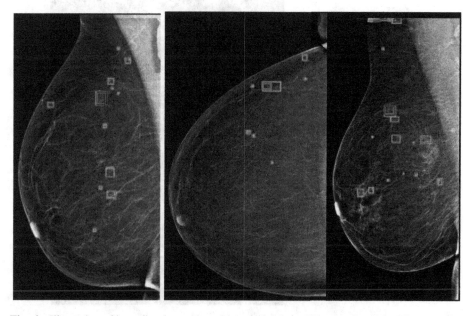

Fig. 4. Illustration of bounding box composition on full breast images. Ground truth annotation is highlighted in green while automatic detection can be viewed in red. (Color figure online)

4   Summary

In this paper we introduced a novel approach for detection and classification of breast tumors based on the state-of-the-art approach of Faster-RCNN. Our preliminary results show the promise of this approach to efficiently and accurately detect and classify

(a) Benign - correctly classified

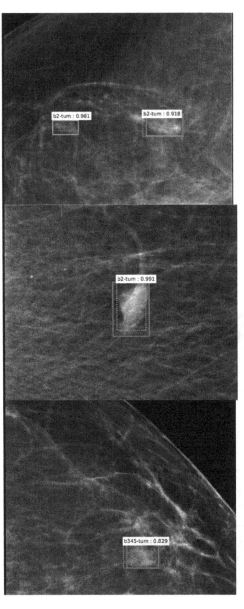

(b)Malignant - wrongfully classified as
benign

(c) Malignant - correctly classified

Fig. 5. Detection and Classification results on parts. We show typical detection and classification results, where benign and malignant masses are in cyan and magenta respectively. Ground truth annotation are marked by a solid line and automatic detection are marked in dashed line. (Color figure online)

breast abnormalities on real up-to-date data. Future work will extend this work to a multi-view approach, take into account associated features, such as breast density, perform segmentation in boxes, and evaluate on publically available dataset.

References

1. Jemal, A., Siegel, R., et al.: Cancer statistics, 2008. CA Cancer J. Clin. **58**(2), 71–96 (2008)
2. American Cancer Society: Cancer facts and figures, Atlanta, GA (2015)
3. Narváez, F., Díaz, G., Romero, E.: Automatic BI-RADS description of mammographic masses. In: Martí, J., Oliver, A., Freixenet, J., Martí, R. (eds.) IWDM 2010. LNCS, vol. 6136, pp. 673–681. Springer, Heidelberg (2010)
4. Krizhevsky, A., Sutskever, I., Hinton, G.: Imagenet classification with deep convolutional neural networks. In: Proceedings of the (NIPS 2012), pp. 1097–1105 (2012)
5. Giger, M.L., Karssemeijer, N., Schnabel, J.A.: Breast image analysis for risk assessment, detection, diagnosis, and treatment of cancer. Annu. Rev. Biomed. Eng. **15**, 327–357 (2013)
6. Oliver, A., Freixenet, J., Marti, J., Perez, E., Pont, J., et al.: A review of automatic mass detection and segmentation in mammographic images. Med. Image Anal. **14**, 87–110 (2010)
7. Carneiro, G., Nascimento, J., Bradley, A.P.: Unregistered multiview mammogram anaysis with pre-trained deep learning models. In: Navab, N., Hornegger, J., Wells, W.M., Frangi, A. F. (eds.) MICCAI 2015. LNCS, vol. 9351, pp. 652–660. Springer, Heidelberg (2015)
8. Arevalo, J., Gonzales, F.A., Ramos-Pollán, R., Oliveira, J.L., Lopez, M.A.G.: Representation learning for mammography mass lesion classification with convolutional neural networks. Comput. Methods Programs Biomed. **127**, 248–257 (2016)
9. Dhungel, N., Carneiro, G., Bradley, A.: Automated mass detection from mammograms using deep learning and random forest. In: DICTA (2015)
10. Girshick, R., Donahue, J., Darrell, T., Malik, J.: Rich feature hierarchies for accurate object detection and semantic segmentation. In: Computer Vision and Pattern Recognition (CVPR), pp. 580–587 (2014)
11. Girshickv, R.: Fast R-CNN. In: Proceedings of the IEEE International Conference on Computer Vision (ICCV), pp. 1440–1448 (2015)
12. Ren, S., He, K., Girshick, R., Sun, J.: Faster R-CNN: towards real-time object detection with region proposal networks. In: NIPS (2015)
13. Ben-Ari, R., Zlotnick, A., Hashoul, S.: A weakly labeled approach for breast tissue segmentation and breast density estimation in digital mammography. In: ISBI (2016)
14. Simonyan, K., Zisserman, A.: Very deep convolutional networks for large-scale image recognition. In: ICLR (2015)
15. Jia, Y., Shelhamer, E., Donahue, J., Karayev, S., Long, J., Girshick, R., Guadarrama, S., Darrell, T.: Caffe: convolutional architecture for fast feature embedding (2014). arXiv:1408.5093
16. Heath, M., Bowyer, K., et al.: The digital database for screening mammography. In: Proceedings of the 5th International Workshop on Digital Mammography, pp. 212–218 (2000)
17. Moreira, I.C., Amaral, I., et al.: Inbreast: toward a full-field digital mammographic database. Acad. Radiol. **19**(2), 236–248 (2012)

Large-Scale Annotation of Biomedical Data and Expert Label Synthesis

Early Experiences with Crowdsourcing Airway Annotations in Chest CT

Veronika Cheplygina[1,2]([✉]), Adria Perez-Rovira[1,3], Wieying Kuo[3,4],
Harm A.W.M. Tiddens[3,4], and Marleen de Bruijne[1,5]

[1] Biomedical Imaging Group Rotterdam, Departments Medical Informatics
and Radiology, Erasmus Medical Center,
Rotterdam, The Netherlands
v.cheplygina@tudelft.nl
[2] Pattern Recognition Laboratory, Delft University of Technology,
Delft, The Netherlands
[3] Department of Pediatric Pulmonology and Allergology,
Erasmus Medical Center - Sophia Children's Hospital, Rotterdam, The Netherlands
[4] Department of Radiology,
Erasmus Medical Center, Rotterdam, The Netherlands
[5] Image Section, Departments of Computer Science,
University of Copenhagen, Copenhagen, Denmark

Abstract. Measuring airways in chest computed tomography (CT) images is important for characterizing diseases such as cystic fibrosis, yet very time-consuming to perform manually. Machine learning algorithms offer an alternative, but need large sets of annotated data to perform well. We investigate whether crowdsourcing can be used to gather airway annotations which can serve directly for measuring the airways, or as training data for the algorithms. We generate image slices at known locations of airways and request untrained crowd workers to outline the airway lumen and airway wall. Our results show that the workers are able to interpret the images, but that the instructions are too complex, leading to many unusable annotations. After excluding unusable annotations, quantitative results show medium to high correlations with expert measurements of the airways. Based on this positive experience, we describe a number of further research directions and provide insight into the challenges of crowdsourcing in medical images from the perspective of first-time users.

1 Introduction

Respiratory diseases are a major cause of death and disability and are responsible for three out of the top five causes of death worldwide [12]. Chest computed tomography (CT) is an important tool to characterize and monitor lung diseases. Quantification of structural abnormalities in the lungs, such as bronchiectasis, air trapping and emphysema, is needed to track disease progression or to predict patient outcomes. We have recently shown that, the airway-to-vessel ratio (AVR) is an objective measurement of bronchiectasis which is sensitive to detect early

© Springer International Publishing AG 2016
G. Carneiro et al. (Eds.): LABELS 2016/DLMIA 2016, LNCS 10008, pp. 209–218, 2016.
DOI: 10.1007/978-3-319-46976-8_22

lung disease [7,11]. Unfortunately, manual measurements of the airways and adjoining arteries suffer from intra- and inter-observer variation and are very time-consuming (8–16 h per chest CT).

Computer algorithms can be used to improve accuracy and efficiency of the measurements. The first step is to extract the airways and vessels from the scan. Machine learning techniques learn from example images which have been manually annotated, and have shown to be very effective for such extraction tasks [4]. However, these techniques require a large amount of annotated images, which is also expensive and time-consuming.

We therefore propose to use the wisdom of the crowd to gather annotations. In crowdsourcing, untrained internet users (knowledge workers or KWs) carry out human intelligence tasks (HITs), such as annotating images[1]. The KWs are unpaid volunteers, or receive a small financial reward for each task. Early research into crowdsourcing for medical images [1,5,6,8] showed that non-expert workers were able to carry out a range of HITs relatively well; our goal is to investigate whether this is true for airway measurement in chest CT.

In this paper we describe our early experiences with crowdsourcing airway measurements in chest CT images. In Sect. 2 we describe how we generate 2D slices, how we collect annotations from the KWs and how the annotations are processed. Section 3 describes the data and the number of annotations collected, followed by a presentation of the results in Sect. 4. We discuss our findings, lessons learnt as first-time users of crowdsourcing and steps for future research in Sect. 5, followed by a conclusion in Sect. 6.

2   Methods

Our main question for this study was whether non-expert workers would be able to annotate airways in chest CT images. By "an airway annotation" we understand two outlines: one of the airway lumen (inner airway) and one of the airway wall (outer airway). Annotating an airway consists of two steps: localizing an airway, and creating the outlines. In this study we focused on the second question only. We therefore acquired annotations using already existing 3D voxel coordinates and orientations as a starting point.

We used 3D voxel coordinates, at which experts have previously annotated airways using the Myrian^{TM} software. As we could not reproduce how this software determines the orientations, we used orientations obtained with an airway segmentation algorithm. This algorithm starts with an initial volumetric segmentation of the airways, rescales it isotropically and uses front propagation to obtain airway centerlines [10], which give us the orientations. Using these 3D coordinates and orientations, we generate 2D slices (described in more detail in Sect. 2.1), which are annotated by the KWs. This allows for a comparison of airway measurements between the experts and the KWs. Figure 1 shows a global overview of our method.

---

[1] We adopt the terminology used by Amazon MTurk platform.

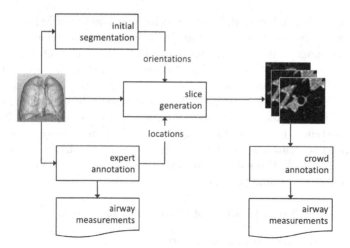

Fig. 1. Overview of the method. A 3D image is annotated by experts. The locations and orientations of the annotations are then used to generate 2D slices of the image, which are then annotated by the workers. Lung image by Noeska Smit.

2.1 Image Generation

Given a 3D location and an orientation vector, we generated a slice of 50×50 voxels, perpendicular to that orientation. Because of possible segmentation errors, an airway was not always visible. We therefore also generated slices in axial, coronal and saggital views, in total generating four different images per airway. We used cubic interpolation and an intensity range between -950 and 550 Hounsfield units for better contrast, as recommended by the experts. An example is shown in Fig. 2.

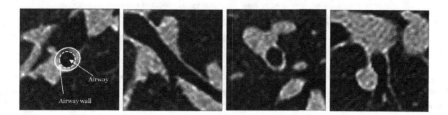

Fig. 2. Slices of 50×50 voxels showing four views of an airway, from left to right: original orientation, saggital, coronal and axial views. An airway cross-section appears as a dark circle (airway lumen, indicated by dashed line) with a light ring (airway wall, indicated by solid line) around it

2.2 Annotation Software

Amazon Mechanical Turk or MTurk [2] is an internet-based crowdsourcing platform that allows untrained internet users, known as knowledge workers (KWs) to perform tasks, known as human intelligence tasks (HITs), for a small (in the order of $0.05) financial reward. To extend the functionality of MTurk to annotation of airways, we integrated a custom-built annotation interface by supplying a dynamic webpage, built with HTML5 and Javascript. The interface originally contained a freehand tool for creating annotations, which was later replaced by an ellipse tool, which more closely resembled the tool used by the experts.

The details of our HIT, which the KWs could see when searching for HITs, are shown in Table 1, and a screenshot of the instructions is shown in Fig. 3. The KWs were instructed to draw two ellipses outlining the airway lumen and the airway wall, or to draw a small circle in the corner of the image, if no airway is visible. For each HIT, the software recorded an anonymized ID of the KW and the coordinates of the annotations.

Table 1. Details of HIT on Mechanical Turk

Title	Save lives by annotating airways!
Description	Draw two contours to annotate an airway (dark circle or ellipse) in image from a lung scan
Keywords	image, annotation, contour, draw, drawing, segmentation, medical

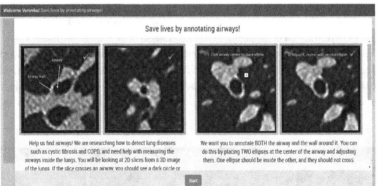

Fig. 3. Screenshot of (part of) the instructions given to the KWs for the task with the ellipse tool. The scrollbar on the right shows that there are more instructions than are visible in one screen. In the second part, incorrect annotations are shown as well.

2.3 Airway Measurement

We applied a simple filtering step to discard unusable annotations. The following annotations are discarded:

– no ellipses
– an odd number of ellipses
– an even number of ellipses, but the distance between centers of paired ellipses (pairs were assigned based on center distance) is larger than 10 voxels

For the remaining usable annotations, we measured the areas of the inner and outer ellipse, in order to compare them to the expert annotations. We perform the comparisons for each KW annotation individually, as well as for a combined measurement of the KWs. To obtain the combined measurements, we used only images with at least three usable annotations, and took the median of the areas.

3 Experiments

3.1 Data

For this preliminary experiment we used 1 inspiratory pediatric CT scan from a cohort of 24 subjects from a study [3,9], collected at the Erasmus MC - Sophia Children's Hospital. In this scan, 76 airways were annotated by an expert using Myrian software. The expert localized an airway, outlined the inner and outer airway, and recorded the measurements of the areas.

3.2 Crowd Annotations

We generated a total of $76 \times 4 = 308$ images using the method described in Sect. 2.1. We randomly created HITs with 10 images per HIT. A KW could request a HIT, annotate 10 images, and then submit the HIT. The KWs were paid \$0.10 per completed HIT. Only KWs who had previously done at least 100 HITs with an acceptance rate of 90 % could request the HITs. We accepted all HITs, i.e. no additional quality control was performed after the HITs were carried out.

We first collected 1 annotation per image with freehand tool. As we will describe in Sect. 4, it became clear that an ellipse tool was needed. With the ellipse tool, we collected 10 annotations per image.

4 Results

4.1 Annotations

We first collected 1 annotation per image with the freehand tool. A selection of the results is shown in Fig. 4 (top). Most of the workers attempted to annotate something in the image (i.e., were not spammers), but many annotations were not usable. For example, many workers misunderstood the instructions, annotated vessels instead of airways, drew only one contour or drew non-ellipsoidal contours. We concluded that this tool allowed too many degrees of freedom, and opted for the more controlled ellipse tool.

With the ellipse tool, we collected 10 annotations per image. However, based on our experience with the freehand tool, to reduce costs we did not gather annotations for all the images. In the end, with the ellipse tool 90 of the 308 images were annotated, resulting in 900 annotations.

A selection of the results with the ellipse tool in shown in Fig. 4 (bottom). Using the tool eliminated the problem of non-ellipsoidal airways. However, the

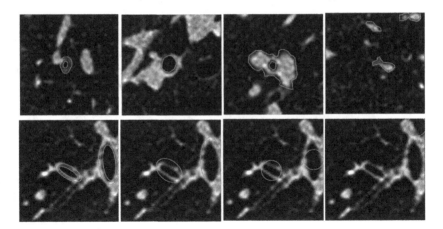

Fig. 4. Top: Annotations acquired with the freehand tool for four different images: correct annotation and three incorrect annotations. Bottom: Annotations acquired with the ellipse for the same image: correct annotations and three incorrect annotations. The incorrect annotations shown here are indicative of worst-case annotations that are presumably not spam

problems of either a single contour, or workers annotating vessels, were still present. While the annotations still were not perfect, we decided to do proceed with an initial analysis of the annotations.

4.2 Airway Measurement

We filtered unusable annotations as described in Sect. 2.3. Out of 900 annotations, 610 were found to be unusable. Of these 610, 133 annotations contained no ellipse, and 445 annotations contained only a single ellipse. For annotations with a single ellipse, there are three possible causes: spam, the worker indicating "no airway visible", or the worker misunderstood the instructions. To better differentiate between these causes, we looked at whether the ellipse was adjusted, indicating that the worker tried to annotate something. This was the case for 244 of the 445 annotations with a single ellipse. Although we do not analyse these annotations in this preliminary study, we note that these annotations still could be used to measure airways.

Next we focus on the the 290 usable annotations, i.e. where the worker placed ellipses in pairs. Of these, 256 annotations contained a single pair, 25 annotations contained two pairs, and a further 6 annotations contained three pairs. For this preliminary study, we only consider the annotations with a single pair for further analysis.

To assess correctness of the annotations, we create expert-vs-worker plots of two quantities: area of the airway lumen and area of the airway wall. We show the annotations for the original orientation in Fig. 5 (top), and the annotations for the saggital, coronal and axial orientations in Fig. 5 (bottom). The correla-

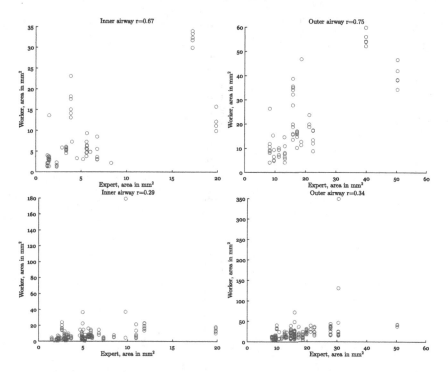

Fig. 5. Scatter plots of expert vs individual worker measurements of the areas. Top: original orientation, bottom: axes-parallel orientations. Left: airway lumen, right: airway wall. r indicates Pearson's correlation.

tions for the original orientations are medium to high, although workers tend to overestimate the airway lumen. The correlations for the other orientations are, understandably, weaker. Possibly here workers annotate other structures that are visible in the images.

Note that analysis above is performed on a per-annotation, not per-image basis. By aggregating the annotations obtained per image, we can get better estimates of the measurements from the crowd. In Fig. 6 we show the median areas for the images for which at least three workers produced usable annotations. The correlations are now medium to high for both types of orientations, although the sample size is lower, because for many images there were too few usable annotations. This motivates collecting more annotations per image in the future.

5   Discussion

Our results show that untrained KWs are able to interpret the CT images and attempt to annotate airways in the images. However, many KWs did not follow the instructions, resulting in unusable annotations. For example, in 244 out of

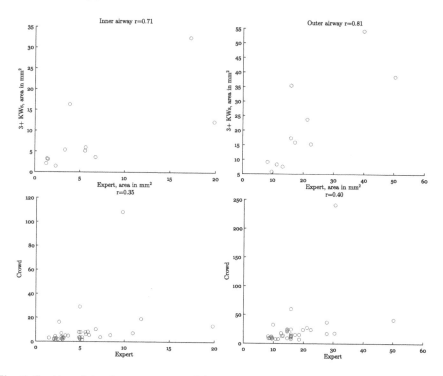

Fig. 6. Scatter plots of expert vs crowd (at least 3 workers) measurements of the areas. Top: original orientation, bottom: axes-parallel orientations. Left: airway lumen, right: airway wall. Left: airway lumen, right: airway wall. r indicates Pearson's correlation.

900 annotations the workers did attempt create an annotation, but only placed a single ellipse in the image. The usable annotations show medium to high correlations with expert measurements of the airways, especially if the worker annotations are aggregated. The results are not convincing enough to say that the workers can annotate the airways as well as experts (as more analysis is needed to test such claims), but the collected annotations could already be useful for training machine learning algorithms. Overall we feel that the results encourage further investigation. The next step is to collect annotations for all 24 subjects in the cohort, after a number of changes we describe below.

Based on our results, the next logical step is to increase the amount of usable annotations per image. There are several ways in which this can be achieved. One possibility is to improve the interface, for example by only accepting annotations that contain two ellipses. Alternatively, we could include a tutorial, showing workers step by step how to create the annotations. However, both of these options require custom-made adjustments to the interface, which is costly/time-consuming for novice users of MTurk such as ourselves.

In the short term, more feasible solutions for us are to simplify the instructions, increase the number of collected annotations per image to 20 (20 is also the choice in other crowdsourcing literature [6,8]), and to improve the postprocessing of the annotations. Here we used very simple rules to filter and aggregate the annotations with reasonable results. An alternative would be to use unsupervised outlier detection, or train a supervised classifier to detect outliers. Such a classifier could be based only on the characteristics of the annotations (such as size of the ellipse), or could also include characteristics of the image.

If our future research demonstrates that the crowd can reliably annotate airways, we will need to address the question of localizing the airways, and of using the annotations in machine learning algorithms. For localizing airways, we could show larger slices, and ask the KWs to click all locations where airways are visible. Such clicks can then be used to learn to recognize good voxel positions, at which airway measurements can be collected. Alternatively, we could use the already collected annotations (both usable and unusable) to learn the appearance of "annotatable" slices, bypassing the localizaton step.

Overall our first experiences with crowdsourcing are positive, but also teach us a number of important lessons: (i) there is more to setting up a crowdsourcing task than we thought, and (ii) the task itself needs to be simpler than we thought. With regard to setting up the task, a challenge was to make a choice between different annotation tools, and how such tools might influence the results. With regard to the task itself, the number and the wording of instructions are likely to affect how well the instructions will be carried out. While it is widely known that the task should be "as simple as possible", it is difficult to estimate the complexity of a novel task in advance, without performing preliminary experiments such as the ones described here.

For both the annotation interface and the instructions, it would be interesting to investigate how exactly different choices influence the final results. However, this "parameter space" is too large, and it is not feasible to explore it. This calls for more "rules-of-thumb" when designing large-scale data annotation tasks, as well as more interaction between researchers in medical image analysis, and researchers in fields where crowdsourcing is a more established technique.

6   Conclusions

We presented our early experiences with setting up a crowdsourcing task for measuring airways in chest CT images. Our results show that the KWs were able to interpret the images, but that the instructions were too complex, leading to many unusable annotations. For the usable annotations, quantitative results show medium to high correlations with expert measurements of the airways, especially if measurements of the KWs are aggregated. Our results are encouraging, we therefore intend to continue this research direction, by simplifying the instructions and collecting more annotations for an in-depth analysis. As beginner users of crowdsourcing, we describe several challenges we encountered during this research, and we hope our experiences will help other researchers in medical image analysis considering crowdsourcing for annotating their data.

Acknowledgements. This research was partially funded by the research project "Transfer learning in biomedical image analysis" which is financed by the Netherlands Organization for Scientific Research (NWO) grant no. 639.022.010. We gratefully acknowledge Dr. Daniel Kondermann of Heidelberg University for his help with crowdsourcing, and the anonymous reviewers for their constructive comments.

References

1. Albarqouni, S., Baur, C., Achilles, F., Belagiannis, V., Demirci, S., Navab, N.: AggNet: deep learning from crowds for mitosis detection in breast cancer histology images. IEEE Trans. Med. Imaging **35**(5), 1313–1321 (2016)
2. Chen, J.J., Menezes, N.J., Bradley, A.D., North, T.A.: Opportunitiesfor crowdsourcing research on Amazon Mechanical Turk. In: CHI workshop on Crowdsourcing and Human Computation (2011)
3. Kuo, W., et al.: Assessment of bronchiectasis in children with cystic fibrosis by comparing airway and artery dimensions to normal controls on inspiratory and expiratory spirometer guided chest computed tomography. In: ECR 2015-European Congress of Radiology (2015)
4. Lo, P., Sporring, J., Ashraf, H., Pedersen, J.J., Bruijne, M.: Vessel-guided airway tree segmentation: a voxel classification approach. Med. Image Anal. **14**(4), 527–538 (2010)
5. Maier-Hein, L., Kondermann, D., et al.: Crowdtruth validation: a new paradigm for validating algorithms that rely on image correspondences. Int. J. Comput. Assist. Radiol. Surg. **10**(8), 1201–1212 (2015)
6. Mitry, D., Peto, T., Hayat, S., Blows, P., Morgan, J., Khaw, K.T., Foster, P.J.: Crowdsourcing as a screening tool to detect clinical features of glaucomatous optic neuropathy from digital photography. PLoS ONE **10**(2), e0117401 (2015)
7. Mott, L.S., Graniel, K.G., Park, J., Klerk, N.H., Sly, P.D., Murray, C.P., Tiddens, H.A.W.M., Stick, S.M.: Assessment of early bronchiectasis in young children with cystic fibrosis is dependent on lung volume. CHEST J. **144**(4), 1193–1198 (2013)
8. Nguyen, T.B., Wang, S., Anugu, V., Rose, N., McKenna, M., Petrick, N., Burns, J.E., Summers, R.M.: Distributed human intelligence for colonic polyp classification in computer-aided detection for CT colonography. Radiology **262**(3), 824–833 (2012)
9. Perez-Rovira, A., Kuo, W., Petersen, J., Tiddens, H., de Bruijne, M.: Automated quantification of bronchiectasis, airway wall thickening and lumen tapering in chest CT. In: ECR 2015-European Congress of Radiology (2015)
10. Petersen, J., Nielsen, M., Lo, P., Nordenmark, L.H., Pedersen, J.H., Wille, M.M.W., Dirksen, A., de Bruijne, M.: Optimal surface segmentation using flow lines to quantify airway abnormalities in chronic obstructive pulmonary disease. Med. Image Anal. **18**(3), 531–541 (2014)
11. Tiddens, H.A.W.M., Donaldson, S.H., Rosenfeld, M., Paré, P.D.: Cystic fibrosis lung disease starts in the small airways: can we treat it more effectively? Pediatr. Pulmonol. **45**(2), 107–117 (2010)
12. World Health Organization: Fact sheet nr 10. Online (2014)

Hierarchical Feature Extraction for Nuclear Morphometry-Based Cancer Diagnosis

Chi Liu[1]([✉]), Yue Huang[2], Ligong Han[1], John A. Ozolek[3],
and Gustavo K. Rohde[1]

[1] Department of Biomedical Engineering,
Carnegie Mellon University, Pittsburgh, USA
chiliu@andrew.cmu.edu
[2] Fujian Key Laboratory of Sensing and Computing for Smart City,
Xiamen University, Xiamen, China
[3] Department of Pathology,
Childrens Hospital of Pittsburgh, Pittsburgh, USA

Abstract. Cell and nuclear morphology, as observed from histopathology microscopy images, have long been known as important indicators of disease states. Due to the large amount of data, obtaining expert pathologists annotations at the individual cell level is impractical in many applications, however. Thus the majority of the approaches currently available for automated classification and cancer detection are based on utilizing the patient label for each segmented cell, and patient classification is performed by classifying single morphological exemplars (e.g. cells or subcellular features) in combination with a majority voting procedure. Here we propose a new hierarchical method for classifying sets of nuclei. The method can be interpreted as a type of multiple instance learning (MIL) method in that it embeds data from each patient into a hierarchical feature space. The feature space, and classification boundary, are alternatively optimized utilizing the support vector machine (SVM) cost function. We demonstrate the application of the method in the diagnosis of thyroid lesions and compare to existing MIL methods showing significant improvements in classification accuracy.

1 Introduction

Cell and nuclear morphology alterations, as observed under light microscopy with routine staining (e.g. H&E), are often associated with tumor progression and visible nuclear changes are the prime interests of pathologists for cancer diagnosis [1]. Numerous approaches for quantitative measurements of cell and nuclear morphology have been reported as powerful tools in automated diagnosis systems for a wide variety of lesion types [2–6]. Though often implicitly, the majority of methods in nuclei-based cancer detection share the assumption that the nuclei are independent to each other and therefore utilize the Naive Bayes model [2–6]. In other words, each cell or nucleus is classified individually and independently. The class label for a patient is then assigned using a majority voting (MV) strategy.

© Springer International Publishing AG 2016
G. Carneiro et al. (Eds.): LABELS 2016/DLMIA 2016, LNCS 10008, pp. 219–227, 2016.
DOI: 10.1007/978-3-319-46976-8_23

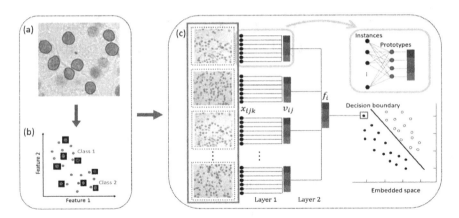

Fig. 1. Illustration of the proposed hierarchical feature extraction framework: (a) cell nuclei segmentation, (b) nuclei feature extraction, and (c) hierarchical feature extraction and label prediction for individual patients. We allow a bag (blue box) to have a set of sub-bags (green boxes) composed of multiple instances (black dots). The upper right window shows how bag level features are extracted via a set of prototypes (red dots). x_{ijk}, v_{ij} and f_i are defined in Sect. 2.1 (Color figure online)

We note two potential limitations of these cancer detection methods. First, the statistical morphology dependencies between nearby cells and nuclei are not fully explored. Intercellular communication between living cells allows cells to work together to perform necessary biological processes [7]. Therefore, it is reasonable to expect that the morphology of one cell nucleus closely depends on its nearby cell nuclei. As shown in [8], neglecting interdependencies between nearby nuclei can lead to sub-optimal classification results. Second, in many important applications, given the difficulties with annotating massive amounts of data, only patient-level labels are available. Thus in many classification approaches [3–5,9] labels for individual nuclei extracted from lesional regions in pathology images are usually propagated from the patient label. However, there are always cell nuclei in the region of interest that don't contain discriminative information about their class, or even contain information about other counterpart classes [10].

Multiple instance learning (MIL) serves as a remedy for such weak supervision problems when only a set of feature vectors (bag) is labeled without knowing the labels for individual feature vectors (instances). In general, existing MIL methods can be categorized into two classes according to how information in the data is extracted [11]. In the first category (instance-space, IS), methods consider the discriminative information at the local, instance-level [12–14]. The goal of these methods is to build an instance-level classifier to predict labels for individual instances. The bag label is usually determined by a voting strategy. In the second category (bagspace, BS), methods consider the global, bag-level information by defining the distance metrics between pairwise bags [8,15] or by extracting bag features by a mapping function summarizing the characteristics of the entire bag [16]. The distance metric between two bags can be generally defined such as aggregation of the instance-level distances, kernel-based comparisons for bags or distances in embedded bag feature space. The bag label is then predicted using distance-based classifiers, e.g. k-NN, SVM.

The MIL framework has been adopted in the domain of medical diagnosis, such as identification of cerebral small vessel disease in CT brain images [17], colon histopathological image classification [18], Barrett's cancer diagnosis [19], to name a few. In nuclei-based cancer detection, data exhibits hierarchical structure where tissue samples under microscopy are composed of image patches taken at different fields of view, which are further composed of many cell nuclei to be analyzed. However, few MIL frameworks in the literature are designed for such hierarchical data structure facilitating classification.

Here we propose a supervised hierarchical feature extraction approach which allows a bag to have a set of sub-bags composed of different numbers of instances. We adapt the MIL idea to include information specific to local neighborhoods of cells in histopathology images, as nearby cells have greater likelihood to be related in morphology than cells far away from each other. Our approach, named mi-hSVM, formulates MIL as a SVM maximum soft-margin problem in a new feature space. It consists of three steps. First, a collection of feature vectors (prototypes) are initialized in the instance feature space with a clustering method. Each of these prototypes represents a subclass of instances. Second, with those prototypes, each bag is hierarchically embedded as a point in a new feature space which is obtained via a nonlinear mapping. This effectively transforms the MIL problem into a standard supervised learning problem. Third, the decision boundary and instance prototypes are jointly optimized by maximizing the soft-margin in the SVM classifier. We apply mi-hSVM along with six widely-used MIL methods in the literature to two thyroid diagnostic challenges. We show that a better performance is possible by capturing hierarchical data structure information and exploiting dependencies among instances in our method.

2   Methodology

2.1   Hierarchical Feature Extraction Model

Given fields of view (windows of a pre-determined size), nuclei from each image patch can be located and segmented as described below. The method we now describe is based on the idea of constructing spatially local bags of nuclear features. Such hierarchical composition provides a way to formulate the patient level diagnosis in MIL framework with two layers of instance-bag relationship. In the first layer, image patches are bags and the detected cell nuclei within them are instances. In the second layer, a bag is defined as the set of image patches pertaining to one patient and individual image patches are instances. The overview of the proposed framework is shown in Fig. 1.

Mathematically, the dataset can be represented as $D = \{P_i, y_i\}_{i=1}^{N}$, where P_i is the ith patient, $y_i \in \{-1, 1\}$ is the class label, and N is the number of patients in the dataset. Each patient P_i consists of n_i image patches, denoted as $P_i = \{I_{ij}\}_{j=1}^{n_i}$, and each image patch I_{ij} has n_{ij} detected cell nuclei, denoted as

$I_{ij} = \{x_{ijk}\}_{k=1}^{n_{ij}}$, where $x_{ijk} \in \mathbb{R}^{d \times 1}$ is a feature vector describing the morphology of a nucleus. The goal of the framework is to learn two layers of prototypes (points in feature space) and the decision boundary that maximizes the soft-margin in the SVM classifier. The algorithm discovers the discriminative prototypes to build the nested function $f_i = \chi(\phi(\cdot))$ for feature extraction, where $\phi(\cdot)$ and $\chi(\cdot)$ are nonlinear mappings and will be defined in the sections below. Assume, momentarily, we have fixed prototypes in two layers, the hierarchical feature extraction proceeds as follows.

Layer 1: The set of prototypes in the first layer is denoted as $U_1 = \{u_t^1\}_{t=1}^{m_1}$, containing m_1 elements $u_t^1 \in \mathbb{R}^{d \times 1}$. Given the image patches $I_{ij} = \{x_{ijk}\}_{k=1}^{n_{ij}}$, the mapping function $\phi(I_{ij})$ returns a vector v_{ij} that is a concatenation of a set of sub-vectors: $v_{ij} = [v_{ij1}^T, \cdots, v_{ijt}^T, \cdots, v_{ijm_1}^T]^T$, where v_{ijt} summaries the attributes of nuclei in I_{ij} corresponding to the tth prototype u_t^1. The similarity between instance x_{ijk} and u_t^1 is measured by the function $h_t(x_{ijk}) \in [0,1]$ defined below. The vector v_{ijt} is the weighted mean of all nuclei feature vectors according to their matching degrees to u_t^1, computed as:

$$v_{ijt} = \frac{\sum_{x_{ijk} \in I_{ij}} h_t(x_{ijk}) x_{ijk}}{\sum_{x_{ijk} \in I_{ij}} h_t(x_{ijk})} \tag{1}$$

where $h_t(x_{ijk}) = e^{-\frac{\|x_{ijk} - u_t^1\|_2^2}{\sigma_1}}$ using radial basis function (RBF) kernel.

Layer 2: Repeating the process outlined above, let the output for patient P_i in the first layer be $O_i = \{v_{ij}\}_{j=1}^{n_i}$. A set of prototypes in the second layer is denoted as $U_2 = \{u_t^2\}_{t=1}^{m_2}$, consisting of m_2 elements $u_t^2 \in \mathbb{R}^{m_1 d \times 1}$. The mapping function $\chi(O_i)$ generates vector f_i that is a concatenation of a set of sub-vectors: $f_i = [f_{i1}^T, \cdots, f_{it}^T, \cdots, f_{im_2}^T]^T$. The vector f_{it} is a linear combination of patch-level features with weights $g_t(v_{ij})$ measuring the similarity to the tth prototype u_t^2, denoted as:

$$f_{it} = \frac{\sum_{v_{ij} \in O_i} g_t(v_{ij}) v_{ij}}{\sum_{v_{ij} \in O_i} g_t(v_{ij})} \tag{2}$$

where $g_t(v_{ij}) = e^{-\frac{\|v_{ij} - u_t^2\|_2^2}{\sigma_2}}$ using an RBF kernel.

2.2   Training and Optimization

The hierarchical feature extraction algorithm described above extracts global information regarding each bag by the nested mapping function $\chi(\phi(\cdot))$ in an explicit way. With bag labels, the method transforms MIL into a conventional classification problem. Our goal is to maximize the pattern margin jointly over two layers of prototypes and the discriminant function. Suppose we have feature representation $f = \{f_i\}_{i=1}^N$ for the training data $D = \{P_i, y_i\}_{i=1}^N$, maximizing the SVM soft-margin equals minimizing the corresponding negative Lagrange dual function $L(D)$ [20]:

$$\min_\beta L(D) = \min_\beta - \sum_{i=1}^{N} \beta_i + \frac{1}{2} \sum_{i=1}^{N} \sum_{j=1}^{N} y_i y_j \beta_i \beta_j \langle f_i, f_j \rangle$$

(3)

$$s.t. \quad \forall i : 0 \le \beta_i \le C, \quad \sum_{i=1}^{N} \beta_i y_i = 0$$

where $\langle f_i, f_j \rangle$ is the inner product between f_i and f_j and C is a regularization parameter. The optimal parameters β^* for the decision boundary in SVM and the prototypes $\{U_1^*, U_2^*\}$ can be jointly optimized by finding the minimum of $L(D)$, $\{\beta^*, U_1^*, U_2^*\} = argmin_{\beta, U_1, U_2} L(D)$.

The optimization problem above is not jointly convex in β and $\{U_1, U_2\}$. Thus we opt to perform a heuristic optimization by two alternating steps: (1) given $\{U_1, U_2\}$ and feature vectors f_i, optimal parameters β^* for the decision boundary can be solved by quadratic programming (QP); (2) given β, prototypes $\{U_1^*, U_2^*\}$ can be updated by minimizing $L(D)$. Therefore, β and $\{U_1, U_2\}$ are alternatively optimized via coordinate descent approach. The minimization of $L(D)$ over $\{U_1, U_2\}$ can be performed using a standard gradient descent scheme.

With β fixed, the gradient of L with respect to u_t^2 can be written using the chain-rule of differentiation:

$$\frac{\partial L}{\partial u_t^2} = \sum_{i=1}^{N} \frac{\partial L}{\partial f_{it}} \frac{\partial f_{it}}{\partial u_t^2}$$

$$\frac{\partial L}{\partial f_{it}} = y_i \beta_i \sum_{j=1}^{N} y_j \beta_j f_{jt} \qquad \frac{\partial f_{it}}{\partial u_t^2} = \begin{bmatrix} \frac{\partial f_{it,1}}{\partial u_{t,1}^2} & \cdots & \frac{\partial f_{it,m_1 d}}{\partial u_{t,1}^2} \\ \vdots & \ddots & \vdots \\ \frac{\partial f_{it,1}}{\partial u_{t,m_1 d}^2} & \cdots & \frac{\partial f_{it,m_1 d}}{\partial u_{t,m_1 d}^2} \end{bmatrix}^T$$

(4)

$$\frac{\partial f_{it,r}}{\partial u_{t,s}^2} = \frac{2 \sum_{v_{ij} \in O_i} (v_{ij,s} - u_{t,s}^2)(v_{ij,r} - f_{it,r}) g_t(v_{ij})}{\sigma_2 \sum_{v_{ij} \in O_i} g_t(v_{ij})}, \quad r, s = 1, \cdots, m_1 d$$

where $f_{it,r}$ and $u_{t,s}^2$ are the rth and s^{th} elements in f_{it} and u_t^2 respectively. Similarly, the gradient of L with respect to u_t^1 can be obtained using the chain-rule.

The initialization of $\{U_1, U_2\}$ are cluster centers by the k-means method performed in instance space across all bags, which was able to yield good results in our experiment. The feature representation of the dataset is recomputed after each update of $\{U_1, U_2\}$, followed by the optimization of the decision boundary. Such alternative steps proceed for a predefined number of iterations n_{iter}.

3   Experiments and Results

Dataset. The performance of our method was tested on two thyroid diagnostic challenges where the goal is to differentiate follicular adenoma (FA) from nodular goiter (NG), as well as follicular variant papillary carcinoma

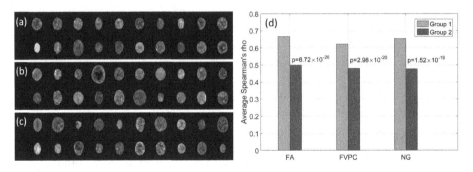

Fig. 2. (a-c) show randomly selected segmented nuclei converted to grayscale from patients diagnosed with FA, FVPC and NG respectively; (d) average Spearman's rho for two groups in three types of thyroid lesions.

(FVPC) vs. NG from nuclear morphology. Under an Institutional Review Board approval, tissue blocks for each type were obtained from the archives of the University of Pittsburgh Medical Center (UPMC). All images in the thyroid dataset were acquired using an Olympus BX51 microscope (100X UIS2 objective and 2 mega pixel SPOT Insight camera) with 0.074 microns/pixel image resolution and $118 \times 89\,\mu m$ field of view. Our study included 78 patients (28 FA, 28 NG, and 22 FVPC) with 609, 584 and 572 fields of view for FA, NG and FVPC respectively. All cases were reviewed by more than one pathologist, and only cases with a clear diagnosis (gold standard) were selected for this study.

Cell Nuclei Segmentation and Feature Extraction. Cell nuclei were segmented using a supervised learning approach [21] from image patches taken at different fields of view. Briefly, the segmentation method constructs a statistical model describing the texture and shape variations of nuclei exemplars selected by users. For any new field of view, each nucleus is segmented by finding the model parameters that maximizes the normalized cross correlation between the model and the local neighborhood. Finally, 28137 cell nuclei were segmented in the dataset, including 10958 nuclei for FA, 6997 nuclei for FVPC and 10182 nuclei for NG. Sample segmented nuclei for each of the thyroid lesions are shown in Fig. 2(a, b, c).

We represented the morphology of each nucleus using a 256-dimensional numerical feature vector described in [9], including 6 morphological features (area, convexity, circularity, perimeter, eccentricity and equivalent diameter), 220 texture features (intensity-based features, Haralick features and Gabor features) and 30 wavelet features. The standard principle component analysis (PCA) technique was then applied to the entire feature set and the top 20 feature directions that captured more than 95 % variations were retained to describe each nucleus.

Existence of Dependency Between Nuclei. The existence of morphological dependency between cell nuclei in the dataset was determined by the correlation degrees in two nuclei groups, including nuclei pairs randomly selected within the same field of view (Group 1) and nuclei pairs randomly selected from two different fields of view (Group 2). The Spearman correlation coefficient was calculated for each group using the first PCA-derived feature direction. The experiment was repeated 100 times and the average Spearman's rho is reported in Fig. 2(d). It can be seen that the correlation degrees are relatively high in both two groups. In addition, the correlation coefficients for Group 1 are higher compared to Group 2 in three types of thyroid lesions, indicating that the correlation degree for nuclei in the same field of view is statistically different (p-$value \approx 0$) from nuclei from two separate fields of view, confirming the hypothesis that nuclei locally close to each other are more correlated in terms of morphology.

Cross Validation. We have utilized a leave one out validation scheme whereby one patient is removed from the dataset and kept as testing data. In the training stage the training data is further split into training and validation sets to search for the optimal parameters of the proposed MIL framework. The usual parameters setting is: $m_1 = 8, m_2 = 3, \sigma_1 = 1.2, \sigma_2 = 1.8$.

Table 1. Evaluation of different approaches on two thyroid diagnosis challenges

Methods	FVPC vs. NG		FA vs. NG	
	Ave. acc	Cohen's kappa	Ave. acc	Cohen's kappa
Naive Bayes+MV [3]	82.00 %	0.6400	69.64 %	0.3928
mi-SVM [12]	72.00 %	0.4427	60.71 %	0.2142
MI-SVM [12]	68.00 %	0.3691	62.50 %	0.2500
Group KNN [8]	75.53 %	0.5211	76.67 %	0.5334
EMDD [13]	74.00 %	0.4849	64.29 %	0.2858
mi-Graph [15]	84.00 %	0.6815	78.78 %	0.5356
mi-hSVM1	82.00 %	0.6434	78.57 %	0.5347
mi-hSVM2	**85.33 %**	**0.7010**	**80.35 %**	**0.6070**

Comparison of Classification Results. We compared the classification performance of our method with six existing approaches, including the frequently used label inheritance plus majority voting strategy (Naive Bayes+MV)[3], mi-SVM [12], MI-SVM [12], Group-KNN [8], EM-DD [13] as well as mi-Graph [15]. In these comparison methods, the entire cell nuclei set belonging to one patient was viewed as a bag and individual segmented nuclei were instances.

For a fair comparison, similar to the proposed method, linear SVM was utilized as the instance-level classifier in Naive Bayes+MV approach. The average accuracy and Cohen's kappa were used to evaluate the classification performance (Table 1). To demonstrate the effectiveness of the hierarchical structure in proposed MIL framework (mi-hSVM2), we also tested the method using one layer (mi-hSVM1) using the same bag-instance definition as the comparison methods.

The proposed method (mi-hSVM2) outperforms other approaches with 85.33 % and 80.35 % average accuracy in FVPC vs. NG and FA vs. NG respectively. From Table 1, we find that mi-hSVM1 provides better accuracy compared to existing methods except mi-Graph in both diagnostic challenges. Moreover, it can be seen that adding another layer will further increase the accuracy and provides the best performance compared to other methods, indicating that the hierarchical structure helps improve the classification performance. In the experiment, the performance of mi-hSVM2 is statistically different from mi-Graph with *p-values* 0.0101 and 0.0366 in FVPC vs. NG and FA vs. NG respectively in 10 runs.

4   Discussion and Conclusion

We have described a novel hierarchical multiple instance learning method for clinical thyroid cancer detection based on cell nuclei morphology. The method provides a solution to the problem of massive nuclei-level diagnostic annotations by pathologists in nuclei-based cancer detection pipelines. Moreover, our method addresses the issue of making use of spatial statistical dependency between instances from the same bag in MIL framework, in addition to showing that if this is done classification results can be improved.

The method extracts hierarchical feature representations for bags to match bag-level labels in a supervised way. In this work, the SVM classifier was utilized to tune the prototypes in each layer for discriminativeness. We note that other types of classifiers can be alternative options in our framework, e.g. neural network classifier for multi-classification appplications.

As far as computational complexity, our method only needs to compute the distance between each instance and each prototype in two layers. Given a patient with m image patches and n nuclei in total, the computational complexities are $O(n_{iter}nm_1)$ and $O(n_{iter}(nm_1 + mm_2))$ for mi-hSVM1 and mi-hSVM2 respectively. For mi-Graph, treating instances within a bag as non-iid, the computation complexity is $O(n(n-1)/2)$ to construct a graph for each bag, which increases quadratically with n.

The proposed method is a general MIL framework that accounts for data structure by being stacked in a repeatable fashion. The better performance of the proposed feature extraction framework compared to other MIL approaches relies on the fact that statistical dependencies among instances are exploited implicitly and hierarchically in supervised feature extraction. The improved performance is likely to manifest itself in other types of pattern recognition tasks.

Acknowledgments. This work was financially supported in part by the National Institutes of Health, grants CA 188938 and GM 090033.

References

1. Zink, D., Fischer, A.H., Nickerson, J.A.: Nuclear structure in cancer cells. Nat. Rev. Cancer **4**(9), 677–687 (2004)
2. Gurcan, M.N., Boucheron, L.E., Can, A., Madabhushi, A., Rajpoot, N.M., Yener, B.: Histopathological image analysis: a review. IEEE Rev. Biomed. Eng. **2**, 147–171 (2009)

3. Ozolek, J.A., Tosun, A.B., Wang, W., Chen, C., Kolouri, S., Basu, S., Rohde, G.K.: Accurate diagnosis of thyroid follicular lesions from nuclear morphology using supervised learning. Med. Image Anal. **18**(5), 772–780 (2014)
4. Basu, S., Kolouri, S., Rohde, G.K.: Detecting and visualizing cell phenotype differences from microscopy images using transport-based morphometry. Proc. Nat. Acad. Sci. **111**(9), 3448–3453 (2014)
5. Daskalakis, A., Kostopoulos, S., Spyridonos, P., Glotsos, D., Ravazoula, P., Kardari, M., Kalatzis, I., Cavouras, D., Nikiforidis, G.: Design of a multi-classifier system for discriminating benign from malignant thyroid nodules using routinely H&E-stained cytological images. Comput. Biol. Med. **38**(2), 196–203 (2008)
6. Irshad, H., Veillard, A., Roux, L., Racoceanu, D.: Methods for nuclei detection, segmentation, and classification in digital histopathology: A review current status and future potential. IEEE Rev. Biomed. Eng. **7**, 97–114 (2014)
7. Loewenstein, W.R., Kanno, Y.: Intercellular communication and the control of tissue growth: lack of communication between cancer cells. Nature **200**, 1248–1249 (1966)
8. Huang, H., Tosun, A.B., Guo, J., Chen, C., Wang, W., Ozolek, J.A., Rohde, G.K.: Cancer diagnosis by nuclear morphometry using spatial information. Pattern Recogn. Lett. **42**, 115–121 (2014)
9. Wang, W., Ozolek, J.A., Rohde, G.K.: Detection and classification of thyroid follicular lesions based on nuclear structure from histopathology images. Cytometry Part A **77**(5), 485–494 (2010)
10. Weinberg, R.: The Biology of Cancer. Garland Science, New York (2013)
11. Amores, J.: Multiple instance classification: review, taxonomy and comparative study. Artif. Intell. **201**, 81–105 (2013)
12. Andrews, S., Tsochantaridis, I., Hofmann, T.: Support vector machines for multiple-instance learning. In: NIPS, pp. 561–568 (2002)
13. Zhang, Q., Goldman, S.A.: EM-DD: An improved multiple-instance learning technique. In: NIPS, pp. 1073–1080 (2001)
14. Zhang, C., Platt, J.C., Viola, P.A.: Multiple instance boosting for object detection. In: NIPS, pp. 1417–1424 (2005)
15. Zhou, Z.H., Sun, Y.Y., Li, Y.F.: Multi-instance learning by treating instances as non-iid samples. In: ICML, pp. 1249–1256 (2009)
16. Chen, Y., Wang, J.Z.: Image categorization by learning and reasoning with regions. J. Mach. Learn. Res. **5**(Aug), 913–939 (2004)
17. Chen, L., Tong, T., Ho, C.P., Patel, R., Cohen, D., Dawson, A.C., Halse, O., Geraghty, O., Rinne, P.E.M., White, C.J., Nakornchai, T., Bentley, P., Rueckert, D.: Identification of cerebral small vessel disease using multiple instance learning. In: Navab, N., Hornegger, J., Wells, W.M., Frangi, A.F. (eds.) MICCAI 2015. LNCS, vol. 9349, pp. 523–530. Springer, Heidelberg (2015). doi:10.1007/978-3-319-24553-9_64
18. Xu, Y., Zhu, J.Y., Eric, I., Chang, C., Lai, M., Tu, Z.: Weakly supervised histopathology cancer image segmentation and classification. Med. Image Anal. **18**(3), 591–604 (2014)
19. Kandemir, M., Hamprecht, F.A.: Computer-aided diagnosis from weak supervision: a benchmarking study. Comput. Med. Imaging Graph. **42**, 44–50 (2015)
20. Bishop, C.M.: Pattern Recognition and Machine Learning. Springer, New York (2006)
21. Chen, C., Wang, W., Ozolek, J.A., Rohde, G.K.: A flexible and robust approach for segmenting cell nuclei from 2D microscopy images using supervised learning and template matching. Cytometry Part A **83**(5), 495–507 (2013)

Using Crowdsourcing for Multi-label Biomedical Compound Figure Annotation

Alba Garcia Seco de Herrera[1][✉],
Roger Schaer[2], Sameer Antani[1], and Henning Müller[2]

[1] Lister Hill National Center for Biomedical Communications,
National Library of Medicine, Bethesda, USA
`albagarcia@nih.gov`
[2] University of Applied Sciences Western Switzerland (HES–SO),
Sierre, Switzerland

Abstract. Information analysis or retrieval for images in the biomedical literature needs to deal with a large amount of compound figures (figures containing several subfigures), as they constitute probably more than half of all images in repositories such as PubMed Central, which was the data set used for the task. The ImageCLEFmed benchmark proposed among other tasks in 2015 and 2016 a multi-label classification task, which aims at evaluating the automatic classification of figures into 30 image types. This task was based on compound figures and thus the figures were distributed to participants as compound figures but also in a separated form. Therefore, the generation of a gold standard was required, so that algorithms of participants can be evaluated and compared. This work presents the process carried out to generate the multi-labels of $\sim$ 2650 compound figures using a crowdsourcing approach. Automatic algorithms to separate compound figures into subfigures were used and the results were then validated or corrected via crowdsourcing. The image types (MR, CT, X–ray, ...) were also annotated by crowdsourcing including detailed quality control. Quality control is necessary to insure quality of the annotated data as much as possible. $\sim$ 625 h were invested with a cost of $\sim$ 870\$.

Keywords: Multi-label annotation · Compound figures · Crowdsourcing

1 Introduction

Probably more than 50 % of the figures in the biomedical literature in PubMed Central (PMC)[1] are compound figures (figures consisting of several subfigures) based on estimations of analysing a subset of the data [11]. In total, PMC in 2016 contains over 4 million images, so the extent of the knowledge stored in compound figures is important. A few simple examples of compound figures are shown

---

[1] http://www.ncbi.nlm.nih.gov/pmc/.

© Springer International Publishing AG 2016
G. Carneiro et al. (Eds.): LABELS 2016/DLMIA 2016, LNCS 10008, pp. 228–237, 2016.
DOI: 10.1007/978-3-319-46976-8_24

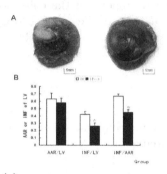
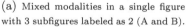
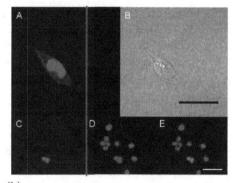

(a) Mixed modalities in a single figure with 3 subfigures labeled as 2 (A and B).   (b) Mixed modalities in a single figure with no visual gaps between most subfigures.

Fig. 1. Examples of compound figures in the biomedical literature.

in Fig. 1 but not all images are as easy to separate. Information indexing and information retrieval (IR) systems for images should be capable of distinguishing the parts of compound figures that are relevant to a given query to deliver focused retrieval results. Identifying the image types of subfigures can help to characterize compound figures, either by using the subfigures separately or the entire compound figure. In addition, image modality is an important piece of information that can be integrated into any retrieval system to enhance or filter its results [12,17]. Therefore, the ImageCLEFmed[2] image classification and retrieval benchmark proposed in 2015 and 2016 a multi-label task aiming at labeling all compound figures with each of the modalities of the subfigures contained without knowing the subfigure separations that are contained in the image [10,11]. It provides a useful scenario to compare the effectiveness of systems to access the detailed content of compound figures. This article presents the work carried out to generate a high quality ground truth for the evaluations in the task.

Image sharing sites like Flickr[3] offer a large number of images often with several tags describing the images added by the user, even though the quality can vary. Sometimes the content of the images is described but sometimes also what the image is about or what the image evokes, for example in terms of feelings. Some studies [14,15] have shown the great potential of crowdsourcing in the context of medical imaging. However, in the medical open access literature almost no meta-data exist for figures and subfigures besides the free text captions.

Work has been done for multi-label annotation in the past. In NUS-WIDE [4], a small set of images from Flickr is manually annotated with 81 concepts. Wang et al. [18] encode each image into a vector and then a sparse label coding based on subspaces is applied to harness multi-label information. Nowak et al. [16] assessed ground truth of 99 multi-label images by using experts and mechanical turk. However, to the best of our knowledge, no previous work deals with multi-label annotation of compound figures or similar images from the medical literature.

---

[2] http://imageclef.org/.

[3] https://www.flickr.com/.

This paper presents the methodology followed to annotated the collection created for the 2016 ImageCLEFmed task. The remainder of the article is organized as follows. Section 2 describes the database and methods used. Results obtained are presented in Sect. 3. The article concludes in Sect. 4.

2   Methods

This section describes the methods used to multi-label compound figures. The Crowdflower[4] platform was used for the crowdsourcing [5].

2.1   Dataset

The database used is a subset of 231,000 images from PMC that contained over 4,200,000 images in 2016. Figure 2 shows that hierarchy of images classes that was used [10,11] to classify all subfigures into types.

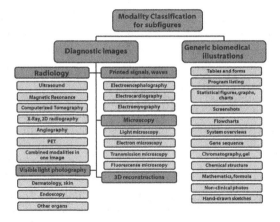

Fig. 2. The image class hierarchy proposed by ImageCLEFmed.

2.2   Overview

To simplify the evaluation of the multi-label annotation of compound figures and optimize the knowledge gained, the task was divided into several subtasks. The following tasks were carried out to evaluate all steps of the process of analysing content in compound figures:

1. automatic compound figure detection (decide whether a figure is a compound or non–compound figure);
2. automatic compound figure separation (find the lines that cut compound figures into their parts);

---

[4] http://www.crowdflower.com/.

3. manual compound figure separation verification (check whether images were correctly separated);
4. automatic subfigure classification (automatic determination of the type of image in a subfigure);
5. manual subfigure classification verification (validate the results of the previous step);
6. manual subfigure classification (manually classify the images incorrectly classified automatically);
7. manual class balancing (assure that all classes are represented);
8. compound figure multi-label assignment.

Details on each of the steps are given below.

Automatic Compound Figure Detection. The procedure described in [6] was used to automatically classify the figures into image types including a 'compound or multipane figure' class. Figures classified as 'compound or multipane figure' were then randomly selected for the next steps in the classification to be able to take as many figures as possible into account.

Automatic Compound Figure Separation. Compound figures were automatically separated into subfigures using the approach proposed by Chhatkuli et al. [3]. Figure 3 shows two compound figures automatically separated into subfigures using this approach. However, not all selected compound figures were correctly separated into subfigures (see Fig. 4 for examples that were incorrectly separated). Both missing lines occurred and additional lines within single subfigures. Therefore, a verification step was implemented to identify incorrect separations and then correct them.

Manual Compound Figure Separation Verification. In this step, a crowdsourcing task was run where the following simple question was proposed:

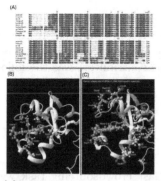 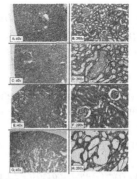

(a) Compound figure containing 3 subfigures. (b) Compound figure containing 8 subfigures.

Fig. 3. Examples of compound figures correctly separated into subfigures automatically. The blue lines show the detected separators (Color figure online).

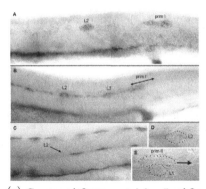 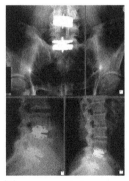

(a) Compound figure containing 5 subfig-   (b) Compound figure con-
ures but separated only into 3 subfigures.   taining 3 subfigures but sep-
                                              arated into 4 subfigures.

Fig. 4. Examples of compound figures incorrectly separated into subfigures automatically.

– Is the compound figure correctly separated?:
  • Yes;
  • No.

The figures marked as correctly separated were used for the following step. Incorrectly separated figures were manually separated in a subsequent step.

Automatic Subfigure Classification. The subfigures obtained using the automatic separation from the previous step were automatically classified into image types using an approach based on k–Nearest Neighbors (k–NN) and multiple visual features (see García et al. [8,9]). On a past database a good performance of 68 % was obtained for the same task.

Manual Subfigure Classification Validation. Similar to [6] a figure classification validation step was carried out to assure the data quality. In this case the subfigures were presented together with the automatically labeled class in a crowdsourcing task. The question asked to the contributors was the following:

– Does the figure correspond to the stated category?:
  • Yes, perfect classification;
  • No, wrong category;
  • Not sure.

Manual Subfigure Classification. One last crowdsourcing task was created to classify the figures not marked as correctly classified in the previous step. This task was slower than the previous steps. Contributors were asked to classify each of the images according to the full hierarchy shown in Fig. 2. A hierarchy was proposed in the interface to simplify the task (see Fig. 5), so more than one click was necessary for the classification, with three levels for diagnostic images and two levels for general illustrations. In a similar task in 2015 we realized for crowdsourcing the contributors used the categories requiring few clicks much more often, which led to changes in the setup. As crowdsourcing pays per annotated image there is a risk to have people use the fastest way to categorize if there are differences. Thus the structure was slightly changed to have the same number of clicks for each of the classes in 2016, which avoided this bias.

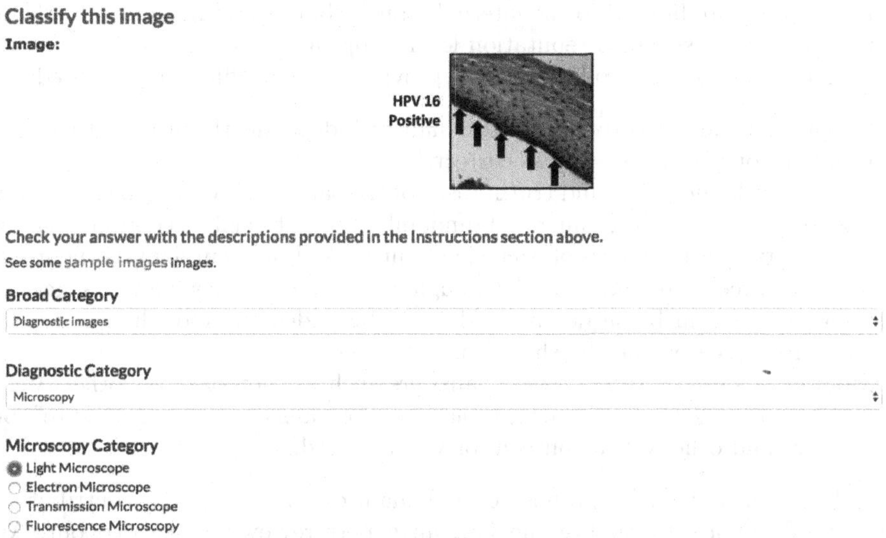

Classify this image
Image:

Check your answer with the descriptions provided in the Instructions section above.
See some sample images images.

Broad Category

| Diagnostic images | ⇕ |

Diagnostic Category

| Microscopy | ⇕ |

Microscopy Category
- ◉ Light Microscope
- ○ Electron Microscope
- ○ Transmission Microscope
- ○ Fluorescence Microscopy

Fig. 5. Screenshot of a crowdsourcing task that aims at classifying biomedical figures from the literature into image types.

Manual Class Balancing. After the previous step several of the classes were not represented or contained only very few images. Therefore, compound figures containing the image types that were underrepresented were manually selected from the database to better represent these classes.

Compound Figure Multi-label Assignment. To finalize the annotation process, each compound figure was assigned with the labels of all subfigures that it contains. Like this we can validate not only images that separate and then classify subfigures but also multi-class labeling based on entire figures.

2.3   Crowdsourcing Quality Control

A quality control (QC) is needed when using crowdsourcing to ensure the success of the annotation task [13], particularly with medical images where some domain knowledge is very benefitial [1]. QC approches were applied during design–time and runtime [2].

First, tasks were designed to be as simple as possible to make sure the persons understand the tasks quickly and correctly. This is the reason to divide the process into several subtasks. Automatic steps were added to limit the manual tasks where possible and reducing the number of figures to be manually classified since this is the most challenging step of the process. A detailed and unambiguous description of the tasks was provided to the participants and in case of doubt the participants could access this description at any moment. In particular, the description included several figure examples of each case or modality. In addition, Crowdflower provides feedback from several experts on the task design. Contributors were limited to the internal team of biomedical imaging experts or contributors with specified reputation level to optimize the quality.

For runtime QC, the following tools provided by Crowdflower were used:

- Output agreement: two contributors had to independently provide the same result to consider an answer as correct.
- Control with known ground truth: tasks of the same type with known answers are proposed at the beginning and randomly during the job execution to check the quality of the answers of each contributor. A 70 % accuracy was the minimum required to be maintained throughout the job as Crowdflower suggests; a few images can be subjective and could be added to more than one class and for this reason the threshold was not stricter.
- Monitor answer patterns: specific answers such as 'not sure' or 'other' were monitored; 17 % was the acceptable range of answers like "Not sure" or "Other" and otherwise a contributor was removed.

Allahbakhsh et al. [2] propose that domain experts check the contribution quality. Therefore, to finalize the QC, an expert review was carried out. An expert in biomedical imaging manually checked the contributions quickly to ensure the high quality of the annotations.

3 Results

This section describes the results obtained in the data classification and annotation steps described in Sect. 2.

15,403 compound figures were initially selected and automatically separated from the ImageCLEFmed 2013 database [7]. After the compound figure separation step, $\sim$ 57 % of the figures were correctly separated based on a manual validation. This task was carried out using the free internal Crowdflower interface that can be used for a known set of people. Eight experts in biomedical imaging verified the separation of the figures in $\sim$ 98 h. A subset was selected to be separated into subfigures and the subfigures were automatically classified. In the subfigure classification validation process $\sim$ 56 % were defined as correctly classified into the correct figure type. More than 100 contributors validated the classification in $\sim$ 49 h with a cost of 396.68$. The incorrectly classified subfigures were manually classified into exact figure types via crowdsourcing. To evaluate the correct design of the task, the first 1,149 subfigures were classified using the internal interface by 5 experts in $\sim$ 5 h. Then, the remaining sub-figures ($\sim$ 9800) were classified by more than 100 contributors in 427 h with a cost of 472.66\$. After this process, a manual expert review was needed to solve subfigure classification mistakes.

As the final selection of subfigures did not contain all figure types and was very unbalanced it was decided to manually add additional compound figures that contain relatively rare subfigure types. 122 compound figures containing the following categories were added and then manually separated and classified: angiography; computerized tomography; magnetic resonance; ultrasound; electroencephalography; mathematics program listing; and combined modalities in one image. Even with this balancing step, the class distribution remains uneven, as it is in the biomedical literature, even though it was slightly more balanced.

In total, 2,651 compound figures were annotated with multiple labels of their subfigures, containing 8,397 subfigures. These figures were distributed for the ImageCLEFmed 2016 multi-label and subfigure classification tasks[5] [11] together with the figure captions. In 2015, 1,568 were distributed for the ImageCLEFmed multi-label task [10]. These figures were distributed as a training set (containing 1,071 figures) and a test set (containing 497 figures). Their subfigures were released for the ImageCLEFmed 2015 subfigure classification task. The training set contained 4,532 subfigures and the test set 2,244 subfigures. In 2016, ImageCLEFmed used all the figures distributed in 2015 as training set and the additional annotated figures were distributed as test set. As a result, 1,568 figures were provided as training set and 1,083 as test set in the ImageCLEFmed 2016 multi-label tasks. The ImageCLEFmed 2016 subfigure classification task contained 6,776 subfigures in the training set and 4,166 subfigures in the test set.

In 2016, ImageCLEFmed proposed 5 tasks: compound figure detection; compound figure separation; multi-label classification; subfigure classification and caption prediction. This work describes the generation of the data for the multi-label classification task and therefore the subfigure classification tasks. The ImageCLEFmed multi-label classification task aims at labeling each compound figure with each of the modalities (see Fig. 2) of the subfigures contained without knowing where the separation lines are. Furthermore, the ImageCLEFmed subfigure classification aims at classifying figures into the 30 image types of the proposed hierarchy.

Research groups could participate in these tasks and compare their research tools with those of other researchers on the same data and the same evaluation scenario. Four groups submitted 15 runs to the ImageCLEFmed multi-label task and ten groups submitted 45 runs to the ImageCLEFmed subfigure classification task. More information can be found in the working notes of CLEF 2016 [11].

4   Conclusions

This article presents the steps used to annotate compound figures from the biomedical literature with figure type information and to separate compound figures

---

[5] http://imageclef.org/2016/medical/.

with separation lines to cut them into all subfigures. As a result 2,651 compound figures were annotated with figure type information and all figures were made available for the ImageCLEFmed 2016 multi-label task. To ensure the quality of the annotation, the process was divided into multiple steps combining automatic tools (e.g. for figure separation and figure modality classification) and manual work to validate or label data. Crowdsourcing was used to accelerate the tasks with a limited cost. Therefore, it was very important to carry out QC. Thanks to the described process it was possible to annotate the figures automatically and thus limit the manual control to verify and correct the annotations. The created resources are now available for the medical image analysis and image retrieval community. This is a manually created gold standard to build tools to create more metadata for the over four million figures in PMC and the likely over 2 million compound figures containing an estimated 6–7 million additional subfigures. Providing detailed metadata for these figures can well help to make the knowledge contained in the figures accessible for research and clinical work.

Acknowledgments. This research was supported in part by the Intramural Research Program of the National Institutes of Health (NIH), National Library of Medicine (NLM), and Lister Hill National Center for Biomedical Communications (LHNCBC).

References

1. Albarqouni, S., Baur, C., Achilles, F., Belagiannis, V., Demirci, S., Navab, N.: Aggnet: deep learning from crowds for mitosis detection in breast cancer histology images. IEEE Trans. Med. Imaging **35**(5), 1313–1321 (2016)
2. Allahbakhsh, M., Benatallah, B., Ignjatovic, A., Motahari Nezhad, H.R., Bertino, E., Dustdar, S.: Quality control in crowdsourcing systems: issues and directions. IEEE Internet Comput. **2**, 76–81 (2013)
3. Chhatkuli, A., Markonis, D., Foncubierta-Rodríguez, A., Meriaudeau, F., Müller, H.: Separating compound figures in journal articles to allow for subfigure classification. In: SPIE Medical Imaging (2013)
4. Chua, T.S., Tang, J., Hong, R., Li, H., Luo, Z., Zheng, Y.: NUS-WIDE: a real-world web image database from national university of singapore. In: Proceedings of the ACM International Conference on Image and Video Retrieval, pp. 48. ACM (2009)
5. Foncubierta-Rodríguez, A., Müller, H.: Ground truth generation in medical imaging: a crowdsourcing based iterative approach. In: Workshop on Crowdsourcing for Multimedia. ACM Multimedia, October 2012
6. de Herrera, A.G.S., Foncubierta-Rodríguez, A., Markonis, D., Schaer, R., Müller, H.: Crowdsourcing for medical image classification. In: Annual Congress SGMI 2014 (2014)
7. Garcia Seco de Herrera, A., Kalpathy-Cramer, J., Demner Fushman, D., Antani, S., Müller, H.: Overview of the ImageCLEF 2013 medical tasks. In: Working Notes of CLEF 2013 (Cross Language Evaluation Forum), September 2013
8. García Seco de Herrera, A., Markonis, D., Joyseeree, R., Schaer, R., Foncubierta-Rodríguez, A., Müller, H.: Semi–supervised learning for image modality classification. In: Müller, H., et al. (eds.) MRMD 2015. LNCS, vol. 9059, pp. 85–98. Springer, Heidelberg (2015). doi:10.1007/978-3-319-24471-6_8

9. Garcia Seco de Herrera, A., Markonis, D., Schaer, R., Eggel, I., Müller, H.: The medGIFT group in ImageCLEFmed 2013. In: Working Notes of CLEF 2013 (Cross Language Evaluation Forum), September 2013

10. Garcia Seco de Herrera, A., Müller, H., Bromuri, S.: Overview of the ImageCLEF 2015 medical classification task. In: Working Notes of CLEF 2015 (Cross Language Evaluation Forum), September 2015

11. Garcia Seco de Herrera, A., Schaer, R., Bromuri, S., Müller, H.: Overview of the ImageCLEF 2016 medical task. In: Working Notes of CLEF 2016 (Cross Language Evaluation Forum), September 2016

12. Kalpathy-Cramera, J., Hersh, W.: Automatic image modality based classification and annotation to improve medical image retrieval. Stud. Health Technol. Inf. **129**, 1334–1338 (2007)

13. Lease, M.: On quality control and machine learning in crowdsourcing. Human Comput. **11**, 11 (2011)

14. Maier-Hein, L.: Crowdsourcing for reference correspondence generation in endoscopic images. In: Golland, P., Hata, N., Barillot, C., Hornegger, J., Howe, R. (eds.) MICCAI 2014. LNCS, vol. 8674, pp. 349–356. Springer, Heidelberg (2014). doi:10.1007/978-3-319-10470-6_44

15. Mitry, D., Peto, T., Hayat, S., Morgan, J.E., Khaw, K.T., Foster, P.J.: Crowdsourcing as a novel technique for retinal fundus photography classification: analysis of images in the epic norfolk cohort on behalf of the UK biobank eye and vision consortium. PLOS ONE **8**(8), e71154 (2013)

16. Nowak, S., Rüger, S.: How reliable are annotations via crowdsourcing: a study about inter-annotator agreement for multi-label image annotation. In: Proceedings of the International Conference on Multimedia Information Retrieval, MIR 2010, pp. 557–566. ACM, New York (2010)

17. Tirilly, P., Lu, K., Mu, X., Zhao, T., Cao, Y.: On modality classification and its use in text-based image retrieval in medical databases. In: 9th International Workshop on Content-Based Multimedia Indexing (2011)

18. Wang, C., Yan, S., Zhang, L., Zhang, H.J.: Multilabel sparse coding for automatic image annotation. In: IEEE Conference on Computer Vision and Pattern Recognition, pp. 1643–1650. IEEE (2009)

Towards the Semantic Enrichment of Free-Text Annotation of Image Quality Assessment for UK Biobank Cardiac Cine MRI Scans

Valentina Carapella[1](✉), Ernesto Jiménez-Ruiz[2], Elena Lukaschuk[1],
Nay Aung[3], Kenneth Fung[3], Jose Paiva[3], Mihir Sanghvi[3], Stefan Neubauer[1],
Steffen Petersen[3], Ian Horrocks[2], and Stefan Piechnik[1]

[1] Radcliffe Department of Medicine, Oxford Centre for Clinical Magnetic Resonance
Research (OCMR), University of Oxford, Oxford, UK
vcarapella@gmail.com
[2] Information Systems Group, Department of Computer Science,
University of Oxford, Oxford, UK
[3] William Harvey Research Institute,
NIHR Cardiovascular Biomedical Research Unit at Barts,
Queen Mary University of London, London, UK

Abstract. Image quality assessment is fundamental as it affects the level of confidence in any output obtained from image analysis. Clinical research imaging scans do not often come with an explicit evaluation of their quality, however reports are written associated to the patient/volunteer scans. This rich free-text documentation has the potential to provide automatic image quality assessment if efficiently processed and structured. This paper aims at showing how the use of Semantic Web technology for structuring free-text documentation can provide means for automatic image quality assessment. We aim to design and implement a semantic layer for a special dataset, the annotations made in the context of the UK Biobank Cardiac Cine MRI pilot study. This semantic layer will be a powerful tool to automatically infer or validate quality scores for clinical images and efficiently query image databases based on quality information extracted from the annotations. In this paper we motivate the need for this semantic layer, present an initial version of our ontology as well as preliminary results. The presented approach has the potential to be extended to broader projects and ultimately employed in the clinical setting.

1 Introduction

UK Biobank is a large scale population study at the national level aimed at improving the understanding, diagnosis and treatment of a wide range of diseases, such as cancer, stroke or cardiac pathologies [1]. In 2006 the recruitment began of 500,000 volunteers aged 40–69 across UK who underwent a number of clinical tests and agreed to have their health followed. UK Biobank is a complex

© Springer International Publishing AG 2016
G. Carneiro et al. (Eds.): LABELS 2016/DLMIA 2016, LNCS 10008, pp. 238–248, 2016.
DOI: 10.1007/978-3-319-46976-8_25

project addressing multiple organs by means of various clinical tests, including different imaging modalities. The outcome of this study will be available to researchers worldwide.

Within UK Biobank, Cardiovascular Magnetic Resonance Imaging (CMR) plays a fundamental role in the assessment of cardiac function. Each volunteer participating to the UK Biobank imaging arm undergoes a series of MRI sequences to image the heart: Cine MRI, tagged MRI, T1-mapping and Phase-contrast imaging [2,3]. A pilot study of 5,000 CMR scans has been released and is shared for data analysis with affiliated researchers analysing Cine MRI, the most common CMR sequence in clinical practice.

The topic of automatic image quality assessment is of particular importance in relation to the management and post-processing of large scale datasets, such as the UK Biobank pilot study, and more generally in clinical research. Consistent image quality assessment provides means to evaluate how reliable the parameters values obtained from the image analysis are. However, image quality assessment is seldom carried out in an organised and structured way. Clinicians and radiographers might repeat a scan if they detect technical problems in real-time, otherwise, the sub-optimal quality goes undetected and is not recorded. In post-processing, image analysts often discard images with technical problems without further feedback to the image acquisition team. In the context of the UK Biobank CMR pilot study, one of the main aims was to address this lack of cross-talk between the acquisition and post-processing phase. Data analysis of the pilot study was in fact based on two key aspects: quality assessment of the imaging data and manual contour delineation. Figure 1 highlights the two components of the analysis. Quality assessment of the Cine MRI scans was carried out through a combination of free-text comments and numerical quality scores. Manual delineation of contours (also known as segmentation) was carried out for the four chambers of the heart, which then results in the computation of fundamental parameters of cardiac function. As per UK Biobank protocols, all such derived data will be returned to UK Biobank for inclusion in the central database, whence they can be disseminated to other groups with appropriate research approvals.[1]

For the purposes of our work, we focus only on the quality assessment data, which is the combination of free-text annotation and numerical quality scores. The quality scores provide a quick overall classification of the images, for example, for statistical purposes. The free-text annotation is rich in information but cannot be processed in an easy and efficient manner as the numerical scores. A promising efficient solution can be sought in the field of Semantic Web. The semantics of the free-text annotations, which describe the quality of the image analysis, will be defined via a structured vocabulary or ontology, which we are going to call *CMR-QA* (Cardiovascular Magnetic Resonance Quality Assessment). An ontology is an explicit specification of a conceptualisation providing an unambiguous and formal representation of a given domain or field of knowledge [4,5]. In other words, ontologies provide a controlled vocabulary about

---

[1] http://www.ukbiobank.ac.uk/register-apply/.

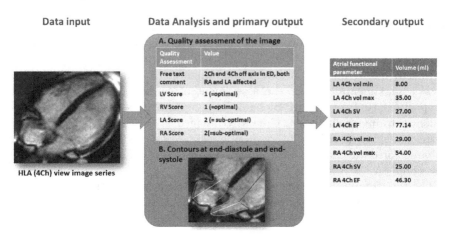

Fig. 1. Example of analysis pipeline restricted to the case of HLA view. Quality scores are 1 = optimal, 2 = sub-optimal and 3 = unreliable or non-analysable.

the relevant terms in that domain and their relationships. Ontologies are extensively used in biomedicine (e.g., [6]) and in other domains like the energy sector (e.g., [7]). There have also been recent efforts in using ontologies to describe the information within a biobank (e.g., [8–11]).

Generating a semantic layer for the annotations provides the means to structure them in a formal and unambiguous way while retaining all the descriptive power of natural language. This semantic layer will provide machine-readable data and will be a powerful tool for (i) fast and efficient processing of the free-text comments; (ii) automatic image quality assessment from such comments and generation of quality scores; (iii) evaluation of the quality of the free-text comments in terms of information completeness, ambiguity and variability; (iv) training purposes (e.g., showing preferred annotation styles for different types of images); (v) efficient semantic access (i.e. database querying) to the images by the UK Biobank target users, such as researchers in the field of automatic segmentation, or clinical researchers who need a specific subset as a control group in their study.

2   Methodological Approach

Data analysis for the 5,000 CMR pilot study was carried out by a team of eight *observers* from two clinical research centres. The observers were professionals experienced in this type of analysis but with different backgrounds and expertise. Quality assessment and general data analysis progress was managed through a shared spreadsheet by the team.

2.1   The Imaging Data

Each individual CMR dataset included in the 5,000 CMR pilot study for the UK Biobank project contains a series of MRI scans of the heart aiming at imaging different aspects of cardiac function and structure. However, for the purposes of the first release of data, only a subset of the images acquired were analysed. Data analysis was initially restricted to the following Cine MRI views: *(i)* Short axis (SA). Left and right ventricle (LV and RV) are contoured in this view at two phases of the cardiac cycle, end-diastole and end-systole. For the left ventricle both endocardial and epicardial contours are drawn. For the right ventricle only the endocardial contour is considered. *(ii)* Horizontal long axis (HLA or 4Ch), also referred to as four chamber view. Left and right atrial (LA and RA) endocardium are contoured in this view at two phases. The first phase is ventricular end-diastole and it provides the minimal atrial volume. The second phase is identified by the opening of the mitral valve, and it is used to obtain the maximal atrial volume. *(iii)* Vertical long axis (VLA or 2Ch), or two chamber view. Only left atrium is contoured at the same phases of the cardiac cycle as HLA.

2.2   Quality Assessment of the Data

The individual dataset for each participant in the pilot study thus contained the three aforementioned Cine MRI views. Data analysis of each dataset was subdivided into two phases, quality assessment and manual contouring of anatomical structures. The quality assessment part is the focus of this paper. Quality assessment addressed the three views individually, as they are acquired separately. Therefore, for example, a good quality SA image can be paired with a poor quality HLA or VLA images. Figure 1, shows the pipeline of data analysis and output for the HLA view.

The observers were required to evaluate each subset of images according to certain aspects likely to affect image quality. The level of detail provided also varied with the experience and background of the observer. For example, those with clinical experience were able to suggest the presence of a specific pathology, only when this was considered to affect the quality of the image. Those with knowledge of MRI physics provided more insight on the nature of artefacts. Figure 2 shows a diagram of the different aspects of quality assessment the observer were taking into account, divided into technical issues (left-side panel) and patient-related issues (right-side panel). Examples of possible issues are provided for each sub-area of quality assessment.

For those images flagged as sub-optimal or unreliable, the observers were asked to write a short free-text comment summarising, for the three imaging views, the reasons for such decision. This resulted in a wide variability in the level of detail provided, but also in the vocabulary employed. In combination to comments, the observers were also asked to provide a numerical score (1 = optimal, 2 = sub-optimal, 3= unreliable) to summarise how reliable the contours of each cardiac chamber was in the light of the quality assessment given to the images.

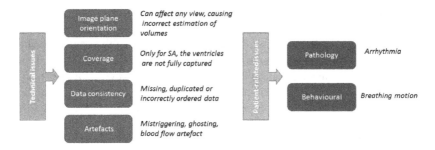

Fig. 2. Quality assessment parameters with examples.

2.3 Definition of the Semantic Layer

We aim at providing a formal description or *semantic layer* for our *domain*, that is the quality assessment (both free-text annotations and quality scores) of the cardiovascular Cine MRI views as performed in the UK Biobank CMR pilot study. The semantic layer will be composed by: *(i)* an *ontology*, containing concepts relevant to our domain (i.e., vocabulary occurring in the free-text annotations or terms relevant to the image analysis) and relationships among those concepts; *(ii) ontology data* which is the re-formulation of the information content of the free-text annotations according to the ontology; *(iii) ontology rules* to infer knew knowledge in combination with the ontology and the ontology data.

Ontology Development. The ontology development is still ongoing and greatly benefits from the close collaboration with the observers involved in the image analysis and quality assessment phase. Given the highly theoretical nature of ontology development, in this section we are only providing some key examples, described in plain text, of the key components of an ontology.

Concepts in biomedical ontologies are typically organised in a hierarchy according to *(i)* a *broader-narrower* relationship, that is classifying concepts from general to more detailed ones, e.g., the heart is an organ; *(ii)* a *part-whole* relationship, e.g., the left atrium is part of the heart. In addition, ontology concepts may also be related to each other by means of other relationships, e.g., arrhythmia affects the heart.

With this framework in mind, we have started developing the *CMR-QA* (Cardiovascular Magnetic Resonance Quality Assessment) ontology to include both general knowledge about the domain and more concrete aspects about the image quality assessment.[2] For example, *CMR-QA* encodes general knowledge about concepts such as *Cine MRI Scan* is a kind of *MRI Scan*; but it also encodes more specific knowledge such as *wrong image plane orientation* is a kind of *technical issue* or *RA off axis* is a specific type of *wrong image plane orientation* (please refer to Fig. 2). Although the relationship specifying that *Cine MRI Scan* is a

---

[2] *CMR-QA* ontology and related assets can be downloaded from https://github.com/ernestojimenezruiz/CMR-QA-Semantic-Layer.

kind of *MRI Scan* may not be seen as an interesting piece of knowledge, this knowledge will not be otherwise known by a computer and thus it should be specified. Furthermore, this top-level knowledge will facilitate the integration with other established domain ontologies that do not contain concepts as fine-grained and specific to our domain as the ones provided in *CMR-QA*.

Concepts and relationships belong to the logical realm. However, non-logical knowledge can also be added to the ontology in the form of lexical information (synonyms, comments, cross-references). For example, *CMR-QA* includes that *LA out of plane* is an alternative label or synonym for *LA off axis*, which captures some of the variability observed in the free-text comments (refer to Table 1 for the complete list of variants).

Ontology Data via Free-text Comment Mining. We are developing *named entity recognition* (NER) techniques to transform the free-text comments into semantically rich data according to *CMR-QA* (see [12,13] for a survey). In other words, each free-text comment is decomposed using text-mining techniques into chunks, which will be then associated to statements or triples in the form of *<subject predicate object>* expressions. For example, suppose we have a composite comment "Basal slice missing, wrong plane RA". The text-mining process identifies two quality issues by breaking the sentence into two parts: "Basal slice missing" and "wrong plane RA". Focussing on the latter, the chunk of text *"wrong plane RA"* in the free-text comment is then associated to the triple: $< issue_i \ rdf{:}type \ RA \ off\text{-}axis>$; this is a computer-friendly representation of the fact that there is a quality issue (the subject), uniquely identified here by *issue$_i$* where i is a counter. This subject belongs to a certain type (the predicate *rdf:type*), the type being *RA off-axis* (the object).

Ontology Rules. Ontology rules are being developed together with the ontology to infer additional knowledge about the data via automatic reasoning (e.g., [14]). The rules are implications between an antecedent and a consequent, that is, whenever the antecedent holds then the consequent must hold as well. For example, if the free-text annotation includes the comment *RA off-axis* (antecedent) then the comment is necessarily referred to the *HLA view* (consequent). Analogously, the free-text comment *basal slice is missing* (antecedent) implies a lack of coverage associated to the *SA view* (consequent). One of the key points of carefully developing such rules in our work is that they can be used to infer numerical quality scores from the comments. For example, the presence of *Lack of coverage* (antecedent) will always lead to a sub-optimal quality score associated to the right and left ventricle (consequent). In addition, we aim to use rules to reveal potential incompleteness or ambiguity. For example, we can classify a comment such as *LA off axis* as incomplete, because neither the imaging view or the cardiac cycle phase are indicated.

Table 1. Variability for the *LA off axis* example in numbers. The synonyms with asterisk take into account variations (abbreviations and most common typos) associated to them.

Synonyms	Occurrence
foreshortened*	2
off axis*	179
off-axis	13
off axis	145
off axes	21
off plane	0
out of axis	26
wrong plane	7

Table 2. Ambiguity in the annotation of HLA (4Ch) when it is not explicitly explained if either left or right atrium or both atria are affected by the off axis technical issue (highlighted in bold in the table).

Off axis subset	Occurrence
Total off axis sentences	515
Only referring to LA	173
Only referring to RA	27
Reference to both atria	53
HLA (4Ch) without reference	**226**
Other annotations	36

3   Preliminary Results

The free-text annotations provide a rich source of information for target users of UK Biobank that goes beyond the simple classification provided by the numerical scores. However, free-text is prone to variability and ambiguity which hinders the efficient use of its information content for querying and access of Cine MRI scans according to the quality assessment outcomes. In this section we provide two examples to motivate the need for a formal structuring of quality assessment by means of the design and implementation of a semantic layer for the annotations.

3.1   Example 1: Variability

Variability is due to natural human variability, for example there is difference in the used terminology or different opinions about the quality of the image. This variability can be limited only in part by the use of a standardised analysis protocol. For example, different observers can correctly flag as *LA off axis*, *LA out of plane*, *wrong LA plane*, *2Ch out of plane*, or *LA foreshortened* an image where the plane chosen to acquire a long axis view was not optimally aligned to measure left atrial (LA) volumes. Table 1 shows the occurrence of the set of synonyms used by the observers for the case of *LA off axis* in a total of 214 comments referring to wrong image plane affecting left atrium. In the development of the semantic layer with respect to this specific example, we made a first decision to define as preferred label *LA off axis*, because it is the most commonly used. Then we have defined as accepted synonyms all the other variants in the table. Figure 3 shows a fragment of *CMR-QA* with the preferred label and a subset of the accepted synonyms of the concept *LA off axis*.

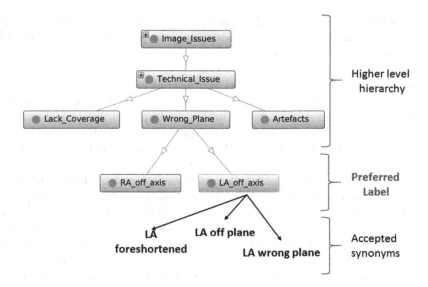

Fig. 3. Example fragment of the *CMR-QA* ontology showing the scope of the concept *LA off axis* and its synonyms.

3.2 Example 2: Ambiguity

Ambiguity is typically due to missing information in the annotations which may lead to an ambiguous interpretation. For example, within the UK Biobank pilot study analysis protocol, the annotation *2Ch out of plane* will always refer to a left atrium that is off-axis since in VLA (2Ch) only the left atrium is contoured. However, *4Ch out of plane* would represent an ambiguous annotation since in HLA (4Ch) both left and the right atria are contoured. Table 2 describes the occurrence of ambiguous HLA (4Ch) related comments, with respect to missing reference about which atrium is affected. On a total of 515 sentences generally relating to off axis issues (could be for any imaging view), 226 address HLA (4Ch) without the explicit reference to LA, RA or atria. Detailed knowledge of the UK Biobank pilot CMR dataset helps addressing such ambiguity, as the observers came to realise that in most of the cases where *4Ch out of plane* applies, the left atrium is most affected. Hence, we have created project-specific ontology rules that *(i)* raise a warning of incompleteness for the comment, and *(ii)* assign *LA off axis* (consequent) as the most likely outcome to such comments where a *wrong plane* is observed in the *HLA view* (antecedent).

4 Discussion

In this paper we have presented the first steps in defining a semantic layer within the quality assessment of UK Biobank Cardiac Cine MRI scans with the main aim of automatically inferring image quality scores from free-text annotations.

In this section we comment on the motivating examples shown in the previous section, summarise the future work and emphasise the likely benefits for UK Biobank users and clinical research.

Motivating Examples. In Sect. 3 we have presented two cases in the evaluation of the quality assessment of image analysis where the benefit of introducing a semantic layer can be appreciated. The first example on the lexical variability naturally encountered in free-text comments demonstrates that adding a semantic layer to complement the free-text annotations would be extremely useful to extract commonalities. In particular, the semantic layer will allow us to *(i)* group annotations that describe the same concept under the same preferred label, and *(ii)* find analogies among similar annotations. The second example is about ambiguity due to incompleteness in the comments. The use of semantics will help find patterns in the annotation procedure and define ontology rules to partially resolve such ambiguity. In the context of these two examples we have also shown how the structured vocabulary associated to the quality assessment information is being designed. Preliminary intuition of the development of domain-specific ontology rules has also been provided.

Related Work. Ontologies are extensively used in biomedicine. Prominent examples are BioPortal, a comprehensive repository containing more than 500 biomedical ontologies [6], and SNOMED CT [15], the reference ontology of choice across National Health Service (NHS) information systems.[3] There have also been recent efforts in adding a semantic layer to describe the information within a biobank. Andrade et al. [8] envisaged the benefits of using ontologies for querying and searching the information in a biobank and across biobanks. Muller et al. [11] presents and updated overview of the state of the art and open challenges for the description and interoperability across biobanks where the use of Semantic Web technologies will play a key role. Examples of concrete Semantic Web-based solutions in biobanks can also be found in [9,10]. Although state-of-the-art ontologies include the description of concepts relevant to our domain, we could not find any ontology meeting all our requirements (e.g., complete description of Cine MRI technical issues) which evidences the necessity of a more specific ontology in this particular domain.

Future Work. As immediate future work, we plan to complete the *CMR-QA* ontology, define the necessary ontology rules and finalise the implementation of the techniques to text mine the comments to extract ontology data. In this way it will be possible to automatically infer numerical quality scores from the annotations. Validation will be carried out by comparing the automatic scores with those manually assigned by the observers as part of their quality assessment. We also aim to design a prototype software for query and retrieval of Cine MRI scans according to certain *semantic* characteristics to be later embedded in the UK Biobank CMR pilot study available tools. Furthermore, we will perform an

---

[3] http://systems.hscic.gov.uk/data/uktc/snomed.

extensive evaluation to analyse the correctness of our approach. In the long-term, the definition of semantics will enable integration at different levels within UK Biobank and with external vocabularies: *(i)* integration with other parts of UK Biobank where different ontologies and controlled vocabularies may be used; *(ii)* integration with other existing biobank ontologies (e.g., [9,10]); and *(iii)* integration with medical vocabularies in order to be compliant with state-of-the-art standards, for example SNOMED CT [15]. The integration with other ontologies will allow the interoperability among different group of experts relying on different ontologies and the creation of a broader semantic layer.

Expected Benefits for Training Purposes. An important related application is the development of training material for future observers analysing clinical imaging data. *CMR-QA* will provide a controlled set of preferred quality assessment comments, together with alternative expressions, so that observers can be more systematically trained in image quality assessment. This will result in a significant reduction of variability and improved quality of the information content of the comments provided.

Expected Benefits of Semantic Access for UK Biobank Users. The use of a controlled vocabulary provided by the *CMR-QA* ontology will ease the retrieval of Cine MRI scans according to their quality and reliability of the analysis outcomes. For example, a clinical researcher interested in building a control group for a study on pathologies affecting the atria, might want to query only for those images whose atrial volumes have been reliably estimated. Therefore, he/she will exclude scans where atria were off axis or the image quality was sub-optimal. A different example coming from the biomedical engineering world: an expert in development of algorithms for automatic contouring of the left ventricle might be interested in testing a newly developed tool on those Cine MRI scans where it was most difficult to define the basal slice. He/she will specifically query for cases whose image analysis was annotated as having difficult definition of the basal slice for the left ventricle.

List of abbreviations

CMR: Cardiovascular Magnetic Resonance imaging **CMR-QA:** Cardiovascular Magnetic Resonance Quality Assessment **HLA:** Horizontal Long Axis **LA:** Left Atrium **LV:** Left Ventricle **MRI:** Magnetic Resonance Imaging **NER:** Named Entity Recognition **NHS:** UK's National Health Service **RA:** Right Atrium **RV:** Right Ventricle **SA:** Short Axis **VLA:** Vertical Long Axis.

Acknowledgements. SEP, SN and SP acknowledge the British Heart Foundation (BHF) for funding the manual analysis to create a cardiovascular magnetic resonance imaging reference standard for the UK Biobank imaging resource in 5,000 CMR scans (PG/14/89/31194, PI Petersen, 6/2015 to 5/2018). SKP, VC and SN were additionally funded by the National Institute for Health Research (NIHR) Oxford Biomedical Research Centre based at The Oxford University Hospitals Trust at the University of Oxford. EJR and IH were funded by the European Commission under FP7 Grant Agreement 318338, "Optique", and the EPSRC projects Score!, ED3 and DBOnto.

References

1. Petersen, S.E., et al.: Imaging in population science: cardiovascular magnetic resonance in 100,000 participants of UK Biobank - rationale, challenges and approaches. J. Cardiovasc. Magn. Reson. **15**(1), 1–10 (2013). http://www.ukbiobank.ac.uk/
2. Petersen, S.E., et al.: UK biobank's cardiovascular magnetic resonance protocol. J. Cardiovasc. Magn. Reson. **18**(1), 8 (2016)
3. Schulz-Menger, J., et al.: Standardized image interpretation and post processing in cardiovascular magnetic resonance: society for cardiovascular magnetic resonance (SCMR) board of trustees task force on standardized post processing. J. Cardiovasc. Magn. Reson. **15**(1), 1–19 (2013)
4. Gruber, T.R.: Toward principles for the design of ontologies used for knowledge sharing? Int. J. Hum. Comput. Stud. **43**(5–6), 907–928 (1995)
5. Guarino, N., Oberle, D., Staab, S.: What is an ontology? In: Staab, S., Studer, R. (eds.) Handbook on Ontologies, pp. 1–17. Springer, Heidelberg (2009)
6. Noy, N.F., et al.: BioPortal: ontologies and integrated data resources at the click of a mouse. Nucleic Acids Res. **37**(Web-Server-Issue), 170–173 (2009)
7. Giese, M., et al.: Optique: zooming in on big data. IEEE Comput. **48**(3), 60–67 (2015)
8. Andrade, A.Q., Kreuzthaler, M., Hastings, J., Krestyaninova, M., Schulz, S.: Requirements for semantic biobanks. Stud. Health Technol. Inform. **180**, 569–573 (2012)
9. Pathak, J., et al.: Applying semantic web technologies for phenome-wide scan using an electronic health record linked biobank. J. Biomed. Semant. **3**, 10 (2012)
10. Brochhausen, M., et al.: Developing a semantically rich ontology for the biobank-administration domain. J. Biomed. Semant. **4**, 23 (2013)
11. Müller, H., Reihs, R., Zatloukal, K., Jeanquartier, F., Merino-Martinez, R., van Enckevort, D., Swertz, M.A., Holzinger, A.: State-of-the-art and future challenges in the integration of biobank catalogues. In: Holzinger, A., Röcker, C., Ziefle, M. (eds.) Smart Health. LNCS, vol. 8700, pp. 261–273. Springer, Heidelberg (2015)
12. Spasic, I., Ananiadou, S., McNaught, J., Kumar, A.: Text mining and ontologies in biomedicine: making sense of raw text. Briefings Bioinf. **6**(3), 239–251 (2005)
13. Bodenreider, O.: Lexical, terminological and ontological resources for biological text mining. In: Ananiadou, S., McNaught, J. (eds.) Text Mining for Biology and Biomedicine, pp. 43–66. Artech House, Boston (2006)
14. Nenov, Y., Piro, R., Motik, B., Horrocks, I., Wu, Z., Banerjee, J.: RDFox: a highly-scalable RDF store. In: Arenas, M., et al. (eds.) ISWC 2015. LNCS, vol. 9367, pp. 3–20. Springer, Heidelberg (2015). doi:10.1007/978-3-319-25010-6_1
15. Schulz, S., Cornet, R., Spackman, K.A.: Consolidating SNOMED CT's ontological commitment. Appl. Ontology **6**(1), 1–11 (2011)

Focused Proofreading to Reconstruct Neural Connectomes from EM Images at Scale

Stephen M. Plaza[(✉)]

Janelia Research Campus, HHMI, Ashburn, VA, USA
plazas@janelia.hhmi.org

Abstract. Identifying complex neural circuitry from electron microscopic (EM) images may help unlock the mysteries of the brain. However, identifying this circuitry requires time-consuming, manual tracing (proofreading) due to the size and intricacy of these image datasets, thus limiting analysis to small brain regions. Potential avenues to improve scalability include automatic image segmentation and crowdsourcing, but current efforts have had limited success. In this paper, we propose a new strategy, focused proofreading, that works with automatic segmentation and aims to limit proofreading to areas that are most impactful to the resulting circuit. We then introduce a novel workflow, which exploits biological information such as synapses, and apply it to a large fly optic lobe dataset. Our techniques achieve significant tracing speedups without sacrificing quality. Furthermore, our methodology makes proofreading more accessible and could enhance the effectiveness of crowdsourcing.

1 Introduction

EM reconstruction is the process of extracting a connectome from an EM dataset. A structural connectome derivable from EM data typically consists of neurons and their connections/synapses. To decipher the intricacy of neuronal structures in a brain, the imaging is at nanometer resolution generating vast amounts of data to be analyzed. Because of this, reconstruction is very time consuming (and costly) and significant advances are needed to handle larger volumes [10].

Two main approaches exist for reconstructing connectomes from an EM dataset: manual skeletonization and refinement of automatic segmentation. Skeletonization requires a proofreader to manually trace the shape of the cell [1,13]. CATMAID [13] achieves some scalability success by making collaborative, web-based tracing very accessible to interested, well-trained biologists. In [1], skeletonization is accomplished through a consensus of, generally, less well-trained students. Segmentation-driven tracing has been successfully deployed in partial reconstructions of the fly optic lobe [16] and mouse retina [4]. Reconstruction is achieved by merging and splitting incorrect segments. In practice, it is much easier to refine an oversegmented label volume than an undersegmented volume. Notably, [16] generates a comprehensive connectome but does not achieve 100 % accuracy. Perfect reconstruction is seemingly unnecessary and also generally untenable due to image ambiguity.

G. Carneiro et al. (Eds.): LABELS 2016/DLMIA 2016, LNCS 10008, pp. 249–258, 2016.
DOI: 10.1007/978-3-319-46976-8_26

Ideally, automatic segmentation would produce a perfect connectome. While recent advances in EM segmentation, such as [8], produce very good results, the segmentations are still far from perfect as shown in Fig. 1. If the initial segmentation is poor, extensive effort must be spent correcting it. This correction effort could be captured by some kind of *nuisance metric*. However, even with 100 % correct segmentation (zero nuisance), verifying correctness on a large dataset could still require thorough inspection by several proofreaders. Better segmentation, alone, will not solve scalability.

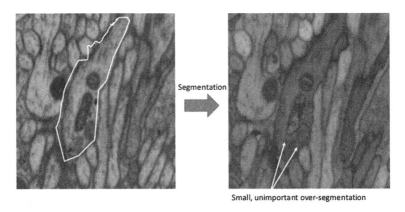

Fig. 1. Automatic segmentation of one image from an EM dataset. While segmentation correctly determines most neuronal profiles, there are still many errors. However, some oversegmentation mistakes in the highlighted neuron are unimportant as it does not significantly alter the shape or connectivity of that neuron.

Crowdsourcing has been pursued in different ways [1,4,13] as a potential solution. However, these strategies are fundamentally unscalable. Traditionally, EM tracing requires a high-level of expertise requiring weeks of training (or more), unreasonable for a general crowdsource community. CATMAID [13] tries to expand the expert base through its accessibility but still requires training to be proficient. Consensus tracing, as in [1] can access a wider pool but requires even more proofreaders to account for errors. Also, an averaged result could lead to a sub-optimal connectome or require extensive expert verification. The approach in [4] attempts to make proofreading accessible to the novice community. Despite tremendous involvement from the community, the efforts were primarily used for validation, and the reconstruction still required a group of trained proofreaders.

To address these scalability challenges, we propose *focused proofreading*. Focused proofreading is a segmentation-driven proofreading that attempts to discern the regions of the segmentation that are both relevant to the connectome and least-likely to be correct. In the process, it distills the task of proofreading to a more digestible series of yes/no decisions. By redefining proofreading, we hope to expand the base of potential proofreaders. Our work has some similarities to the uncertainty-driven proofreading suggested in [11]. However, we propose a more practical approach that uses efficiently computed local constraints to guide proofreading rather than a global strategy. Furthermore, we exploit synapse information and other biological priors to greatly enhance proofreading efficiency and the quality of the final reconstruction. We apply focused proofreading techniques to comprehensively reconstruct seven medulla columns in the Drosophila optic lobe [15]. Our best estimates indicate 3–5x speedup in reconstruction with improved accuracy compared to similar efforts [16]. As datasets get bigger and manual effort dominates connectomic budgets, focused proofreading could yield significant financial savings. Figure 2 shows our high-level workflow.

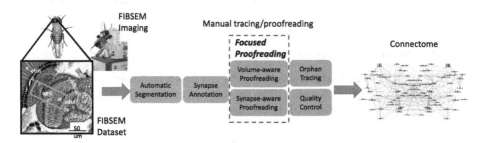

Fig. 2. Connectome reconstruction methodology with focused proofreading. Fixing disconnected (orphan) fragments and final validation ensure a good final result.

2 Uncertainty-Driven Focused Proofreading

We consider the case where a proofreader is given segmentation S and must revise it to S', so that it is reasonably close to a ground truth G. The differences between S and G can be quantified with the variation of information (VI) [5]:

$$VI(S, G) = H(S|G) + H(G|S) \tag{1}$$

where H is the entropy function. The first term, $H(S|G)$ gives the information of the underlying segmentation compared to ground truth and indicates over-segmentation. Likewise, $H(G|S)$ indicates under-segmentation. 0 information means high similarity. Compared to other similarity metrics, such as Rand Index [2,12] and Warping Index [3], VI is both simple to compute and has interpretability advantages as highlighted by the authors in [6].

Since image segmentation is generally tuned to limit under segmentation, we assume, for simplicity, that a proofreader is restricted to merge-only operations. Therefore, we consider the proofreading problem as an assignment of *yes* or *no* for edges in S, where an edge connects two neighboring s. In practice under-segmentation errors occur but are often easily detectable during or after proofreading. We can define an optimal similarity (sim) after m decisions as:

$$sim(m) = min_{S_{\pi(m)}}(H(S_{\pi(m)}|G)) \tag{2}$$

where $\pi(n)$ denotes an optimal ordering of m yes, no decisions. Since we are starting from an oversegmented S, $\pi(m)$ consists of an ordering of only m no (merge) decisions (yes decisions will not change the current segmentation). We define m^* as the optimal number of decisions to achieve some desired level of completeness or accuracy.

We do not attempt to solve $\pi(m)$ optimally. Instead we favor greedy-based orderings that have the greatest impact on $H(S|G)$. However, simple, greedy-based approaches have two problems. First, explicit G is unavailable for measuring impact. Second, an impactful edge decision might not exist until a less impactful merge is first performed. We address these concerns in the following two sections.

2.1 Prioritizing Decisions

Greedy-based ordering without ground truth requires a formulation of the impact and likelihood of a given decision. The impact or information associated with a yes/no between segments a_i and a_j is given by:

$$Impact(e_{(i,j)}) = -|a_i|log_2(\frac{|a_i|}{|a_i| + |a_j|}) - |a_j|log_2(\frac{|a_j|}{|a_i| + |a_j|}) \qquad (3)$$

$|a_i|$, and $|a_j|$ could represent the number of voxels or synaptic connections in a_i, and a_j respectively (we do not normalize by total volume for convenience).

We define the risk associated with a given edge as:

$$Risk(e_{(i,j)}) = P(\neg e_{(i,j)})Impact(e_{(i,j)}) \qquad (4)$$

The riskiest edges define the edges that will likely have the greatest impact on this segmentation. To determine $P(\neg e_{(i,j)})$, we first train a classifier on the edges of an oversegmented volume. The resulting prediction determines the confidence in the edge. This classifier is trained similarly to those discussed in [6,8]. We chose the random forest classifier since it achieves good segmentation results [8], while being fast and easy to deploy. We will evaluate the quality of confidence predictions in Sect. 4.1.

2.2 Focused Proofreading Algorithm

We define *focused proofreading* as the examination of a subset of edges where $Risk(e_{(i,j)}) > k$, where k is parameter empirically determined for a given dataset and segmentation. However, the greedy-based strategy introduced previously is flawed since two labels s_i and s_j might belong to the same neuron but have no direct edge. As in [11], we avoid this problem by considering the probability that a set of edges connect s_i and s_j:

$$P(\neg E_{(i,j)}) = \Pi_{\neg e_{k,l} \in E_{i,j}} P(e_{k,l}) \qquad (5)$$

where $P(\neg E(i,j))$ is the probability of a path existing between s_i and s_j. Greedily examining risky paths allows for more global awareness.

Input: Segmentation: S, Threshold: k
Output: Proofread Segmentation: S
foreach $s_b \in S'$ **do**
  $S_E = $ findNeighbors(s_b);
  foreach $s_a \in S_E$ **do**
    if risk($E(s_a, s_b)$) $> k$ **then**
      result = decide($E(s_a, s_b)$) ;
      S ← result ;
      $S_E = $ findNeighbors(s_b);
    end
  end
end

Algorithm 1. Focused proofreading algorithm.

We can now present a strategy for proofreading an oversegmentation (Algorithm 1). The algorithm starts by iterating through all segments considering the *largest* first. Then, all potential segments connected to this body (within some uncertainty threshold) are determined through function findNeighbors. The proofreader is given edges along the riskiest path in decide. After each decision, the graph and list of candidate edges are updated.

If the segmentation is good, focused proofreading can still perform poorly. If the uncertainties favor false merging, the algorithm will lead to inefficiency, as many true edges will be examined. If the uncertainties favor false splitting, errors will occur in the final segmentation. Errors are mitigated by our risk measure since very impactful sites can still be examined even if the true edge probability is high. The next section discusses how this algorithm is deployed in practice.

3 Workflow to Reconstruct a Large Connectome

In practice, there are many challenges to reconstruction. (1) The initial segmentation will falsely merge some regions. (2) Focused proofreading will miss some important areas. (3) Proofreaders will make errors. To address these concerns, we describe the workflow shown in Fig. 2 and used in [15].

We first divide a large dataset in several subvolumes to simplify data management (though the following could be applied over the entire dataset). For each subvolume, proofreaders first annotate synapses as described in [9] and then proofread. Three rounds of proofreading are performed: (1) volume-threshold focused proofreading, (2) synapse-threshold focused proofreading, and (3) orphan (small-body) tracing. The first two rounds closely follow the algorithm in the preceding section where the size of segment is either the number of voxels or synaptic connections. The orphan (small-body) tracing is a quality control that has the proofreader examine disconnected segments that either contain synapses or are of at least a certain size. Therefore, orphan tracing ensures *important* areas are examined even if focused proofreading missed them. We also add some synapse connectivity constraints to eliminate unnecessary work. For instance, in the synapse focused proofreading pass we ignore edges that would result in a rare autapse (a reflexive connection where a neuron drives itself).

A final, accurate connectome is produced after various quality controls. While proofreading these subvolumes, proofreaders note areas of false merging. These areas are split in a separate pass after focused proofreading. The subvolumes are then stitched to create a global segmentation. We then look for large-scale anomalies of cell shape or connectivity. A reconstruction is generally considered accurate if most voxels are segregated into a set of neurons that contain most of the synaptic connections, where each neuron is considered correct by spot checking and matching to available priors.

4   Experiments

In the following sections, we first evaluate the effectiveness of focused proofreading, in terms of achieving the best accuracy with the fewest decisions, against other proofreading strategies on a small dataset. We then highlight the role of focused proofreading in a practical setting on a large-scale, multi-year reconstruction of the fly optic lobe [15]. This dataset contains around $27,000\,\mu m^3$ of proofread neuropil containing hundreds of partial neurons and several hundred thousand synaptic connections.

We implement the focused algorithms in a publicly available C++ tool called *NeuroProof* (https://github.com/janelia-flyem/NeuroProof). The initial segmentation is generated using Ilastik [14] for voxel prediction and algorithms described in [8]. The synapses were semi-manually annotated before segmentation as in [9]. All proofreading, including focused yes-no decisions, was performed with the open-source tool Raveler [7].

4.1   Validation of Focused Proofreading

In this section, we show that the proposed focused proofreading strategies are more efficient than other proofreading strategies. The results are collected for a 500^3 volume with $10 \times 10 \times 10$ nm voxel resolution from [15]. The difficulty of producing near-pixel perfect ground truth limits our ability to validate on more datasets. We effectively increase our test set by running many of the experiments on 10 random initial segmentations. Segmentation training is performed on two smaller, disjoint volumes. Before we show the effectiveness of the focused proofreading strategies, we validate the quality of uncertainty prediction, as shown Fig. 3. Lower confidence predictions are generally accurate; higher confidence predictions underestimate the number of true edges, which will result in more proofreading work.

We now evaluate the trade-off between proofreading effort and proofreading quality using different focused proofreading heuristics in Fig. 4. We consider only the over-segmentation VI since the under-segmentation error is small and minimally impacted by our merge-only technique (fixing under-segmentation

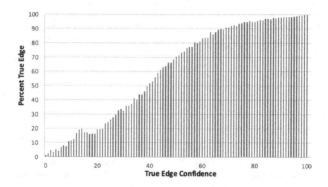

Fig. 3. Accuracy of the predicted edge confidences. This plot shows the percentage of true edges (y-axis) for a given classifier confidence (x-axis).

will be discussed in the next section). For these tests, proofreading effort is determined by the number of automatic decisions made.

In Fig. 4a, we show volume VI trends. As expected, the focused strategy that uses synapses for guidance does not do a good job improving the volume VI. The two volume-guided focused strategies, volume-local and volume-path, do much better. Volume-local only considers local bodies when making a decision. Both perform similarly though volume-path has a slightly lower VI because of a longer cut-off. We compared these approaches to a straightforward strategy of only using edge probabilities. The most confident false edges are chosen first, producing slightly worse, but comparable, results under 2000 decisions. But more improvements are possible if one is willing to examine more edges.

Does this suggest that simple edge ordering is potentially sufficient? First, focused proofreading explicitly chooses a stopping condition that trades-off errors. The simplistic stopping condition for just using edge probability could result in a lot of unnecessary work. Second, it appears that edges between big bodies (presumably where there is more boundary evidence) have more confidence. This is apparently not the case for the smaller processes often important in tracing synapses. The synapse VI plot in Fig. 4b, shows that the synapse-guided mode is much better than all of the other techniques. We note that random decision heuristics (not shown) perform significantly worse than the above strategies.

4.2   Validation of Production Proofreading

We used focused proofreading to help reconstruct seven columns of Drosophila medulla optic lobe [15]. The focused proofreading work described here was primarily completed within 6 months with a staff of 5–10 trained proofreaders. We note that multiple proofreaders on an example subvolume agreed on over 98 % of yes/no decisions. The high consistency is motivation for using only one proofreader per subvolume for focused proofreading. Subsequent quality control and spot check by senior biological experts ensure an accurate final result.

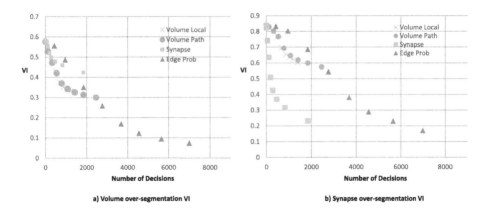

a) Volume over-segmentation VI   b) Synapse over-segmentation VI

Fig. 4. Improvements in VI over-segmentation similarity metric as a function of proofreader decisions. Four ordering strategies are considered. (a) Shows slightly faster improvement using volume-based decision compared to using only edge confidence when considering volume VI. (b) Shows significantly faster improvement to synapse VI using synapse-based decisions.

We report the time to proofread the seven column medulla in Table 1. Proofreading was performed over 216 subvolumes each 125 cubic microns and assigned randomly to the proofreaders. The column `session hrs` gives the amount time taken to complete the task. `working hrs` gives the amount of time that the proofreader interacts with the proofreading tool (attempts to account for normal work distractions and circumstances where a proofreader needs to ask for help). The ratio of working hours to session hours gives the `efficiency`. In general, 100 % efficiency is only possible for a robot. Frustratingly challenging tasks tend to have a lower efficiency. This could also be seen as a *frustration factor*. `microns/day` gives a rate based on session time.

We show results for the following tasks: `focused proofreading` (also includes the effort for orphan tracing), `synapse QC`, and `body split`. `synapse QC` has proofreaders review synaptic connections that seem suspicious, such as autapses. `body split` shows the time required to fix under-segmentation errors

Table 1. Breakdown of proofreading effort in [15] (ignores synapse annotation time and downstream quality control). Focused proofreading includes both volume and synapse focusing, as well as, orphan tracing. Synapse QC involves verifying and fixing some local connectivity anomalies observed in the data. Body split fixes under-segmentation.

Task	session hrs	working hrs	efficiency	microns/day
Focused proof	3374	2934	87 %	64
Synapse QC	226	198	88 %	956
Body split	756	495	66 %	286
Average				**49.6**

detected while proofreading. Despite each subvolume requiring only 10 s of splits, the task is time-consuming and has lower efficiency. While focused proofreading alone is insufficient to produce a connectome, it is a significant time component.

We assess the reconstruction speedup due to focused proofreading against a previous reconstruction [16], which did not use focus proofreading but a more proofreader-directed approach. A comparison is difficult since the quality of initial segmentation differs. The rate for proofreading subvolumes in [16] is around 10–20 microns per day (unpublished correspondence). We believe the proofreading in this paper to be more comprehensive and results in a rate 3–5 times faster. While much of the improvement likely stems from improved segmentation, our methodology is more focused, systematic, and likely less *frustrating*.

5   Conclusions

The time-consuming nature of EM reconstruction stymies our ability to understand larger, complex neurological systems. This paper introduces a strategy called focused proofreading to greatly improve reconstruction speed allowing the analysis of much larger regions. We demonstrated the effectiveness by reconstructing a complete connectome from a region of the Drosophila optic lobe, the largest such reconstruction ever performed. The proposed workflow is amenable to large-scale, crowdsourcing efforts.

This work is one of the first to focus on the quality of the uncertainty estimates of the segmentation engine, rather than just the resulting segmentation. Future work should be directed at optimizing these confidence intervals. Furthermore, this work pioneers efforts at using biological priors and synaptic connectivity to guide proofreading process. We believe exploiting more biological rules or priors can lead to great speedups. Finally, this work emphasizes the need to decompose a complex task (proofreading) into a series of digestible decisions. Additional work on improving visualization and making the task accessible to an even larger workforce should be explored.

Acknowledgments. We thank Zhiyuan Lu for sample preparation; Shan Xu and Harald Hess for imaging; Pat Rivlin, Shin-ya Takemura, and the FlyEM proofreading team (Roxanne Aniceto, Lei-Ann Chang, Shirley Lauchie, Mathew Saunders, Christopher Sigmund, Satoko Takemura, Julie Tran) for reconstruction efforts; Donald Olbris for Raveler development; Toufiq Parag for generating segmentation classifiers; Louis Scheffer for useful discussions and suggestions.

References

1. Helmstaedter, M., Briggman, K., Turaga, S., Jain, V., Seung, H., Denk, W.: Connectomic reconstruction of the inner plexiform layer in the mouse retina. Nature **500**(7461), 168–174 (2014)
2. Hubert, L., Arabie, P.: Comparing partitions. J. Classif. **2**(1), 193–218 (1985)

3. Jain, V., Bollmann, B., Richardson, M., Berger, D., Helmstaedter, M., et al.: Boundary learning by optimization with topological constraints. In: CVPR, pp. 2488–2495 (2010)

4. Kim, J., Greene, M., Zlateski, A., Lee, K., Richardson, M.: Spacetime wiring specificity supports direction selectivity in the retina. Nature **509**(7500), 331–336 (2014)

5. Meilă, M.: Comparing clusterings by the variation of information. In: Schölkopf, B., Warmuth, M.K. (eds.) COLT-Kernel 2003. LNCS (LNAI), vol. 2777, pp. 173–187. Springer, Heidelberg (2003). doi:10.1007/978-3-540-45167-9_14

6. Nunez-Iglesias, J., Kennedy, R., Parag, T., Shi, J., Chklovskii, D.: Machine learning of hierarchical clustering to segment 2D and 3D images. PLoS One **8**(8), e71715 (2013). doi:10.1371/journal.pone.0071715

7. Olbris, D., Winston P., Plaza S., Bolstad M., Rivlin P., Scheffer L., Chklovskii D.: https://openwiki.janelia.org/wiki/display/flyem/Raveler

8. Parag, T., Chakraborty, A., Plaza, S., Scheffer, L.: A context-aware delayed agglomeration framework for electron microscopy segmentation. PLoS One **10**(5), e0125825 (2015)

9. Plaza, S., Parag, T., Huang, G., Olbris, D., Saunders, M., Rivlin, P.: Annotating synapses in large EM datasets. In: arXiv.org (2014)

10. Plaza, S., Scheffer, L., Chklovskii, D.: Toward large-scale connectome reconstructions. In: Current Opinion in Neurobiology, pp. 201–210 (2014)

11. Plaza, S., Scheffer, L., Saunders, M.: Minimizing manual image segmentation turnaround time for neuronal reconstruction by embracing uncertainty. PLoS One **7**(9), e44448 (2012). doi:10.1371/journal.pone.0044448

12. Rand, W.: Objective criteria for the evaluation of clustering methods. J. Am. Stat. Assoc. **66**(336), 846–850 (1973)

13. Saalfeld, S., Cardona, A., Hartenstein, V., Toman, P.: CATMAID: collaborative annotation toolkit for massive amounts of image data. Bioinformatics **25**(15), 1984–1986 (2009)

14. Sommer, C., Straehle, C., Koethe, U., Hamprecht, F.: Ilastik: interactive learning and segmentation toolkit. In: Proceedings of the IEEE International Symposium on Biomedical Imaging, pp. 230–233 (2011)

15. Takemura, S., Xu, S., Lu, Z., Rivlin, P., Parag, T., et al.: Synaptic circuits and their variations within different columns in the visual system of Drosophila. PNAS **112**(44), 13711–13716 (2015)

16. Takemura, S., Bharioke, A., Lu, Z., Nern, A., Vitaladevuni, S., et al.: A visual motion detection circuit suggested by Drosophila connectomics. Nature **500**(7461), 175–181 (2013)

Hands-Free Segmentation of Medical Volumes via Binary Inputs

Florian Dubost[1,2]($\boxtimes$), Loic Peter[1], Christian Rupprecht[1,3],
Benjamin Gutierrez Becker[1], and Nassir Navab[1,3]

[1] Computer Aided Medical Procedures,
Technische Universität München, Munich, Germany
floriandubost1@gmail.com
[2] Biomedical Imaging Group Rotterdam, Erasmus MC,
Rotterdam, The Netherlands
[3] Computer Aided Medical Procedures,
Johns Hopkins University, Baltimore, USA

Abstract. We propose a novel hands-free method to interactively segment 3D medical volumes. In our scenario, a human user progressively segments an organ by answering a series of questions of the form *"Is this voxel inside the object to segment?"*. At each iteration, the chosen question is defined as the one halving a set of candidate segmentations given the answered questions. For a quick and efficient exploration, these segmentations are sampled according to the Metropolis-Hastings algorithm. Our sampling technique relies on a combination of relaxed shape prior, learnt probability map and consistency with previous answers. We demonstrate the potential of our strategy on a prostate segmentation MRI dataset. Through the study of failure cases with synthetic examples, we demonstrate the adaptation potential of our method. We also show that our method outperforms two intuitive baselines: one based on random questions, the other one being the thresholded probability map.

1 Introduction

The segmentation of medical images or volumes is a key research topic in medical image analysis. The segmentation of objects of interest - e.g. organs or tumors - is a key process for operation planning, navigation or design of personalized prosthesis. Interactive segmentation is often a well-suited framework as it allows the user to actively participate in the segmentation process and correct possible mistakes or refine the segmentation. However this interactive aspect can rise issues when the segmentation has to be made during surgery: (i) the process of zooming and navigating through slices can be overwhelming and time-consuming, (ii) the hands of the clinicians are already busy with the operation itself. The use of hands-free techniques can thus be handy and is in general appreciated by clinicians [1,2] as they significantly reduce the labelling effort for medical data.

In many popular methods for interactive segmentation the user gives indications - scribbles, bounding boxes - as an input to the algorithm [3,4]. Once the

© Springer International Publishing AG 2016
G. Carneiro et al. (Eds.): LABELS 2016/DLMIA 2016, LNCS 10008, pp. 259–268, 2016.
DOI: 10.1007/978-3-319-46976-8_27

indications are given, the algorithm runs autonomously without new input from the user. A example of a hands-free technique in this framework would be Eyegaze [5] which is based on eye tracking. However this technique still involves much navigation and zooming and needs a calibration.

Another way to perform interactive segmentation is to build an algorithm which iteratively includes the indications of the user, following a refinement technique. The simplest way to handle this is to display the resulting segmentation after each interaction. Each input of the user will then be seen as a hard constraint [6]. Another general idea of this framework is to use the answers already provided by the user to hint for areas of high uncertainty and guide the user in the search. One possible way to locate such areas is through segmentation sampling. State of the art methods of segmentation sampling can be based on Markov Chain Monte Carlo (MCMC) [7,8] or Gaussian Process [9]. Both methods [8,9] proved to be effective in 2D but encounter - because of the use of Geodesic Distance Transform - high running time when performed on 3D data.

In this paper, we propose a novel hands-free interactive segmentation method. In our scenario a human user segments an object of interest from a 3D medical volume only by answering questions of the type "*Is this voxel inside the object to segment?*". These answers are binary interactions - "yes" / "no" - and can be easily recorded trough a pedal or voice recognition system. They provide a set of positive and negative seeds to compute the final segmentation. In order to choose the question voxels we sample candidate segmentations thanks to a MCMC framework. This sampling process relies on an adaptive weighting between a probability map learnt off-line and the consistency with previous answers. If the probability map is misleading, the algorithm detects it and changes accordingly. The answer of the user halves then the space of the sampled candidate segmentations, following a dichotomic search in this space. We propose a diagram (Fig. 1) summarizing our technique. We evaluated the performance of our method on a 3D MRI prostate segmentation dataset. Through the study of failure cases generated with synthetic examples, we demonstrate the adaptation potential of our method. Our results demonstrate that our technique can correct inaccurate annotations or ameliorate imprecise ones in a reasonable time.

2   Methods

In the following paragraphs we start by briefly explaining the learning of the probability map (Sect. 2.1). In the next section we detail the core of our method and contribution for the segmentation sampling of the MCMC technique (Sect. 2.2). Our idea consists in combining a relaxed shape prior, a learnt probability map and the consistency with previous answers. One of our main contributions is the adaptation capability of our algorithm, which can identify misleading probability maps and adapt accordingly. The last paragraphs briefly review how to propose questions voxels from the sampled segmentations (Sect. 2.3) and how to compute the final segmentation of the algorithm, once all K questions have been answered (Sect. 2.4).

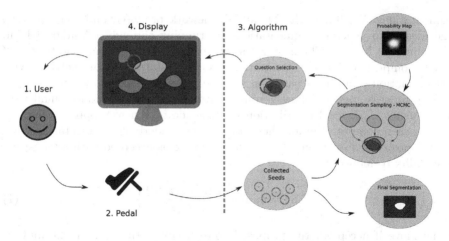

Fig. 1. Diagram summarizing the processes of our method. The user (1) communicates for instance via a pedal (2) with the algorithm (3) which outputs question voxels to the user (4). Using a probability map learnt offline (Sect. 2.1) and previous answers from the user, the algorithm samples several segmentations (Sect. 2.2) and finds the area where they disagree the most. The question voxel is taken within this area (Sect. 2.3). The question is of the form "*Is this voxel inside the object to segment?*". The answer of the user provides a seed which halves the space of candidates segmentations. The final segmentation is computed from the set of seeds provided by the user and by running a last segmentation sampling procedure (Sect. 2.4).

Let $\Gamma = \{1, ..., H\} \times \{1, ..., W\} \times \{1, ..., D\}$ be a three-dimensional lattice and V a volume defined on Γ. We call S the space of segmentations, i.e. the set of functions $\mathbf{s} : \Gamma \mapsto \{0, 1\}$. If the voxel $v(x, y, z)$ is inside the segmented object then $\mathbf{s}(x, y, z) = 1$, otherwise $\mathbf{s}(x, y, z) = 0$.

2.1 Probability Map

Our method uses as prior knowledge a probability map π defined over Γ. This probability map is obtained with a classifier trained offline. $\pi(v)$ is an estimation of the probability that the voxel $v(x, y, z)$ belongs to the targeted object. We have no prior information on the quality of this probability map.

To obtain π, we use an AdaBoost classifier [10] based on Haar features [11], which we more precisely defined and sampled as in [12]. We denote the stumps h_t for $t = \{1, ..., T\}$, where T is the number of boosting iterations. We compute the decision function H as the sum of the h_t. In order to rescale the output values so that $0 < \pi(x, y, z) < 1$ we apply a sigmoid function to the score H [13].

2.2 MCMC Framework

We would like to generate segmentations to approximate the space of probable segmentations and then use the answer of the user to halve this space, following a dichotomic search. In this section we present our technique to sample candidate segmentations. We follow the MCMC framework proposed and used in [7,8]. The idea is to generate segmentations by running through a Markov Chain. We define the Markov Chain over a state space $\mathcal{X}$ so that from a state $\mathbf{x} \in \mathcal{X}$ we can compute a unique segmentation $\mathbf{s}(\mathbf{x})$. The states are parametrized with transformation coefficients based on a shape prior (see next paragraph).

The process goes as follows: from a current state $\mathbf{x}$, we induce small variations using a proposal distribution Q to generate a new proposed state $\mathbf{x}'$. We can then compute the likelihood of the new underlying segmentation $\mathbf{s}(\mathbf{x}')$ using a posterior probability P. The new state $\mathbf{x}'$ is accepted with a transition probability α defined as

$$\alpha(\mathbf{x}'|\mathbf{x}) = \min\left\{1, \frac{P(\mathbf{x}')Q(\mathbf{x}|\mathbf{x}')}{P(\mathbf{x})Q(\mathbf{x}'|\mathbf{x})}\right\}. \tag{1}$$

If the move if accepted, the proposed state becomes the current one and we reiterate the process. Otherwise we come back to $\mathbf{x}$ and a new state is proposed.

Parametrization of Segmentations. The objective is here to explain how segmentations are represented. We decided to use shape models for it allows us to generate 3D segmentations with a very low running time. Following a similar idea than in [14] we define a relaxed notion of shape based on signed distance functions. Given a training set of m relaxed shapes $\mathcal{Y} = \{y_1, ..., y_m\}$, we can calculate the mean μ and the n first eigenmodes $\psi_1, ..., \psi_n$. To create a new relaxed shape we compute

$$y = \mu + \sum_{i=1}^{n} b_i \psi_i, \tag{2}$$

where $b_1, ..., b_n$ are the eigencoefficients of the shape prior. To widen the space of segmentations we allow as well resizing and rigid transformations such as translation and rotation. Therefore a state $\mathbf{x}$ is defined by $7 + n$ parameters, as $\mathbf{x} = (a, t_x, t_y, t_z, \alpha, \beta, \gamma, b_1, ..., b_n)$, where a is the size parameter, t_x, t_y and t_z translation parameters, α, β and γ rotation parameters and $b_1, ..., b_n$ the eigencoefficients of the shape prior. The resulting segmentation $\mathbf{s}(\mathbf{x}) \in S$ is computed as $y(\mathbf{x})$ thresholded at 0.

Posterior Probability. This probability is encoding how likely a state $\mathbf{x}$ - and its underlying segmentation $\mathbf{s}(\mathbf{x})$ - is, given the already provided answers Σ and the probability map π. We denote it as $P(\mathbf{x}|\Sigma)$ and compute it as

$$P(\mathbf{x}|\Sigma) \propto \frac{1}{1 - L(\mathbf{x}) + \beta_k g(\mathbf{x})}, \tag{3}$$

where $L(\mathbf{x})$ denotes the likelihood between the probability map π and the proposed segmentation $\mathbf{s}(\mathbf{x})$, $g(\mathbf{x})$ is a penalty term including the k previous answers from the user, and β_k a weighting parameter between these two objectives after k questions. By doing so, we consider as likelier the segmentations that are close to the probability map and compatible with the user responses. The relative weighting β_k of these two terms is adjusted after each question by checking the compatibility of the posterior with the provided answers. Thereby, if the posterior probability is mistaken, its impact is gradually decreasing. The next paragraphs expose our model for L, β_k and g.

Likelihood - Probability Map. To evaluate whether a candidate segmentation is close to the probability map, we use a maximum likelihood scheme. To simplify the following notations, we write $v(x, y, z) = v(t)$ where t is a parameter spanning the whole volume. For a given voxel $v(t)$ we assume $\mathbf{s}(t)$ follows a Bernoulli distribution $B(\pi(t))$. If we consider $\mathbf{s}(1), ..., \mathbf{s}(|\Gamma|)$ iid samples, the weighted log-likelihood is given by

$$L(\mathbf{x}) = \frac{1}{|\Gamma|} \log(\mathcal{L}(S = \mathbf{s}|\pi)) = \frac{1}{|\Gamma|} \sum_{t \in \Gamma} \mathbf{s}(t) \log(\pi(t)) + (1 - \mathbf{s}(t)) \log(1 - \pi(t)). \quad (4)$$

This quantity is always negative and reaches its maximum - $L(\mathbf{x}) = 0$ - when perfect match occurs.

Penalty Term. We introduce a penalty term $g(\mathbf{x})$ to include the information provided by the k previous answers of the user in the estimation of the posterior probability P. This way, we would like to penalize a candidate segmentation $\mathbf{s}(\mathbf{x})$ which is not compatible with the given answers. We model the answers as a seed location $\sigma = \{x_\sigma, y_\sigma, z_\sigma\}$ and a corresponding label $a(\sigma) \in \{0, 1\}$. We denote Σ_{err} the set of m seeds violated by the candidate segmentation, with $m \leq k$. We consider that a segmentation violates a seed σ when its prediction for this seed does not match the label provided by the user $a(\sigma)$.

Following the definition of signed distance functions, $|y(\mathbf{x}, \sigma_{err})|$ gives a measure of the distance between the violated seed σ_{err} and the border of the proposed segmentation $\mathbf{s}(\mathbf{x})$. We compute therefore the penalty term as

$$g(\mathbf{x}) = \sum_{\sigma \in \Sigma_{err}} |y(\mathbf{x}, \sigma)|. \quad (5)$$

Adaptive Weighting Parameter. For the weighting parameter β_k between the two objective functions L and g we propose an automatic adaptable setting. The idea consists in updating β at each question to progressively verify whether the probability map π can be trusted and adapt the loss function $-L(\mathbf{x}) + \beta g(\mathbf{x})$ accordingly. If the probability map is accurate, β should stay close to 0, otherwise beta should increase. The setting is inspired from online transfer learning [15]. β is initialized to β_0 and a new value β_{k+1} is computed after each question k according to

$$\beta_{k+1} = \max(\beta_{max}, \beta_k * e^{-\epsilon \mu l(1/2, \pi(\sigma))}), \quad (6)$$

where μ is a parameter encoding the amplitude of the update, i.e. the learning rate, β_{max} a parameter encoding the maximum value for beta to avoid divergence, ϵ is the agreement between the answer of the user and the probability map and l a loss function encoding the confidence of the probability map in its prediction. In our case we chose $l(x, y) = |x - y|$ to measure the distance between the neutral answer $1/2$ and the probability $\pi(\sigma)$. The closer to $1/2$ the probability $\pi(\sigma)$ is, the less it influences the update of β.

Our definition for ϵ is led by the one of the Dice similarity coefficient. We do not consider true negative seeds informative. Let $\pi_{threshold}$ be the probability map thresholded at 0.5. We set $\epsilon = 1$ if $\pi_{threshold}(\sigma) = a(\sigma) = 1$; $\epsilon = -1$ if $\pi_{threshold}(\sigma) \neq a(\sigma)$ and $(\pi_{threshold}(\sigma) = 1$ or $a(\sigma) = 1)$; and $\epsilon = 0$ if $\pi_{threshold}(\sigma) = a(\sigma) = 0$ which is considered as uninformative and therefore does not update the value of beta.

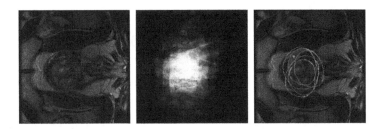

Fig. 2. Illustration of the steps of our algorithm on a MRI image of the prostate. From left to right: original image; probability map obtained from boosting; overlapping of the candidate segmentations for the question selection during the MCMC. The question voxel (green) is taken on the centroid of the selected region (red). (Source of the original image: Prostate Segmentation Challenge MICCAI09) (Color figure online)

2.3   Question Voxel

In order to compute the question voxel from the sampled segmentations, we follow the same framework as [8]. By superposing the accepted sampled segmentations, we divide the volume into several regions. We choose the voxel question as the centroid of the most unsure of these regions (Fig. 2).

2.4   Final Segmentation

After K question have been asked and the K corresponding seeds have been collected, we now compute the final segmentation $\mathbf{s}_f$. We sample candidate segmentations reusing the MCMC framework and compute their posterior probability $P(\mathbf{x})$ according to Eq. (3). During this step the weighting parameter is fixed to β_K, i.e. the lastly updated β_k. The final segmentation is taken as the one maximizing $P(\mathbf{x})$.

3   Experiments

Our experimental evaluation was performed on the dataset of the Prostate Segmentation Challenge MICCAI09. This dataset is a collection of 15 3D MRI annotated images coming each from a different patient. The voxel resolution is $0.55 \times 0.55 \times 5 \, \text{mm}^3$. The images have an average voxel size of $256 \times 256 \times 32$. We used the T2-weighted images for our experiments.

3.1   Experimental Settings

We follow a 5-fold cross-validation framework, where the training set is used to learn the probability maps and shape models. To generate new shapes, we retain only the $n = 3$ first eigenmodes of the shape, which defines our state space $\mathcal{X}$ with 10 dimensions. Concerning the weighting parameter β_k, we set $\beta_0 = 1$, $\mu = 3$ and $\beta_{max} = 4$. During the MCMC we perform a burn-in step of 100 iterations and run 25 iterations between each sampled segmentation. The total number of sampled segmentations at each question is $N = 15$. During the exploration of the states $\mathbf{x} \in \mathcal{X}$ in the segmentation sampling, the proposal distribution Q draws the parameters of $\mathbf{x}$ from Gaussian distributions centered on their current value. We use the Dice Similarity Coefficient (DSC) [17] to evaluate the performance of our algorithm. We implemented our algorithms in C++ and ran the experiments on a Intel i7-4702MQ 2.20GHz CPU. The computation time between each question is low enough to allow an interactive use of the algorithm. We performed an experiment to study the time statistics over the dataset. Over 165 questions - 45 per patient - the computation time between two questions was in average 4.2 s, in median 3.9 s and had a standard deviation of 1 s.

3.2   Results

Synthetic Probability Map. In our first experiments we demonstrate the adaptation capability of our method through the automatic setting of parameter β_k. Instead of using the learnt probability maps we create synthetic ones to cover the two extreme case scenarios: (1) the probability map is almost perfect and can be trusted, (2) the probability map is inaccurate and shouldn't be considered to generate segmentations. To simulated these probability maps, we use for (1) the blurred ground truth and for (2) the translated blurred ground truth such that the dice overlap with the original ground truth is zero. In Fig. 3 we plot respectively for (1) and (2) curves showing the evolution of the dice similarity coefficient (DSC) according to a manual setting of β ranging from 0 to 7. On the same plot we show the result obtained using the automatic adaptable setting of beta detailed in Sect. 2.2.

Learnt Probability Map. To assess the quality of our segmentations we compute the DSC after 30 questions. We compare our technique with two intuitive baselines: the first one corresponds to probability map from boosting thresholded at 0.5. The second one consists in asking the questions at random voxels instead

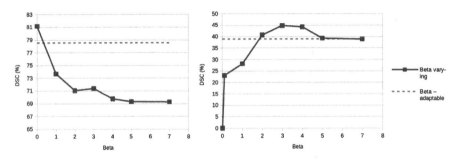

Fig. 3. Evolution of performance of our algorithm on synthetic data with different values of a fixed β. The straight line shows the performance obtained using the automatic setting of β. On the left, we use the blurred ground truths as probability maps (1). We notice that if the probability maps are already performing well, the answers of the user do not increase the performance. This can be detected in a very few questions looking at the automatic setting of beta. The segmentation can then be considered as already too accurate to be improved by our algorithm. The DSC is capped to 81 % because of the lack of freedom of our shape model. On the right, we use misleading probability maps (2). We notice that increasing beta correlates with a significantly better performance in this scenario. Note that β has much more influence over the performance in this case than in (1). Here our algorithm learns to identify and ignore inaccurate probability maps.

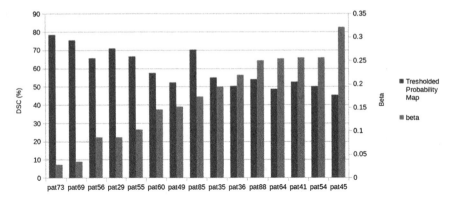

Fig. 4. Automatic setting of β after 30 questions in comparison the Dice score of the tresholded probability map. The results are displayed for each patient individually. In this experiment we use the learnt probability maps. As expected, we notice a trend of the coefficient β to adapt to the quality of the probability maps. Low beta for trustworthy ones, high beta for the ones of poorer quality. This fits to the expected behaviour of the coefficient β.

of trying to find the most unsure area with the MCMC framework. The results are shown in Figs. 4 and 5. If we look more closely, we notice that our algorithm performs better than the random questions baseline for the patients for which the probability map performed the worst. This fits well our motivation to

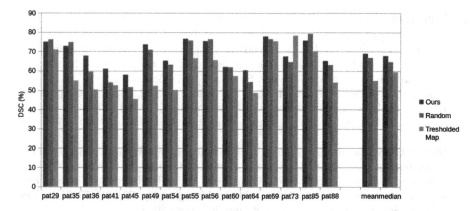

Fig. 5. Comparison of Dice scores on the prostate dataset. Comparison between our method (blue) and two baselines: random questions (red) and the thresholded probability map (yellow). The last two columns are the mean and median over patients. As pictured in Fig. 3 the use of shape models bounds the DSC to 80 % in average. (Color figure online)

retrieve poor segmentations. However we notice for instance that for patient 73, the thresholded probability baseline performs better than both our method and the random questions baseline. This could be resulting from a lack of freedom of our shape-model which therefore impede the mimic of unusual shapes as the one in patient 73. The algorithm proposed by [8] cannot be applied here because 3D GDT is not feasible in real time. Dowling et al. [16] report results on the same dataset and have more heterogeneous results. Our initial model - the probability map - is in average not as accurate as theirs and we expect better results if this component is improved via the use of more sophisticated learning techniques. However, our contribution here is mainly to illustrate the interactive scenario with a restriction to binary inputs and our initial model has not been optimized for this specific task. We also believe that there is room for more accurate shape models on this dataset, since the number of training volumes for this task was limited here.

4   Conclusion

We presented an interactive hands-free method to segment objects of interest in medical volumes. Experiments demonstrate the potential of our method to retrieve inaccurate and misleading segmentations. Using a probability map and a shape prior we are able to locate informative areas to ask questions. The use of shape models to generate segmentations allows a quick computational time between each question. We provided an automatic adaptable setting for weighting the influence of the probability map. This method could be useful in surgery, to allow for instance last minute corrections of incorrect segmentations. Future work could include interactive updates of the probability map with the answers of the user, combining it for instance with an unsupervised model.

References

1. Liu, Y., Bauer, A.Q., Akers, W.J., Sudlow, G., Liang, K., Shen, D., Berezin, M.Y., Culver, J.P., Achilefu, S.: Hands-free, wireless goggles for near-infrared fluorescence and real-time image-guided surgery. Surgery **149**(5), 689–698 (2011)
2. Miller, E.C., Wang, C.N., Gunday, E.H., Juergens, A.M.: Stryker Corporation. Eyewear for hands-free communication. U.S. Patent 6,729,726 (2004)
3. Grady, L.: Random walks for image segmentation. TPAMI **28**(11), 1768–1783 (2006)
4. Rother, C., Kolmogorov, V., Blake, A.: Grabcut: Interactive foreground extraction using iterated graph cuts. ACM Trans. Graph. (TOG) **23**(3), 309–314 (2004)
5. Sadeghi, M., Tien, G., Hamarneh, G., Atkins, M.S.: Hands-free interactive image segmentation using eyegaze. In: SPIE Medical Imaging, pp. 72601H–72601H. International Society for Optics and Photonics, February 2009
6. Gauriau, R., Lesage, D., Chiaradia, M., Morel, B., Bloch, I.: Interactive multi-organ segmentation based on multiple template deformation. In: Navab, N., Hornegger, J., Wells, W.M., Frangi, A.F. (eds.) MICCAI 2015. LNCS, vol. 9351, pp. 55–62. Springer, Heidelberg (2015). doi:10.1007/978-3-319-24574-4_7
7. Tu, Z., Zhu, S.C.: Image segmentation by data-driven Markov chain Monte Carlo. TPAMI **24**(5), 657–673 (2002)
8. Rupprecht, C., Peter, L., Navab, N.: Image segmentation in twenty questions. In: CVPR, pp. 3314–3322 (2015)
9. Lê, M., Unkelbach, J., Ayache, N., Delingette, H.: GPSSI: gaussian process for sampling segmentations of images. In: Navab, N., Hornegger, J., Wells, W.M., Frangi, A.F. (eds.) MICCAI 2015. LNCS, vol. 9351, pp. 38–46. Springer, Heidelberg (2015). doi:10.1007/978-3-319-24574-4_5
10. Freund, Y., Schapire, R., Abe, N.: A short introduction to boosting. J. Japan. Soc. Artif. Intell. **14**, 771–780 (1999)
11. Viola, P., Jones, M.: Rapid object detection using a boosted cascade of simple features. In: CVPR, vol. 1, pp. 511–518 (2001)
12. Peter, L., Pauly, O., Chatelain, P., Mateus, D., Navab, N.: Scale-adaptive forest training via an efficient feature sampling scheme. In: Navab, N., Hornegger, J., Wells, W.M., Frangi, A.F. (eds.) MICCAI 2015. LNCS, vol. 9349, pp. 637–644. Springer, Heidelberg (2015). doi:10.1007/978-3-319-24553-9_78
13. Niculescu-Mizil, A., Caruana, R.: Obtaining calibrated probabilities from boosting. In: UAI, p. 413, July 2005
14. Cremers, D., Schmidt, F.R., Barthel, F.: Shape priors in variational image segmentation: convexity, lipschitz continuity and globally optimal solutions. In: CVPR, pp. 1–6 (2008)
15. Zhao, P., Hoi, S.C., Wang, J., Li, B.: Online transfer learning. Artif. Intell. **216**, 76–102 (2014)
16. Dowling, J., Fripp, J., Freer, P., Ourselin, S., Salvado, O.: Automatic atlas-based segmentation of the prostate: a MICCAI prostate segmentation challenge entry. In: MICCAI Worskshop (2009)
17. Sørensen, T.: A method of establishing groups of equal amplitude in plant sociology based on similarity of species and its application to analyses of the vegetation on Danish commons. Biol. Skr. **5**, 1–34 (1948)

Playsourcing: A Novel Concept for Knowledge Creation in Biomedical Research

Shadi Albarqouni[1]([✉]), Stefan Matl[1], Maximilian Baust[1], Nassir Navab[1,2], and Stefanie Demirci[1]

[1] Chair for Computer Aided Medical Procedure (CAMP),
Technische Universität München (TUM), Munich, Germany
shadi.albarqouni@tum.de

[2] Johns Hopkins University, Baltimore, MD, USA

Abstract. Being considered as a valid solution to the lack of ground truth data problem, crowdsourcing has recently gained a lot of attention within the biomedical domain. However, available concepts in life science domain require expert knowledge and thereby restrict the access to only very specific communities. In this paper, we go beyond state-of-the-art and present a novel concept for seamlessly embedding biomedical science into a common game canvas. Besides introducing the visual saliency concept, we thereby essentially eliminate the requirement for prior knowledge. We have further implemented a game to evaluate our novel concept in three different user studies.

Keywords: Gamification · Crowdsourcing · Aggregation · Annotation

1 Introduction

With the recent rise of powerful machine learning techniques opening up incredible potential in the biomedical field, crowdsourcing has become a valid option for creating large amount of annotated image data [11,12]. Two major challenges have been identified with this strategy: (i) how to adapt state-of-the-art machine learning methods to learn models from noisy annotations, and (ii) how to motivate the crowd to work on highly specialized datasets [2]? Whereas Albarqouni et al. [1] have recently introduced a novel adaptation of a convolutional neural network (CNN) that directly integrates label aggregation into the learning process, the second challenge has been addressed only very little in the literature.

The conventional strategy of crowdsourcing as implemented by most web-based platforms, considers each user as a worker who is reimbursed financially. Even though this concept has worked well for commercial purposes, it has been questioned whether its adoption in the field of biomedical sciences yields sufficient interest for players to get seriously involved [1,2]. The immense success

---

S. Albarqouni and S. Matl—contributed equally towards this work.

© Springer International Publishing AG 2016
G. Carneiro et al. (Eds.): LABELS 2016/DLMIA 2016, LNCS 10008, pp. 269–277, 2016.
DOI: 10.1007/978-3-319-46976-8_28

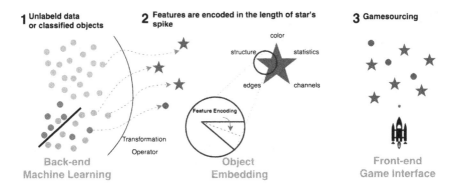

Fig. 1. Playsourcing framework: Unlabeled data or already classified objects go through a transformation process to be ready for game space embedding.

of playsourcing games such as Foldit [3], MalariaSpot [9], The Cure [6] and Dr. Detective [4] have brought up the idea of gamification and game-play in combination with crowdsourcing. Still, it has been shown that readily available game designs are not suitable for playsourcing. Besides, most of these games require a certain degree of *prior* knowledge in life sciences which restricts the access to these games to only specific communities.

In order to eliminate the requirement for this *prior* knowledge, we introduce a novel visual saliency concept for seamlessly embedding biomedical science, i.e. detection and classification, into a common game canvas. Afterwards, we try to answer the following questions: (i) is it possible to transform a medical image to a visual salient game object?, (ii) does the gamification positively influence the annotation and performs better than a crowdsourcing platform?, (iii) does the feature representation influence the saliency of the embedded game object, and therefore affect the classification performance?

As a proof-of-concept, we have designed and implemented an online game for detection and classification of mitotic figures in breast cancer histology images. In the remainder of this paper, we will first introduce our general embedding concept before stating details on our actual game implementation. The manuscript is concluded by reporting on three different test cases evaluating the effect of our game and discussing potential future endeavors.

2   Methodology

Our Playsourcing framework depicted in Fig. 1 is based on the idea to augment previously learned models from only a few expert annotations with crowdsourcing labels [1]. Reducing the amount of "noisy" annotations to a minimum and having a positive impact on the crowds' motivation, our playsourcing concept allows collecting annotations for unlabeled data as well as to refine already detected and miss-/classified objects for high-sensitive applications. We propose to embed the data into a star shape, employing extracted or previously learned features, and place resulting star objects into a common games canvas.

2.1 Object Embedding

Given a database of N RGB images of dimension n, i.e. $X = \{x_1, x_2, ..., x_N\} \in \mathbb{R}^{n \times N}$, each image can be represented by a d-dimensional feature vector $f_i = \phi(x_i)$, where $\phi(\cdot)$ is the feature extraction operator. This operator can vary from simple hand-crafted features (i.e. color, texture, or shape) to more sophisticated ones (i.e. deep learned features).

Next, we aim at embedding these d-dimensional features into a known game object preserving the homogeneity and heterogeneity of our features. We propose a parametric k-spikes star object, carefully designed to be in line with well-known necessary games engineering requirements regarding orthogonality, similarity perception [5] and gestalt perception laws [15], including symmetry, continuity, proximity and past experience.

In order to encode features into the k-spikes star object, we employ a transformation (embedding) operator

$$\mathbf{T} : \mathbb{R}^d \to \mathbb{R}^k$$
$$s_i = \mathbf{T}(f_i), \quad \text{s.t.} \quad 0 \le s_i^j \le 1.$$

Here, $s_i \in \mathbb{R}^k$ is the star's parameters vector, and s_i^j represent the length of spike j of star s_i. Ideally, the transformation operator should embed the features into an orthogonal and lower dimensional space preserving the similarity between homogeneous features and increasing the separability among heterogeneous ones.

Dimensionality reduction techniques like Principal Component Analysis and Sparse Coding techniques [13] can be further applied to reduce the amount of parameters to only a few. However, obtaining a distinct set of parameters relies mainly on the features per se, i.e. embedding the deep learned features into three dimensional space shows better separability than embedding handcrafted features. In this paper, we incorporate feature selection techniques (i.e. Laplacian score, Fisher score) to select a few distinct features.

To this end, features are transformed and embedded into rather distinct star shapes that can be collected easily, i.e. positive samples have sharp and lengthy spikes, however, negative ones show fatty and short spikes (c.f. Fig. 2).

2.2 Game Canvas

The following key requirements have been incorporated into our gaming platform: learning, problem-solving, collecting unpaid annotation, entertainment and competition.

Introduction and Learning. The game starts with a demo phase (c.f. Fig. 2) introducing the game objectives, settings and the visual saliency concept. Players get to steer a plane inside an infinite tunnel, where 3D star objects appear in regular intervals. For each star object, a corresponding patch is displayed to provide the original image to the crowd. Gamers are supposed to make a distinction between correct and wrong stars and collect the relevant stars only,

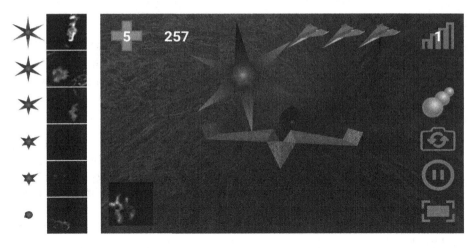

Fig. 2. Star representation: Six different patches (left), game interface showing status bar and buttons for user actions, a plane flying towards the star and a corresponding patch at the bottom left corner (right). As this is the first level, star centers indicate the ground truth by showing a greenish or reddish center. Additional buttons allow to change game settings like fullscreen or camera view or even pause the game.

while avoiding or even actively pushing away the other ones. During the first levels, hints are given to the players to build a better understanding of the relevant stars, i.e. showing a greenish or reddish center for the positive or negative class respectively. Here, ground truth from respective expert annotations is employed, initiating learning and knowledge transfer. For every classification, immediate visual feedback is given to the crowd, additionally supporting the learning process.

Levels and Entertainment. To keep the players engaged, we design multiple levels associated with ascending difficulty (c.f. Fig. 3), that includes increasing the number of stars gradually per level, showing fewer hints, advancing the speed of the plane and increasing the tunnel length and curvature. If hints are not displayed, a gray center indicates the user to make a decision.

The player is initially equipped with five bullets, recharging frequently, allowing to push away the irrelevant stars. Further, three backup planes are provided, allowing the player to resume the game whenever the plane has crashed into the tunnel wall. A new plane is rewarded after every completed level.

Scoring and Competition. Correct decisions are rewarded with a score, otherwise a penalty is given. The scoring strategy is defined as follows:

$$p(y_i^j | y_i^*, level) = \begin{cases} fixed\ score & new\ patch \\ score \times level & y_i^j = y_i^* \\ -score \times level & otherwise \end{cases}$$

where y_i^j is the gamer's decision for star s_i. Depending on its availability, y_i^* can be either the ground truth y^{GT} or the aggregated label from the crowds, referred to as crowd truth y^{CT}, for the corresponding star. Right now, the crowd truth was computed offline for validation purpose, therefore, a fixed score has been assigned online for every decision on the testing dataset. As indicated above, for new patches in the testing set, no labels are available and consequently a fixed score is assigned.

Users don't know if the upcoming star has been labeled already, hence their decision should be straightforward and solely based on the presented data, i.e. star and corresponding patch. In order to reduce spammers, players may only enter a higher level, if they have a certain balance accuracy γ for the training set in the current level. Since higher levels lead to a higher score, this presents an additional incentive to make the correct decision. In order to raise the competition among players, a scoring board is presented on the game website, listing players with their user name, reached level and score.

2.3   Aggregation

We assume that the players have better balance accuracy scores than their mates in the crowdsourcing platforms, which should positively influence the aggregation. Therefore, the weighted majority voting (WMV) algorithm [8] is employed to aggregate the labels:

$$y^{CT} = p(y|Y, \Gamma) = \frac{\sum_{j=1}^{G} \gamma^j y^j}{\sum_{j=1}^{G} \gamma^j},$$

where $Y = \{y^1, ..., y^G\} \in \mathbb{R}^{N \times G}$ is the players-votes matrix, $\Gamma = \{\gamma^1, ..., \gamma^G\} \in \mathbb{R}^{1 \times G}$ is the accuracy score matrix, and G is the number of players. It should be noted that the crowd truth y^{CT} becomes the simple majority voting (MV) when the players are handled equally.

3   Experiments and Results

We have validated our proposed methodology on a subset of the publicly available MICCAI-AMIDA13 challenge dataset[1], containing 311 annotated histology images from 12 breast carcinoma patients [14]. Before extracting patches for classification, images were stain-normalized [10].

Test Cases and Datasets. Three different test cases were constructed (c.f. Table 1). Patches in the first one contain either a mitotic figure or random background and can be considered simple. For the remaining two test cases, the

---

[1] http://amida13.isi.uu.nl/.

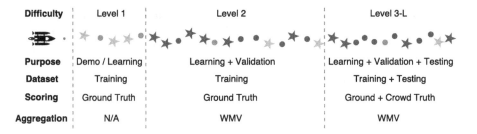

Difficulty	Level 1	Level 2	Level 3-L
Purpose	Demo / Learning	Learning + Validation	Learning + Validation + Testing
Dataset	Training	Training	Training + Testing
Scoring	Ground Truth	Ground Truth	Ground + Crowd Truth
Aggregation	N/A	WMV	WMV

Fig. 3. Gameline shows the purpose, used datasets, scoring and aggregation per level.

Table 1. Description of test cases

Test case	Dataset Difficulty	Features	Patches
TC1	Simple	Handcrafted (HC)	6160
TC2	Challenging	Deep Learned (DL)	3496
TC3	Challenging	Handcrafted (HC)	3496

challenging crowdsourcing dataset appeared in [1] was chosen. For every test case, a subset of five features was selected.

While we differentiate between training and testing dataset (ground truth is still known for evaluation purposes), it should be noted that patches can have three different functions. In the training dataset, a patch can serve for learning purpose, i.e. the ground truth is always displayed to the user. Otherwise, a patch is used for validation, meaning that immediate feedback will be given after the user has made a decision. Patches in the testing dataset always fulfill the testing purpose. They are considered unlabeled data intended for augmentation.

Implementation. For immediate accessibility, we have implemented a web-based game interface, platform-independent, using PHP language on the server side, and JavaScript and WebGL 1.0 on the client side. Since every game action can be done by pressing certain keys or by tapping a respective button, the game can be easily used on mobile devices as well. Our server hosts calculated features and patches. Once a user visits the website and plays the game, a unique user id is assigned and kept for return. Decisions made by the crowd are uploaded in regular intervals during the game and stored on the server.

Evaluation Metrics. We compute different evaluation metrics such as balance accuracy $\gamma = \frac{1}{2} \cdot (\frac{TP}{TP+FN} + \frac{TN}{TN+FP})$ and F_1-score $= \frac{2 \times TP}{FP+FN+2 \times TP}$, with TP being true positives, FP false positives, and FN false negatives. Further, we plot the Receiver Operating Characteristic (ROC) curve together with computing the area under the curve (AUC).

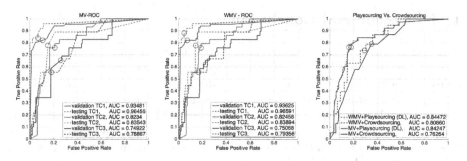

Fig. 4. A comparison between the ROC results of aggregated labels using MV (left) and WMV (middle). A comparison of playsourcing against crowdsourcing (right). The black circles refer to the operating point (threshold) at 0.5.

Results. Within about three weeks, we have collected around 14000 votes, distributed among our three test cases, from 86 users with a collective playing time of 14 hours. Users have been invited through mailing lists and social media channels. We did not provide any other incentive than having a lot of fun. To ensure enough votes for aggregation, i.e. three votes per patch, around 3900 votes and related users were removed. The remaining votes were part of training (learning and validation) and testing sets (c.f. Table 2).

We have employed both WMV and MV as aggregation strategy, for a comparison purpose, on the different test cases as shown in Fig. 4. Simple MV cannot reduce the "noisy" decisions made by spammers. In contrast, employing WMV shows a good impact on the AUC and consistently improved for all test cases. This proves the validity of our carefully designed qualitative test together with the strong assumptions made in Sect. 2.3. As expected, TC1, a simple dataset, performed best. For the challenging dataset, TC2, with deep learned features yields an improvement in AUC of 10 % and 6 % compared to TC3 for validation and testing votes respectively. Hence, the feature representation significantly influences the visual perception. Next, playsourcing votes are compared with the crowdsourcing votes (c.f. Fig. 4). It is obvious that the playsourcing performs better than crowdsourcing with a relative gain up to 10 % in AUC. Similar to the previous comparison, the WMV consistently improves the performance.

Table 2. Distribution of remaining player votes

Test case	Total	Learning	Validation	Testing	Patches
TC1	1524	348	812	364	251
TC2	3883	801	2008	1074	534
TC3	4791	864	2517	1410	658

4   Discussion and Conclusion

In this paper, we have introduced a novel concept for playsourcing in biomedical context. Our playsourcing framework is designed to embed different features into a visual salient game object that can be integrated easily into a game canvas, efficiently eliminating any requirements for *prior* knowledge.

The deep learned features show a better embedding than the handcrafted ones for the challenging patches, however, it has been demonstrated that the concatenation of both features could improve the performance [16]. Although we use few ground truth labels for learning and scoring purposes, this can be replaced by crowd truth for obvious tasks [4].

We have further compared our proposed playsourcing against the crowdsourcing platforms showing a relative gain up to 10 % in the AUC. In addition, it has been shown that playsourcing reduces the cost (i.e. unpaid annotation), time and false positives. Based on this result, we can answer the question raised by Hamari et al. [7], *"Does gamification work?"*, and conclude that *"Yes, it works"*.

Acknowledgment. We would like to thank all anonymous players who participate in our game. We are also grateful to Dr. Mitko Veta for giving us the permission to use the AMIDA13 dataset in our research.

References

1. Albarqouni, S., Baur, C., Achilles, F., Belagiannis, V., Demirci, S., Navab, N.: Aggnet: deep learning from crowds for mitosis detection in breast cancer histology images. IEEE Trans. Med. Imaging **35**(5), 1313–1321 (2016)
2. Aroyo, L., Welty, C.: The three sides of crowdtruth. Hum. Comput. **1**(1), 31–44 (2014)
3. Cooper, S., Khatib, F., Treuille, A., Barbero, J., Lee, J., Beenen, M., Leaver-Fay, A., Baker, D., Popović, Z.: Foldit players: predicting protein structures with a multiplayer online game. Nature **446**, 756–760 (2010)
4. Dumitrache, A., Aroyo, L., Welty, C., Sips, R.J., Levas, A.: Dr. detective: combining gamication techniques and crowdsourcing to create a gold standard in medical text. In: Proceedings of the 1st International Conference on Crowdsourcing the Semantic Web-Volume 1030, pp. 16–31. CEUR-WS. org (2013)
5. Fuchs, J., Isenberg, P., Bezerianos, A., Fischer, F., Bertini, E.: The influence of contour on similarity perception of star glyphs. IEEE Trans. Vis. Comput. Graph. **20**(12), 2251–2260 (2014)
6. Good, B.M., Loguercio, S., Griffith, O.L., Nanis, M., Wu, C., Su, A.I.: The cure: design and evaluation of a crowdsourcing game for gene selection for breast cancer survival prediction. JMIR Serious Games **2**(2), e7 (2014). doi:10.2196/games
7. Hamari, J., Koivisto, J., Sarsa, H.: Does gamification work?-a literature review of empirical studies on gamification. In: 2014 47th Hawaii International Conference on System Sciences (HICSS), pp. 3025–3034. IEEE (2014)
8. Littlestone, N., Warmuth, M.K.: The weighted majority algorithm. Inf. Comput. **108**(2), 212–261 (1994)

9. Luengo-Oroz, M.A., Arranz, A., Frean, J.: Crowdsourcing malaria parasite quantification: an online game for analyzing images of infected thick blood smears. J. Med. Internet Res. **14**(6), e167 (2012)
10. Macenko, M., Niethammer, M., Marron, J., Borland, D., Woosley, J.T., Guan, X., Schmitt, C., Thomas, N.E.: A method for normalizing histology slides for quantitative analysis. In: ISBI, vol. 9, pp. 1107–1110 (2009)
11. Maier-Hein, L., Ross, T., Glocker, B., Bodenstedt, S., Stock, C., Heim, E., Wirkert, S., Kenngott, H., Speidel, S., Maier-Hein, K., et al.: Crowd-algorithm collaboration for large-scale endoscopic image annotation with confidence
12. Maier-Hein, L., Kondermann, D., Roß, T., Mersmann, S., Heim, E., Bodenstedt, S., Kenngott, H.G., Sanchez, A., Wagner, M., Preukschas, A., Wekerle, A.L., Helfert, S., März, K., Mehrabi, A., Speidel, S., Stock, C.: Crowdtruth validation: a new paradigm for validating algorithms that rely on image correspondences. Int. J. Comput. Assist. Radiol. Surg. **10**(8), 1201–1212 (2015)
13. Mairal, J., Bach, F., Ponce, J., Sapiro, G.: Online learning for matrix factorization and sparse coding. J. Mach. Learn. Res. **11**, 19–60 (2010)
14. Veta, M., Van Diest, P.J., Willems, S.M., Wang, H., Madabhushi, A., Cruz-Roa, A., Gonzalez, F., Larsen, A.B., Vestergaard, J.S., Dahl, A.B., et al.: Assessment of algorithms for mitosis detection in breast cancer histopathology images. Med. Image Anal. **20**(1), 237–248 (2015)
15. Wertheimer, M.: Untersuchungen zur lehre von der gestalt. ii. Psychologische Forschung **4**(1), 301–350 (1923). http://dx.doi.org/10.1007/BF00410640
16. Zheng, Y., Liu, D., Georgescu, B., Nguyen, H., Comaniciu, D.: 3D deep learning for efficient and robust landmark detection in volumetric data. In: Navab, N., Hornegger, J., Wells, W.M., Frangi, A.F. (eds.) MICCAI 2015. LNCS, vol. 9349, pp. 565–572. Springer, Heidelberg (2015). doi:10.1007/978-3-319-24553-9_69

Erratum to: Automated Retinopathy of Prematurity Case Detection with Convolutional Neural Networks

Daniel E. Worrall$^{(\boxtimes)}$, Clare M. Wilson, and Gabriel J. Brostow

Department of Computer Science, University College London, London, UK
d.worrall@cs.ucl.ac.uk

Erratum to:
Chapter "Automated Retinopathy of Prematurity Case
Detection with Convolutional Neural Networks" in:
G. Carneiro et al. (Eds.)
Deep Learning and Data Labeling for Medical Applications, LNCS,
DOI: 10.1007/978-3-319-46976-8_8

In the original version of the chapter 'Automated Retinopathy of Prematurity Case Detection with Convolutional Neural Networks', Acknowledgement section was revised. The erratum chapter have been updated with the changes.

The updated original version of this chapter can be found at DOI: 10.1007/978-3-319-46976-8_8

© Springer International Publishing AG 2016
G. Carneiro et al. (Eds.): LABELS 2016/DLMIA 2016, LNCS 10008, p. E1, 2016.
DOI: 10.1007/978-3-319-46976-8_29

Author Index

280   Author Index

Printed in the United States
By Bookmasters